NURSING MANAGEMENT AND EDUCATION
A Conceptual Approach to Change

Nursing Management and Education: A Conceptual Approach to Change

MICHAEL P. BOWMAN
BEd, MEd, SRN Nurse Tutor Diploma (Lond.), RNT, MBIM

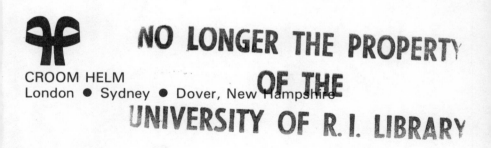

CROOM HELM
London • Sydney • Dover, New Hampshire

© 1986 Michael P. Bowman
Croom Helm Ltd, Provident House, Burrell Row,
Beckenham, Kent BR3 1AT
Croom Helm Australia Pty Ltd, Suite 4, 6th Floor,
64–76 Kippax Street, Surry Hills, NSW 2010, Australia

British Library Cataloguing in Publication Data

Bowman, Michael P.
    Nursing management and education: a conceptual
    approach to change.
    1. Nursing service administration
    I. Title
    610.73'068   RT89
    ISBN 0-7099-3234-0

Croom Helm, 51 Washington Street, Dover, New Hampshire, 03820 USA

Library of Congress Cataloging in Publication Data

Bowman, Michael P., 1930–
    Nursing management and education

    Includes index
    1. Nursing service administration. 2. Nursing — Study
    and teaching. 3. Nursing service administration —
    Great Britain. 4. Nursing — Study and teaching —
    Great Britain. 5. National Health Service (Great Britain)
    I. Title. [DNLM: 1. Education, Nursing — Great
    Britain. 2. Nursing — Great Britain. 3. Nursing Care —
    organization & administration.
    WY 105 B787n]
    RT89.B69 1986   610.73'07'1141   85–30004
    ISBN 0-7099-3234-0 (pbk.)

Filmset by Mayhew Typesetting, Bristol, England
Printed and bound in Great Britain by Mackays of Chatham Ltd, Kent

CONTENTS

Foreword *Professor R.W. Revans*

Acknowledgements

Preface   1

1. Innovation and Change   5

2. The National Health Service: The Continuing Search
   for Better Management   28

3. Nursing: Structure and Functions   48

4. Patients and their Needs   81

5. The Management of Care: Meeting Patients' Needs   89

6. Professionalism in Health Care and Nursing   106

7. Standards and Quality of Care in Nursing   126

8. Information, Manpower and Productivity   150

9. Stress   178

10. Interpersonal Skills: Relevance to Nurse Management
    and Patient Care   187

11. Continuing Education: Perspectives and Options   224

12. Legislation and Key Reports: A Framework for
    Changing Nursing Education and Nursing Management   251

Index   281

To my wife Kay and my son Michael
and to the many individuals who have
influenced my professional development

FOREWORD

In the last few years a handful of people have started to ask if the river of history is bearing us the truth. Is it still enough to know all that is written in the books in order to get the best jobs, leaving it to the un-lettered to get on with the physical tasks? There are several reasons why such questions as this must be asked today, even though it might not have been necessary to pose them yesterday.

The first, and most obvious, is that the world is changing more rapidly today than at any other period of its known history. Today the changes within the same decade mean that no individual can expect to be doing the same job at forty as he was doing at thirty; he may even be lucky to continue in any kind of job at all. Thus, what is printed in the books of one generation may be completely out of date in the next. In times of impetuous change one must have the ability not merely to quote from the books, but to challenge the value of what they are on about. Britain has reached this point, and those who live by the book are alarmed; the universities are uniting to oppose their challengers.

The second is that the social ascendency of the scribe is no longer quite so conventionally accepted. The trouble is that, the more the author-ity of the scribes is manifested the more the basis of that authority will come up for wider debate. Changes of today are not only to magnify technology still more and more; they are also in the relations between those who give orders and those supposed to obey them.

The third lies in the remaining dimension of human experience — personal, as distinct from social and technical. It touches upon learning itself, the virtues within the individual enabling him or her to accom-modate to the changes that now descend like avalanches in every quarter. Our views upon teaching and learning are no longer what once they were. It is not still so firmly held that the pupil simply sits at the feet of the master and, like a parrot, mouths over and over again that which is first uttered from above. It is now believed (although not yet by all) that learn-ing is a symbiotic activity, so that both master and pupil must learn afresh from their common experience. In this respect we need systems for help-ing the young (and also for helping ourselves) that, first, seek to adjust to unexpected change; second, continuously improve relations between those where the work is done; and, third, not only recognise but also build upon the spontaneity of personal development at the here-and-now challenge of the work itself.

Nowhere are the difficulties of cultural change likely to be more vigorously triumphant than in the field of caring for the sick. When human life — or even well-being — is to be protected, those who carry the final responsibility must steadfastly resist the charlatan and even the enthusiast through his own untested beliefs. It may even be that one substantial reason for the hospitals and other arms of our health services to be under such apparent stress is the inflexibility of their training systems.

Thus it is that, breaking forth from time to time upon the pages of this chronicle, we read the message for tomorrow . . . 'How can the local training centre, committed to prepare the future nurse to carry the heavy and responsible burden of her vital task, not only communicate to her sufficiently, but also bring out from within herself all that is needed, first, to face the unexpected when on duty; second, to keep up with the unforeseeable moves made by her colleagues; and, third, to recognise *that it is from within herself* (helped, perhaps, by colleagues who are also helped in the effort) rather than from the scribes and from the teachers that all true learning must derive?' . . .

Thus, if the present book has been written to be sold, it must necessarily uphold both the central thesis that books are good things for preparing the bosses and it must support the scholarly brotherhoods who have turned out the stuff that now fills the books by the thousand. To do other than this would display that lack of micropolitical judgement that is the undoing of so many other innovators. Mr Bowman has made a most complete review of our present methods of training those who take responsibility for what goes on at the bedside; he also calls forward the necessary accounts of the syllabuses and of the researches upon which those methods are said to be based. From time to time he gives us his personal evaluation of how these may work in practice, for he is not only a teacher and an observer, but also one who has long carried the personal responsibility, not only at the individual patient's bedside, but for the whole ward and even wider . . .

But, for those who claim to have made a particular study of what goes on at the points where the health service meets its patients (whether in the hospital or at home), the most interesting parts of the present book are those recited by the voice of the author expressing what he sees to be needed.

All who have tried to influence management education and other professional training in this country must often feel like giving up entirely and for good. Of what use is it, one may well ask, to throw paper darts against the foundations of the citadel? . . . Much depends, of course, upon the message any particular dart may carry. And some darts may even manage to skim the fortress walls. They may then be read, and, from time to time, even understood. Some of us are coming round to believe that, so long as those inside the fortress can persuade others that the message they picked up from the dart was really their own original inspiration, there will be hope for the citadel as a whole. Let us all wish that this book becomes the Super Dart that bears the three-fold tidings.

Reg Revans,
Former Professor of Industrial Administration,
University of Manchester.

ACKNOWLEDGEMENTS

In writing a book of this nature inevitably the author is obliged to refer to many sources of information and to draw upon the expertise of other authors who, over the years, have contributed immeasurably to the development of management knowledge.

The help afforded me by the many writers and publishers both in the United Kingdom and abroad has been unstinted. I am additionally indebted to Professor Revans for writing the foreword to the book and for offering guidance on the text. My sincere thanks also to Ms Taket of the DHSS Operational Research Service and to Mr Goldstone, School of Health Studies, Newcastle Polytechnic, for useful comments on the chapter 'Nurse Manpower' and to Mr D Rye, Director of Professional Activities at the Royal College of Nursing of the UK, for his comments on the chapters, 'Continuing Education' and 'Legislation and Reports'. I would also like to thank Croom Helm for giving me the opportunity to write the book, and Mrs I. Lawson for typing the manuscript.

I am especially grateful to the following statutory and professional bodies and organisations for their unstinted help, advice and support:

The Department of Health and Social Security
The Office for Official Publications of the European Communities
The English National Board for Nursing, Midwifery and Health Visiting
The Controller of Her Majesty's Stationery Office
International Publishing Corporation (*Nursing Mirror*)
Macmillan Journals Ltd (*Nursing Times*)
The National Staff Committee (N & M)
Newcastle upon Tyne Polytechnic Products Ltd
Office of Health Economics
The Royal College of Nursing of the United Kingdom
The Scottish Home and Health Department
The United Kingdom Central Council for Nursing, Midwifery and Health Visiting
World Health Organisation

The following is a list of the principal sources used in the preparation of the text for which permission to publish is much appreciated:

Allan Gay, W.A. and Cameron, D. (1967) *A Manager's Casebook*, Heinemann, London

Binsted, D. (1982) *Learning to Cope with Change in the 80s*. (Special Paper) 1982. Centre for the Study of Management Learning. University of Lancaster

Cole, G. A. (1982) *Management Theory and Practice*. D. P. Publications, Eastleigh, Hants

Cooper, C. L. (1981) *Psychology and Management: A Text for Managers and Trade Unionists,* Macmillan, London

Davey, W., Jefferies, T., Skipp, R. and White, D. (1978) *Management Development Options in the NHS*. Occasional Paper No.14, April, 1978. Health Services Management Centre, University of Birmingham

Department of Health and Social Security (Operational Research Service) (1982) *Nurse Manpower: Approaches and Techniques*, HMSO, London

Fearns, P. (1980) *Business Studies: An Integrated Approach*, Hodder and Stoughton, London

Fulmer, R. (1983) *The New Management*, 3rd edn, Macmillan, New York

Hersey, P. and Blanchard, K. (1982) *Management of Organizational Behaviour: Utilizing Human Resources*, 4th edn, Prentice Hall, USA

Herzberg, F. (1966) *Motivation to Work* (5th Printing), Wiley, New York

Jelinek, R. and Dennis, R. (1976) *A Review and Evaluation of Nursing Productivity*, US Department of Health and Human Services (Division of Nursing), USA

Lancaster, J. and Lancaster, W. (1982) *Concepts for Advanced Nursing Practice,* C. V. Mosby Co, St Louis

Mauksch, H. and Miller, M. H. (1981) *Implementing Change in Nursing*, C. V. Mosby Co, St Louis

Mayeroff, M. (1971) *On Caring*, Harper and Row, New York

Pines, A. M., Anderson, E. and Kafry, D. (1981) *Burnout: From Tedium to Personal Growth*, Macmillan, New York

Revans, R. W. (1982) *The Origins and Growth of Action Learning* Chartwell-Bratt, Bromley

Revans, R. W. (1983) *The ABC of Action Learning*, Chartwell-Bratt, Bromley

Roberts, J. N., White, D. K. and Thompson, D. J. C. (1981) *Change Strategies for Health Authorities: The Contribution of Organisational Development*. (Special Paper) May 1981. Health Services Management Centre, University of Birmingham

Rowbottom, R. *et al.* (1973) *Hospital Organisation*. Heinemann, London

Taylor, D. (ed.) (1984) *Understanding the NHS in the 1980s*. Office of Health Economics, London

Williams, D. (1969) *The Administrative Contribution of the Nursing Sister. Journal of Public Administration, XLVII*, 307–28

PREFACE

Management education and training for nurses and other health care professionals has, since the advent of the Salmon (1966) and Mayston (1969) reports, incurred large investments of resources — money, time, personnel and effort — by the DHSS.

The literature underlining different approaches to education and training in management skills and management knowledge, together with its alleged relevance to the integrity of the service through staff development and the provision of quality care, is vast and varied.

However, despite this deluge of information, there continues to be some doubt as to the suitability of certain management structures (Patients First, para, 1, p.1) and the reliability of some management practices and procedures (Griffiths paras. 2, 4, 8 and 15, pp. 10, 11, 12 and 17) to ensuring the effective and efficient delivery of health care. Despite some disparaging comments by observers, a recent report states: 'If the NHS record is examined in terms of delivering technically adequate care and relieving the population of financial stress in times of illness, then its performance has been more than satisfactory.' (OHE, 1984).

Change

The National Health Service has undergone three major changes during the past decade (1974, 1982, 1983). In addition, nursing has undergone major changes during the past two decades, notably in 1966, 1969, 1974, 1979, 1982, 1983.

The changes that have taken place in nursing have many roots, which include the EEC Nursing Directives (1977), the *National Health Service Acts* of 1972 and 1980 together with the *Nurses, Midwives and Health Visitors Act* 1979, and more recently the NHS Management Inquiry Report (1983) which includes changes to be introduced by the end of 1985. In addition to the influence of reports and legislation in precipitating change in nursing management and nursing education, additional factors have prefaced the need for urgency in preparing health care professionals in general and nurses in particular, who are able to cope with changing public attitudes, values and aspirations together with a better

1

informed and more demanding clientele, which properly is well aware of its rights and needs.

Environment of Care: Stress

Nurses work in an environment which is 'cradled in anxiety' (Revans, 1964). The stress that inevitably results is due in part to nurses' constant striving to maintain standards in the face of increasing odds (Nurse Alert, 1984). Recent research indicates that nurses' stress may be accentuated 'because the standards they set for themselves and are set by others are perhaps too high' (Hingley, 1984).

In the context of the role of the nurse, the inordinate level of their responsibility together with the demands of their accountability, seem to be wholly disproportionate to the extent of their authority — and autonomy — to make nursing decisions. This disbalance in the central elements of role poses many educational and managerial problems for nurses in relation to their day-to-day work; also it limits the chances of nurse educators to provide suitable curricula to meet nurses' training needs.

The functions of the qualified nurse embrace behavioural, statutory and legislative as well as organisational elements (NSC, 1980).

Professionalism

Nurses continue to question the validity of their professionalism. Basic to this questioning issue is the uncertainity of the professional education, development and updating of nurses, not only in 'professional' knowledge and skills; but most important, in managerial knowledge and skills. The management education of nurses has its roots mainly in the philosophies of the Salmon (1966), Powell (1966) and Mayston (1969) reports. However, despite stringent attempts over the past two decades to get nurses to 'accept' the validity of, and the reasons for management education, results have been less than favourable. Many reasons underlie this apparent failure. My own research (Bowman, 1980) indicated that senior nurses see their principal role as 'nurse'. In addition, research carrried out by Williams (1969) underlines the fact that 'sisters are patient orientated': a point which is confirmed by other studies (Haywood, 1968). Also, Williams' work shows that, 'a resistance to "management" by sisters is founded on an inadequate understanding of the meaning of the term'. To compound this resistance, 'courses devoted to management training did not allow enough time for the communication of practical information about the workings of the various departments of the hospital'. And, most important, 'sisters found some management concepts difficult to understand and to apply to their own roles'.

It is against this complex and complicated background that the rationale of this textbook is based.

The philosophy underlying the text is based on thorough and extended discussion with nurses at all levels of management, education and practice, that, to be effective, management theory and management practice must be seen to be closely related not only to meeting the organisational needs of the service and those of nurses' job satisfaction and career aspirations; but, most important, it must be seen to be appropriate and relevant to meeting patients'/clients' needs. To help the reader engage more closely in and relate more effectively to the text, each chapter includes 'Advised Further Reading' as well as specific references. In addition to aid the reader with the chapter on Interpersonal Skills, a series of tapes is available entitled "The Nurse in the 1980s", published by Graves Audiovisual Library.

Finally, I hope that, even in a moderate way, the book affords satisfaction, pleasure and usefulness to the reader by focusing on the key issues underlying the changing of nursing management and nursing education.

References

Bowman, M. P. (1980) The Management Education and Training Needs of First-line Nursing Officers in the Gateshead Area Health Authority. Unpublished MEd. Thesis. University of Newcastle upon Tyne

DHSS (1969) Report of the Working Party on Management Structure in the Local Authority Nursing Service (Mayston) DHSS, London

——— (1972) Management Arrangements for the Reorganised National Health Service (Grey Book). HMSO, London

——— (1979) Patients First. Consultative Paper on the Structure and Management of the NHS in England and Wales. HMSO, London

——— (1983) NHS Management Inquiry (Griffiths). DHSS, London

European Economic Community (1977) Legislation. *Official Journal of the European Communities, 20,* no. L176

Haywood, S.C. (1968) The unwilling managers. *British Hospital Journal, LXXVIII* (4061), 297–8

Health Services Act 1980. (Chapter 53). HMSO, London

Hingley, P. (1984) Stress: A Report of King Edward Hospitals Fund. *Nursing Standard, 352,* 3

Ministry of Health Central Services Council (1966) The Post-certificate Training and Education of Nurses (Powell). HMSO, London

Ministry of Health Scottish Home and Health Dept (1966) Report of the Committee on Senior Nursing Staff Structure (Salmon). HMSO, London

National Staff Committee for Nurses and Midwives (1980) Foundation Management Training, NSC

Nurses, Midwives and Health Visitors Act 1979 (Chapter 36), HMSO, London

Revans, R. W. (1964) *Standards for Morale: Cause and Effect in Hospitals.* Oxford University Press, Oxford

Royal College of Nursing (1984) A Report on the Effects of the Financial and Manpower
    Cuts in the NHS (Nurse Alert). RCN, London
Taylor, D. (1984) *Understanding the NHS in the 1980s*. Office of Health Economics, London
Williams, D. (1969) The administrative contribution of the nursing sister. *Journal of Public
    Administration, XLVII* (307), 307-28

Global Aims

The global aims of the book are:

1. To examine the nature of nursing management and nursing education.
2. To discuss changes in nursing management and nursing education.
3. To interpret the relevance of changes in nursing management and nursing education
   to the role and functions of the nurse.
4. To elucidate the implications of key reports, papers and legislation for nursing management and nursing education.
5. To relate changes in nursing management and nursing education to meeting the needs
   of patients and clients.

Global Objectives

The principal objectives include:

1. To enable nurses to understand relevant concepts in management and education.
2. To assist nurses to appreciate the significance of changes in nursing management and
   nursing education to improving the performance of their role.
3. To help nurses apply management skills, management knowledge and educational principles and philosophy to meeting the needs of patients and clients.

1 INNOVATION AND CHANGE

Aims

The aims of this chapter are:

1. To examine the concepts of innovation and change.
2. To discuss some theories of change.
3. To discuss the main precipitating influences of change in nursing education and nursing management.
4. To explore the problems associated with introducing innovation and change in organisations.

Learning Objectives

The purpose of this chapter is to enable the reader to:

1. Understand the concept of change.
2. Appreciate theories of change.
3. Appreciate the climate and conditions conducive to introducing change.
4. Understand some of the problems associated with introducing change in large organisations.

Background to Change

Nursing and the National Health Service as a whole, has been the subject of continuing change over the past two decades.

As the theme of this book is about change — changing nursing education and nursing management — it seems appropriate, at this point, to outline the main events, reports, papers and legislation which, over the past two decades, have attempted to initiate and/or influence change (Table 1.1). (Further amplification of these reports and legislation is given in the subsequent chapters.)

Nursing, both in the context of the hospital and the community has been subjected to change since the advent of the Platt Report (RCN, 1964) which had the ambiguous title of *A Reform of Nurse Education*. The Platt Committee had been entrusted to consider the whole field of nurse education and training in the light of developments since the Nursing Reconstruction Committee (RCN, 1943). Its recommendations which

5

Table 1.1: Changing Nursing Education and Nursing
Management — Legislation, Reports and Papers

Legislation:
EEC Nursing Directives, 1979
Nurses, Midwives and Health Visitors Act, 1979
Nurses, Midwives and Health Visitors Rules Approval Order, 1983, No. 873
Trade Union and Labour Relations Act, 1974
Ibid. (Amendment) 1976
Employment Protection (Consolidation) Act, 1978

Reports and Papers:
Platt, 1964
Revans, 1964
Salmon, 1966
Mayston, 1969
Management Arrangements for the Reorganised NHS, 1972
Briggs, 1972
Merrison, 1979
Consultative Paper, Patients First, 1979
Towards Standards, 1981
Continuing Education for the Nursing Profession in Scotland, 1981
Griffiths, 1983
Towards a New Professional Structure for Nursing, 1983
Körner, 1982, 1983, 1984
Commission on Nursing Education, 1985

---

were numerous and far-reaching and included vital issues, some of which today remain unresolved yet crucial to the profession, as the independence of schools of nursing of the hospital service, the creation of a realistic educational standard of entry to nursing, the age of entry of nursing students to the profession, the pattern of post-registration nursing education, the inadequacy of the existing pattern of nursing education in meeting present day needs, together with the difficulty of meeting demands for skilled nursing care within the context of a rapidly developing and increasingly complex service, and the effect on nursing of social change.

In 1964, the results of a comparative study of student nurse wastage (*Standards for Morale: Cause and Effect in Hospitals*) which was carried out by a small group at Manchester College of Science and Technology, directed by Professor Revans, concluded that the extent to which student nurses find their work intelligible is an indication of their security: where they feel that they may be, beyond a reasonable limit, expected to take responsibility for matters they cannot understand, there is a significant likelihood that they will abandon their training. In addition, the study underlined that dissatisfaction of staff centres around staffing, pay, hours worked, training, promotion, communication, social relations and personal security. The study particularly indicated that insecurity and uncertainty generate anxiety which is exacerbated by communication failure, which in itself is impaired by a poor understanding of personal roles, knowledge, status and inaccurate or unhelpful self images. It is interesting, through predictable, that reference to the study should again be made in a recent report (RCN, 1984).

Clearly, any attempts to change nursing education and nursing management, in a meaningful way, must take cognisance of these central issues otherwise the change will only be of cosmetic value.

The Salmon Committee (HMSO, 1966) was set up to advise on the senior nursing staff structure in the hospital service, the administrative functions of the grades and the methods of preparing staff to occupy them. In its recommendations it advised making the jobs of senior nurse administrators less burdensome by relieving them of the control of services for the management of which nursing expertise is not necessary. Also, the committee recommended that the jobs of senior nursing staff should be graded according to the quality of the decisions to be taken. The committee emphasised that in the partnership of nursing with medical and non-nursing administration, nursing appeared to occupy a secondary position: a position which stems from the incoherence of nurses and their apparent inability to assert the rights of their profession.

The Mayston Committee (DHSS, 1969) was set up to consider the extent to which the principles of the Salmon report were applicable to the Local Authority services and to advise any changes necessary. The principal recommendations made by the committee included the appointment of a chief nursing officer to co-ordinate health visiting, home nursing and domiciliary midwifery services and to provide a single channel of communication on policy matters. The committee also recommended that staff at each level of management should have clearly defined responsibilities and spheres of authority.

These early reports of the 1960s prefaced or precipitated change. Even though their philosophy and intentions were sound, the structures which were developed to implement change in their wake, were not always satisfactory in meeting the needs of the service, the staff, the patients and clients, and thus failed to effect necessary change. Examples of the less effective reports particularly relate to those of Salmon which, even though intending to effect very positive changes particularly in relation to the management of nursing, in some respects undermined the real authority and autonomy of first-line nurses, particularly ward sisters/charge nurses. Also the role of the Unit Nursing Officer, in retrospect, proved unsuccessful insofar as its design and philosophy failed to provide the role occupant with job-satisfaction.

The Briggs Report (HMSO, 1972) reviewed the role of the nurse and midwife and advised on the education and training required for that role, to ensure the best use of manpower to meet the needs and demands of an integrated health service. Regrettably it took two years following the publication of the report before it was officially acknowledged by the DHSS. The General Nursing Council for England and Wales was un-happy about the implementation of its major recommendations until it was given assurance that the conditions underlying the training of nurses could be met, e.g. the provision of an adequate tutorial service.

The Briggs Report, even though very sound in its philosophy and recommendations, was kept 'in abeyance' for nine years before the enact-ment of the legislation of *The Nurses, Midwives and Health Visitors Act* 1979, which substantially reflected the report's recommendations.

The EEC Nursing Directives (1977) together with the *Nurses, Mid-wives and Health Visitors Act, 1979*, are serious attempts through legisla-tion to initiate change with the structures within which nursing education and nursing practice operate in the quest for an improved standard and quality of care.

The EEC Nursing Directives, which attempts to regularise nursing education and nursing practice in Europe by establishing a common prac-tice of nursing through the agency of regulating basic nurse education, training and practice throughout the community, even though sound in its concept, has some shortcomings, notably in relation to the employ-ment of the general trained nurse, enabling 'free movement', albeit sub-ject to certain regulations being met, throughout member States. Apart from the language (communication) problems there may also exist pro-blems in relation to the interpretation of the nursing legislation, what nurses are permitted to do legally in different States, and most impor-tant there exist problems relating to the standard and quality of service practised. In this respect, prior to Britains's membership of the EEC, statutory bodies in the UK did not wholly recognise, on an equivocal basis, the standard of nurse training and nurse practice of some current EEC countries.

The National Health Service has undergone major change in 1974 to 1982 and is currently undergoing further change following the publica-tion of the Griffiths Report in 1983 (DHSS, 1983). The 1974 reorganisa-tion of the NHS had as its major aims the integration of the major limbs of the Health Service, i.e. the hospitals, general practitioner and local authority services, to enable an improved service for patients and clients by ensuring that every aspect of health care be provided as far as possible locally and with due regard to the health needs of the community as a whole.

The concept and principle of an integrated and management-orientated NHS was difficult to accept, particularly as the contracts and organisation of clinicians working in hospitals and in general practice were different. In this respect, a separate committee was set up (by the AHA) to administer the contracts of the general practitioners. The committee dealt directly with the DHSS and was separately financed. In addition, both consultants and general practitioners were allowed to exercise clinical autonomy and were consequently their own managers. However, to promote improved efficiency in the organisation of medical work, various Cogwheel Reports (DHSS, 1967, 1972, 1974) gave advice. Had the Cogwheel philosophy been grasped fully in its implementation, it would have subscribed considerably to improving the image — and the role — of the clinician in the NHS. Regrettably, the reorganisation failed in that 'it did not provide the best framework for the delivery of care' *(Patients First* (DHSS, 1979) para.1, p.1), and in 1982 further change took place, on this occasion by removing the area tier of management. However, continued problems plagued the service and in 1983 with the publication of the Griffiths Report further change was strongly advised: change of a far-reaching nature which must be fully implemented by the end of 1985.

The Merrison report and the White Paper, *Patients First*, highlight many problems and advise new approaches to change the structure within which health care is delivered.

The Griffiths Report (1983) focuses on many weaknesses of the existing structure for delivering health care and recommends major change particularly in the context of the management of the National Health Service.

The various reports of the Körner Working Groups (NHS/DHSS 1982, 1983, 1984), highlight problems in relation to the deficit, acquisition and use of information in such critical areas of importance as Hospital Clinical Activity (1982), Community Health Services (1983), Patient Transport Services (1984b), Paramedical and Maternity Services (1984), Services For and In the Community (1984c), The Collection and Use of Information (1984d), and the Collection and Use of Information on Manpower (1984a).

In addition, reports, such as *Towards Standards* (RCN, 1981) invite nurses to change and adopt a systematic framework to ensure a more appropriate approach to patient care. Also, the report *Towards a New Professional Structure for Nursing* (1983) is a response to concerns expressed by nurses at the inadequacies of the current nursing structure and explores ways in which it might be improved.

Finally, a major report, *Continuing Education for the Nursing Profession in Scotland* (Scottish Home and Health Dept, 1981), has as its main philosophy the rationalisation of courses intended to meet the management education needs of nurses in order to use resources more efficiently, and prepare them to cope with developments in nursing, medical and technological services and to enable them to meet the demands of patients and clients.

This brief resume of the principal reports, papers and legislation highlights the many changes (attempted or actual) to which nursing and the National Health Service as a whole has been subjected — and which either have succeeded or failed. No doubt other reports and legislation will follow in the never ending quest for success in the management of patient/client care. These reports when implemented demand that nurses — and other health care professionals — change, to secure, or at least to attempt to secure, a measure of change and some success.

Nature of Change

Change makes many demands on staff. Therefore, their proper preparation ensuring, as far as possible, their ability to cope with change can either spell success or disaster for the organisation, the staff and the consumer. The problems are immense but not insurmountable. Central to all change in the health care profession, is that of securing a better deal for patients and clients. In essence, securing a quality service.

The following account is intended to explore the ways, theories and strategies, the problems, and the coping behaviours which are central to all major change.

'Nurses must change nursing education not to please others but to produce competent practitioners capable of exercising autonomous moral judgements.' (McFarlane, 1984).

As chronicled, nursing education, nursing management and nursing practice have, despite some continuing problems due to traditional entrenchment which affect nurses' attitudes, values, education and practice, undergone significant change since the beginnings. This has been more noticeable during the past forty years and more significant during the past two decades, climaxing in more recent change which is influenced by the EEC Nursing Directives, the *Nurses, Midwives and Health Visitors Act* 1979 and the much discussed changes in the role of the nurse.

Nurses and nursing are constantly faced with change. This change, especially change of a major nature, usually has marked effects on the behaviour of nurses who often are not suitably prepared for change and its effects, and who sometimes, for personal reasons, may not be interested in change. For these, and other reasons, change in nursing has not always been effective. However, despite disinterest, the consequences of change will ultimately affect all nurses, the interested and the disinterested.

In the early, formative years of nursing, nurses were identified (in fact in many instances still are) as occupying a purely passive role — accepting the orders of doctors and other health care professionals and nursing the patient in a ritualised way, without using their abilities, skills and knowledge and without using their intelligence and/or creative abilities. In those early days (and regrettably still) some nurses rarely initiated nursing interventions. This abnormal and disproportionate dependence by nurses on doctors has many roots, but was recently exemplified to me when a senior ward sister said: 'If I want to know how good my nursing care is, the doctors will tell me'. This example of course is not a true reflection of nurses' thinking in general — hopefully!

The changes with which nurses are faced in the 1980s are many and include those relating to their own professionalism, particularly in the context of the role and functions, the authority, responsibility, accountability and autonomy to make and take nursing decisions. In addition, changes in nursing practice are precipitated through technical advance generally, developments in the field of medicine, as well as through major scientific discoveries which precipitate change. As a logical sequence to these developments the management of illness, of patients and clients, is becoming more technical, more complex and more demanding and requires up-to-date nursing skills and nursing knowledge, to cope with the panorama of new medical techniques, new drugs, surgical innovations and interventions and the now regular use of complex monitoring and computerised approaches to the management of care.

Changes in the knowledge level, understanding, attitudes and the demands of a better educated and more informed society, make it additionally necessary for change in nursing. Mauksch and Miller (1981) summarise the precipitating factors for change in nursing in the context of 'societal demands, interprofessional expectations and demands, intraprofessional decisions and an overall climate of change in society'.

What is Change?

Essentially the process of change is going on all the time. Change may be effected without our conscious awareness. It may take some time to effect or it may be effected promptly. Examples of the pace at which change occurs can be exemplified by focusing on two major reports. The Briggs report was originally published in 1972 but, for reasons unknown, remained dormant for seven years. Conversely, the Griffiths Report was published in 1983 and its recommendations were to be fully implemented by June 1985. There are clear instances where a change agency, the Government, in the first instance, possibly for political reasons did not want to change the nursing organisation; but, in the second instance, clearly urgently wanted to change the target population, particularly the organisations in which nurses and doctors practice as well as other health care professionals.

Organisational and personal life is continually undergoing change. Change involves a series of assumptions which include:

> The individual can be provided with new insight or knowledge; these will provide some altered motivation with respect to the organisational role; these insights and motivation will persist when the individual leaves the special circumstances in which they were acquired and returns to his or her accustomed role in the organisation; they will be adapted as necessary to that role or it to them; and they will be persuaded to make complementary changes in their own expectations and behaviour. (Katz and Kahn, 1966)

Change in the NHS and in nursing, which has been frequent over the past decade, necessitates staff learning new behaviours and a new role; but most important, necessitates the unlearning of some existing behaviours together with their existing role. In this situation, to obviate problems and insecurity, the potential and/or actual problems associated with the role changes, with which nurses are very familiar, e.g. expanded role and practitioner role, must be made known, i.e. the need to unlearn old/existing behaviours before new behaviours can be learned. In addition, staff must be given opportunities to discuss pertinent issues related to the change and in particular their own fears, anxieties and insecurity about their potential role, together with affording them emotional support and security during and following the transition stage. Most important, according to Ullrich and Wieland (1980), 'staff must be provided with role models, and/or a description of their new role, which is integrated and makes sense in terms of the nurses' training, skills and function in the hospital'.

In this respect, nursing must be in harmony with technological and societal developments and change its practice as deemed necessary, if it is to fulfill its vital role in the health care system.

Currently, nursing education is, perhaps, at its most exciting for many years; the opportunities for nurses to develop and secure the recognition and viability of their profession are at their greatest. Hopefully, this realisation will become a reality and a forward thrust of nursing into the next century can be achieved particularly through the agency of the EEC Nursing Directives and the *Nurses, Midwives and Health Visitors Act* 1979, whose prime purpose is to educate and develop nurses, by re-shaping the structures and re-defining the philosophy which traditionally have been the roots of nursing, thereby enabling them more realistically to meet patients' needs as well as enhancing their own status, security and job satisfaction. In this context, the opportunity to change — redefine and revitalise — nursing education is great, with nurses themselves being the chief agents.

The legislation and the reports on nursing and the NHS are important precipitators of change by emphasising the more controversial issues which are related to securing a quality nursing service, the improved educational development of the nurse, clarification of the nurse's role and in this way by nurturing the professionalisation of nursing.

Some observers suggest that since organisational stability ensures the maximum results at a given moment, any change will affect the productivity of the organisation, certainly until new behaviours are learned and new roles are established. However, the succession of organisational changes in the NHS and their subsequent effects on the health care professions, has probably limited their intention to improve the service to patients and clients, substantially because nurses were managerially unprepared and educationally inadequate, due to lack of communication and information on their part in the change, and, most important, because nurses were bewildered because of the frequency and rapidity of change and its monumental demands emotionally, physically and socially.

Change Agencies and Change Agents

'Managers must be aware of individual and organisational behaviour so that ultimately they are able to understand the needs of people at work, identify problem areas and take action to change or minimise adverse work environments' (Cooper, 1981).

From time to time a Government department, e.g. the Department of Health and Social Security, together with some statutory and/or professional body may become a change agency and in this way attempt to alter the authority structure and attitudes of a target population, nurses and/or doctors. As indicated earlier, many examples are given of government and other reports and legislation which have as their target a special group of professionals, and have as their main intention changing the structure within which the professionals operate as well as influencing their behaviour to encourage them to perform differently; ostensibly more effectively, in the quest for improved patient/client care.

Change Agents

A change agent is 'a professional who influences innovation decisions in a direction deemed desirable by a change agency' (Rogers, 1961).

A change activity is 'an attempt to influence one or more people in a desired and preplanned direction' (Kramer, 1974).

The assumption underlying change is that some system (organisational) states are preferable to others, i.e. the present system in its organisation, values and goals may not be operating in an efficient and effective way, therefore it is proposed to move — change from the present to the preferred state.

Initiators of organisational change should deal with three questions: What is the present state of the organisation? What is the preferred state? (Katz and Kahn, 1966). These authors also emphasise that attempts to change organisations by changing individuals 'tend to be inadequate theoretically and fail practically' as they 'stem from a disregard of the systematic properties of organisations and from the confusion of individual changes with modification in organisational variables'.

Change in an organisation is precipitated by the perception of a gap, usually by senior management (in the case of the National Health Service, by the Secretary of State and his advisers), between planned, desired goals and performance, and achieved, actual goals and performance. Even though, through the agency of monitoring programmes together with various other pertinent information, a gap is perceived between planned and actual performance, there may not be consensus about the real need for change. The reason for this may be that 'because organisations pursue a number of goals most salient to managers and the accuracy with which performance toward them can be measured, conflict may arise' (Ullrich and Wieland, 1980).

Nurses at all levels operate almost constantly as change agents. In this respect senior nurses (top-line and middle management) may attempt to influence front-line nurses to adopt a different approach to the management of patient care. The introduction of the nursing process is one example of an attempt to change the attitudes of nurses (nationally and internationally) in the belief, hopefully right, that a systematic and planned approach to patient care will ultimately prove beneficial to the patient and also enable greater self-actualisation of nurses by encouraging their use of the problem-solving approach to care and by utilising their skills, abilities, knowledge, intelligence and creativity to the full. In addition to securing more effective patient care, this approach could also have an important side-effect, enabling improved job satisfaction through their self-actualisation.

Rogers (1972) states that for nurses to be effective as change agents: 'The target group must be aware of the innovation; it must be persuaded of its value; it adopts the innovation; and it continues to use the innovation after its initial adoption'. And, to be successful in their goal to introduce innovation, nurses must be able to:

Develop the ability to calculate potential risks surrounding the implementation of the change and decide whether these risks are worth taking; have a commitment to the efficacy of change; and be competent in nursing knowledge, nursing practice and interpersonal relationships and communication skills. (Mauksch and Miller, 1981)

Approaches to Change

Change may be planned, where the outcomes are well thought out: it is, in effect, predictable, intentional and deliberate. However, despite this, not all professionals may subscribe to it. For example the change envisaged may increase the workload of nurses, underlined by the RCN in relation to the possible implementation of the third Körner Report on Health Services Information (NHS/DHSS, 1984). The RCN's view is that demands on nurses' time in collecting information may result, which could adversely affect the quality of nursing care.

It is the view of Bennis *et al.* (1976) that many people have difficulty foreseeing the outcome of planned change. Also, staff may not want the stated or envisaged outcomes of change, or indeed may not subscribe to the view that the envisaged change will bring certain benefits in its wake. This is certainly borne out by the somewhat pessimistic view of some health care professionals in relation to the alleged benefits that repeated change to the National Health Service would bring to patients, clients and staff. As well, some nurses have doubts as to the real benefits to nurses of rationalising nursing education through the agency of the EEC Nursing Directives and the *Nurses, Midwives and Health Visitors Act* 1979. In fact, four years following the implementation of the 1979 *Nurses Act*, the Chief Executive Officer to the UKCC said: 'After the distribution of much information on the UKCC, some nurses say: 'We have not heard of you'. (*Nursing Mirror*, Oct. 1983).

Unplanned change is change that occurs even though it is not deliberately planned — nor wanted. As a result, the outcomes are largely unpredictable and unintended. This is certainly true of the changes which followed the introduction of the Salmon Report (1966) which, even though largely benefiting the profession, also produced some unacceptable outcomes, individually and organisationally. These were depicted in the development of an unclear role at nursing officer (NO) level and in an alleged reduction of the real authority and autonomy of the ward sister/charge nurse. Currently, there seem to be problems associated with the introduction of the nursing process and the extended/expanded role of the nurse, which has resulted in some conflict and ambiguity principally among nurses and doctors, which emanates largely from lack of planning, lack of understanding, together with a lack of useful dialogue between doctors and nurses on the pertinent issues.

Theories of Change

There are many theories which help the understanding and the implementation of change. They include the 'conflict' theory, 'systems' theory, and 'individual' theories. Despite this, a number of observers including Olsen (1978) conclude: 'Most social changes are preceded by conflicting forces seeking to prevent change'. In this context, it follows that change may be resisted by opposing professional groups and/or professionals from the same group within the organisation. This seems to be the case with the changes intended to take place through the implementation of the Griffiths Inquiry. Some professionals favour the recommendations because they see advantages for their career progression, others e.g. nurses, on the whole do not because they see patient care being manipulated and jeopardised.

The 'systems' theory of change is based on the notion that:

The state of the elements that enter the system and of the mutual relationships between them is such that any choice in one of the elements will be followed by changes in the other elements tending to reduce the amount of that change. (Homans, 1950)

All systems have arrangements of their elements which are interrelated and interdependent. This interrelationship of the elements of the system is important to its proper functioning. Any alteration, change in one part, will result in a change in some other part of the system. If this change is of an adverse nature, this will result in a dysfunction of the system.

Individual change theories relate to change taking place in the attitudes and behaviour of people. In this respect, senior nurse managers and nurse educationists may attempt to promote efficiency either through introducing new practices or by altering the approach to existing practices. In addition, nurses frequently attempt to change the behaviour of their patients/clients and attempt to motivate them away from practices which are deemed to be harmful to their health towards those practices which are deemed to be beneficial to them. However, changing attitudes will not always result in changing behaviour. It is not a perfect match. Even though 'attitudes predispose behaviour, their expression also relates to the individual's social situation. Much depends on what is appropriate or approved in a particular instance.' (Hollander, 1976).

Lewin (1951) identified three main phases in the process of change, including 'unfreezing', 'cognitive redefinition' and 'refreezing'.

'Unfreezing' is a 'thawing out' phase where the organisation or group recognise the need for change, identify — or at least attempt to identify — the underlying problem and attempt to resolve it. Clearly this is a vital phase in the change process and the group should be encouraged, supported, and 'motivated in the direction of the desired change'.

The phase of 'cognitive redefinition' is characterised by the group moving towards 'a new level of behaviour' which is based upon the group having 'adequate information — and understanding about the need and the way to alter their own attitudes and behaviour'. Lewin says, 'that the ability of leader — through his authority and influence to get accepted appropriate change strategies', contributes substantially to the success of this phase.

The third phase, which is that of 'refreezing', includes 'the integration and personalising of the newly acquired behaviour' into the participants' personalities. To ensure this integration and personalising of behaviour necessitates using various forms of reinforcement, particularly through feedback, support and encouragement of individuals and groups.

Innovation and Change in Clinical Practice: The Real Issues

Currently, nurses are having to cope with new problems arising out of
the introduction of new technology, restricted resources, manpower issues
— increased specialisation, increased Government intervention, new approaches to work and work practices — and new legislation. Change
in nursing may also be precipitated by altered public opinion which may
affect the views of Government, on such issues as abortion, contraception and euthanasia. In this respect, changing morals and taboos may
ultimately affect nurses' work. Other factors which may contribute to
change in nursing relate to the abilities, weaknesses and scarcity of the
available professional manpower. In addition, the environment in which
nurses and other health care professionals work is 'turbulent' — much
of the change is discontinuous. A time of turbulence is a 'dangerous time,
its greatest danger being a temptation to deny reality which may be due
to an inability to interpret the signals, make sense or even notice new
signals as well as previous experience and learning, leading to a misinter-
pretation of the signals' (Binsted, 1982).

In view of the turbulence, and its effects, it is vital that nursing
managers, nurse teachers and clinical nurses know how to effect change
and, most important, that they are able to appreciate the events that signal
change ensuring the personal side-effects of change are reduced or obviated, for patients, clients and staff.

Innovations, virtually by definition are concerned not only with
unlearning, but most important with increased learning, on an individual
or group basis. This increased learning is central to understanding the
new role the nurse will fulfil and in this respect through job confidence,
security and educational enlightenment, enhance the quality of care.

Innovation and change is about how to introduce new ideas — per-
sonally, organisationally, managerially, educationally and clinically —
and to change existing structures and philosophies. Change may be intentional and sudden: there is a growing awareness that there is movement into a stage which is characterised by increasing or decreasing
stability.

Innovation and change in the NHS, nursing and the health care professions, has the explicit intention of improving quality and standards
of care. In fact usually the many reports concerned with innovations and
change make this explicit, e.g. Merrison (HMSO, 1979) and Griffiths
(DHSS, 1983).

Some nurses may feel inadequate either to initiate or influence change
in a positive way, because of their position in the organisation and/or

because of their lack of knowledge, skills or expertise: or because of their total disinterest.

Nurses, doctors and other health care professionals have experienced change, to a greater or lesser extent, virtually continuously over the past two decades. The focus of this change for nurses was the Salmon (HMSO, 1966) and Mayston (DHSS, 1969) reports together with the EEC Nursing Directives and the *Nurses, Midwives and Health Visitors Act* 1979. Health care professionals generally have been subject to change following the reorganisation of the NHS in 1974, 1982 and 1983.

Change in itself may be necessary, as exemplified by altering the structure of the NHS to effect improved decision making and to simplify its structure thus making it more accommodating to staff in facilitating the effective and efficient performance of their work thus enabling them to meet more readily the needs of patients and clients.

Pointers to Introducing Change

Regrettably, sometimes the reasons underlying change may not be made known to staff — or if they are known they may not seem to be relevant to their improved efficient working or productivity. Also, little if any preparation of staff may have taken place, thus accentuating this bewilderment as well as possibly increasing their stress due to their apprehension from or anxiety of the nature of the intended change together with its consequences for them, i.e. apprehension about their changing role, new demands physically and emotionally, loss of status and possible redundancy.

Before introducing change in nursing certain factors need to be considered. For example, the legal constraints must be regarded seriously in relation to introducing an expanded role of the nurse. In this instance, the tasks and functions included in the expansion of the nursing role may not necessarily be in accord with legal requirements in so far that the nurse is properly trained and has the necessary statutory authority to undertake those tasks and functions (Finch, 1981; Martin, 1981). In this context, strategies which are adopted to implement change must be legally correct and acceptable. Also, before attempting to implement change, social-professional norms must be considered. This particularly applies to any change which relates to the hospital environment, where many professionals operate, and which, by its very nature, is rigid, each professional group having fairly fixed boundaries. In this context, some nursing change has already caused problems with doctors, e.g. following the introduction of the nursing process and the adoption of the extended role of the nurse (Mitchell, 1984). A third major constraint regarding the introduction of change in nursing is that of resources, both human and material. Today, because of financial cutbacks in the NHS, change requiring even modest resourcing, is unlikely to be met.

Effecting Change in Clinical Practice

Change in clinical practice is intended to mean any alteration that occurs within the field of the NHS in general, and in nursing, i.e. the total and/or particular environment in which health care is delivered, or 'any attempt to influence the behaviour of others in a nursing subculturally desirable direction' (Kramer, 1974).

Change may be attitudinal — changing the attitudes of nurses towards their patients; technical — introducing a new approach to the checking of drugs; communicational — improving the flow of information to patients; and procedural — introducing the nursing process.

Change in nursing may be precipitated by such things as technological developments, increased medical knowledge, as well as being associated with new medical and nursing specialisms that demand techniques and observations about which nurses need to be informed to ensure proper care of patients, e.g. intensive nursing care practices. In addition, new nursing legislation, as well as the changing structure within which nursing is practised, demands new approaches to the way nurses are trained and educated. These new approaches which are pointing nursing towards the next century, have their roots in the EEC Nursing Directives, the *Nurses, Midwives and Health Visitors Act* 1979 and the recent RCN report on Nursing Education (1985).

Central to introducing 'change' is an attempt to influence the behaviour of people preferably in a desired and planned way. Therefore it is wise for management to recognise and consider important aspects such as: communication — 'change is influenced considerably by the knowledge people have of the change attempted' (Kramer, 1974). Participation — people follow their own decisions best; 'autonomy and trust gained through leadership coupled with honesty and interest in the staff' (Fulmer, 1983); and the intended change must be seen to be relevant and essential to the improved functioning of the organisation.

In Fulmer's view, 'one must be prepared and motivated for the experience of change where it is necessary to eliminate, or unfreeze present attitudes so that a vacuum can be created for new ones'. And, internalisation which includes 'the person identifying with another who has the desired attitude, which will facilitate the willingness to change'. For this reason, he concludes, 'it is important for managers to look for opinion leaders as change agents'.

Resistance and Constraints to Change

Research carried out on organisational crisis and change (Fink *et al.*, 1971) describes certain phases, as a human system adapts to a crisis situation. These phases include that of an initial state of 'shock', a situation which is characterised by the immobility of the organisation — an inability to plan, reason, and make decisions. This phase is usually followed by that of 'defensive retreat' — an inability and/or unwillingness to acknowledge the situation — to face the reality of the problem. This phase may also include trivialisation of the disruption. This is followed by the phase of 'acknowledgement' — the reality of the change begins to show: there is an examination of the problems and a search for a solution. Finally, there is the phase of 'adaption' — change is evident — there is modification and adaption to the new situation — the organisation begins to function as a whole.

The resistance to change may occur for many reasons, of which innovators must be aware and if possible obviate or diminish. The many impediments to change include inconvenience — the working environment may be made more difficult — new ideas and attitudes have to be acquired and new information effected possibly through new learning or unlearning: uncertainty — new approaches are full of uncertainty and individuals feel threatened; relationships — social and working relationships may be affected through new staff adopting different approaches; and resentment — if the change comes solely from management without involving staff, resentment with an accentuating of resistance to the change may result. Therefore careful thought and planning, and discussion with colleagues and staff ultimately to be affected by the change, are paramount to success.

In view of the potential resistance of staff to change — irrespective of its nature and magnitude, it is incumbent upon management to take cognisance of certain factors which will reduce and/or obviate its potential side-effects and enhance its acceptance. Therefore, in view of the many potential problems associated with introducing change certain strategies can be used to obviate or diminish resistance as well as to ensure causing the least possible emotional trauma to the recipients of the change.

The process of planned change involves a change agent, a client system, i.e. 'the individual personality, face-to-face group, and the organisation' and, 'the change agent must be more than a man of action, he must be a professional who draws on a body of scientific knowledge' (Bennis, 1970). Change agent activity is 'any attempt to influence the behaviour of others in a desirable direction'. In nursing 'there has to be evidence that the desired change will potentially benefit nursing and/or patient care, that preplanning had been done, and that the activity of influence involved more than just the change initiator' (Kramer, 1974).

Effecting Change: Introducing Innovation: Some Research Findings

In the mid 1960s a survey of eighteen studies of organisation change particularly looking for similarities and differences was conducted by Greiner (1967). He identifies eight major patterns in the evolution and effecting of change. They include:

> top managment is under pressure — external and internal, for improvement: this is signalled by low productivity performance and morale; a consultant — known for his ability to introduce improvements, joins the organisation; the new consultant encourages a re-examination of past practices and current problems; the head of the organisation and his subordinates become directly involved in this re-examination; top management engages different levels of the organisation to identify current problems — fact-finding; the consultant provides members with new ideas and methods for developing situations; the solutions and decisions are developed and tested for solving problems on a small scale, before an attempt is made to widen the scope of change to larger problems; and, the change spreads with each success experience — management support grows.

Research by Binsted (1982) highlighted key factors affecting catastrophe/non-catastrophe situations as they relate to the chemical industry. He found 'some differences between those companies who had experienced and survived a catastrophe, and those who by deliberate action seemed to have avoided it'. Five factors were significant of Binsted's work. These were:

> Recognising the signals as the environment became more turbulent and as the changes in it became discontinuous (new factors not

experienced before); attitudes to change; perceptions of change; positive effects of catastrophe; (the catastrophe unlocked the situation inside the organisation e.g. with the unions); and collusion (collusion between a number of parties was terminated by catastrophe).

The research highlights two key challenges for managers, i.e. avoiding discontinuous change or if it has already happened surviving it. The authors say that managers may have to make considerable adjustment to their career expectations or their future role as well as having to undergo the painful processes of unlearning — and insecurity.

Innovation

Introducing something new — making changes successfully — depends 'on how clearly the ideas are explained to the involved parties'. In essence, 'an innovation is brought to a receptive social (client) system by a change agent' (Lancaster and Lancaster, 1982).

Participants tend to evaluate the innovation according to:

relative advantage — the degree to which the new idea is superior to the old one: compatibility — the degree of congruence between the innovation and existing values, habits and needs of the participants: complexity — the amount of difficulty that the participants have in understanding and subsequently using the innovation: trialability — the degree to which the new idea can be pretested or tried on a limited basis: and observability — how visible the innovation is to participants and onlookers. (Rogers and Shoemaker, 1971)

'An anticipated change will be resisted to the degree that the organisation possesses little or incorrect knowledge about the change and has comparatively low influence in controlling the nature and direction of change.' (Bennis, 1966)

Introducing innovation and change into clinical practice is both complex and demanding on the innovators (the managers) as well as the staff. It must include leaders who are creative and innovatory and who encourage and support their staff. The climate created must enable staff to 'be free to probe, to be creative, and to work together with mutual respect' (Kilbrick, 1972). Leaders and managers must develop an understanding and perceptiveness; but, most important, they must use appropriate behaviours based on these. In the final analysis, leaders and managers must 'listen to ideas and convert them into innovative reality' (Drucker, 1980).

To effect change in nursing, the organisation (nurses) should have as much understanding of the change and its consequences, as much influence in developing and controlling the fate of the change, and as much trust in the initiator of the change as is possible. Despite the fact that everything possible may be done by nurse managers and initiators to effect change in a harmonious and untraumatic way, nevertheless individuals and organisations may undergo certain effects.

Effects

Innovation and change offer both a challenge to one's creativity, inventiveness and managerial prowess, and a threat to one's personal security. In this way both innovation and change can be emotionally taxing and traumatic for those responsible for providing the innovation and masterminding the change, as well as the recipients of change.

The whole process of managing major change requires the skills of planning, motivating and educating staff as well as the skill of managing change. In addition, it requires knowledge, tact, interest, commitment, support — and the perseverance of managers and staff. For the change intended to be accepted, and most important sucessful, requires a determined and conscious effort by innovators to get relevant information to staff thereby ensuring their effective learning of new skills, attitudes and new knowledge as well as their unlearning of redundant skills and the displacement, and substitution, of appropriate attitudes and goals. Most important, 'the degree to which the change agent is trusted and respected whithin the organisation will influence the acceptance of the idea' (Lancaster and Lancaster, 1982).

> Roles demanding innovative problem-solving activities are a major source of role conflict and tension to the extent that such roles place one (change agent) in conflict with those who stand to profit from maintaining the status quo. Furthermore, change agents experience conflicts arising from their involvement in non-routine activities, as this involvement competes with their routine, administrative activities. (Ullrich and Wieland, 1980)

> Episodes which constitute serious crisis and which arise because organisations strive for outstanding success, or seek to contribute something new to society, may actually be occasions for renewed organisational growth. For such growth to occur, first of all necessitates an understanding of the psychology of human reactions to such events. Also, leaders and managers must develop insights into

the processes of adaption by getting to know and understanding the kinds of actions which facilitate adaption. (Fink *et al.*, 1971)

In the final analysis, change is more likely to be accepted and be successful 'if the driving forces for change outweigh the restraining forces,' (Lancaster and Lancaster, 1982). And

Unless the client to be changed is aware of the stress that the attempt to change the organisation may bring upon him, and that in this attempt he may be obliged to recognise his own need to be changed, it is useless to proceed. And, any permanent change to the organisation, to any marked degree, merely by fraternisation among those in the lower ranks, although senior management may be less reluctant to take a disagreeable line of action if it is assured that its subordinates are more united in support of it than had been expected, cannot occur. (Revans, 1971)

References

Bennis, W. G. (1966) *Changing Organizations*. McGraw-Hill, New York
———— (1970) Beyond Bureaucracy. in W. C. Bennis (ed.) *American Bureaucracy*. Aldine, Chicago, pp. 3–16
———— *et al.* (1970) *The Planning of Change*, 2nd edn, Holt, Rinehart and Winston, New York
———— (1976) *The Planning of Change*, 3rd edn, Holt, Rinehart and Winston, New York
Binsted, D. (1982) Learning to Cope with Change in the 80s. (Research paper). Centre for the Study of Management Learning. University of Lancaster, pp. 1–16
Cooper, C. L. (1981) *Psychology oand Management*. Macmillan, London.
DHSS (1967/72/74) Organisation of Medical Work in Hospitals. (Cogwheel). HMSO, London
———— (1969) Report of the Working Party on Management Structure in the Local Authority Nursing Service (Mayston). DHSS, London
———— (1972) Management Arrangements for the Reorganised National Health Service (Grey Book). HMSO, London
———— (1979) Patients First (Consultative Paper in the Structure and Management of the NHS in England and Wales). HMSO, London
———— (1983) NHS Management Inquiry (Griffiths), DHSS
Drucker, P. F. (1980) *Managing in Turbulent Times*. Pan Books, London
EEC (1977) Legislation. *Official Journal of the European Communities, 20*, no.L176, July
———— (1981) Legislation. *Official Journal of the European Communities, 24*, no.L385, Dec.
———— (1981) Advisory Committee on Training in Nursing (Report of the Training of Nurses Responsible for General Care). April
Finch, J. (1981) The law and learner. *Nursing Mirror, 152* (18), 30
Fink, S. C. *et al.* (1971) Organizational crisis and shock. *Journal of Applied Behavioural Science, 7*, 15–34

Fulmer, R. M. (1983) *The New Management*, 3rd edn, Macmillan, New York
Greiner, L. E. (1967) Pattern of organizational change. *Harvard Business Review, 3*, 119–30
HMSO (1966) Report of the Committee on Senior Nursing Staff Structure (Salmon). Ministry of Health Scottish Home and Health Dept, HMSO, London
———— (1972) Report of the Committee on Nursing (Briggs). Cmnd. 5115, HMSO, London
———— (1979) Royal Commission on the National Health Service (Merrison), Cmnd. 7615, HMSO, London
Hollander, E. P. (1976) *Principles and Methods of Social Psychology* 3rd edn. Oxford University Press, New York
———— and Hunt, R. G. (eds.) (1976) *Current Perspectives in Social Psychology*, 4th edn. London University Press
Homans, G. C. (1950) *The Human Group*. Harcourt Brace Janovich, New York
Katz, D. and Kahn, R. L. (1966) *The Social Psychology of Organizations*, 2nd edn. Wiley, New York
Kilbrick, A. (1972) Leadership. *American Journal of Nursing, 72*, 1451–2
Kramer, M. (1974) *Reality Shock*. C. V. Mosby, St Louis
Lancaster, J. and Lancaster, W. (1982) *Concepts for Advanced Nursing Practice: The Nurse as a Change Agent*. C. V. Mosby, St Louis
Lewin, K. (1951) *Field Theory in Social Science*. Harper and Row, New York
Macfarlane, Baroness (1984) Still a long way to go before image meets reality. Fifth Annual Royal Marsden Hospital Lecture. *Nursing Mirror, 159* (10), 6
Martin, A. (1981) Easy does it! *Nursing Mirror, 152* (18), 30
Mauksch, I. and Miller, M. H. (1981) *Implementing Change in Nursing*. C. V. Mosby, St Louis
Mitchell, J. R. A. (1984) Is nursing any business of doctors? A simple guide to the 'Nursing Process' *British Medical Journal, 288*, 216–19
NHS/DHSS (1982/84) Steering Group on Health Services Information: A Report on the Collection and Use of Information about Hospital Clinical Activity in the NHS. (First Report) (Körner). HMSO, London
———— (1984a) Steering Group on Health Sevices Information: A Report on the Collection and Use of Information about Manpower in the NHS. (Third Report) (Körner). HMSO, London
———— (1984b) Steering Group on Health Services Information: A Report on the Collection and Use of Information about Patient Transport Services in the NHS. (Second Report) (Körner), HMSO, London
———— (1984c) Steering Group on Health Services Information: A Report on the Collection and Use of Information about Services for and in the Community in the NHS. (Fifth Report) (Körner), HMSO, London
———— (1984d) Steering Group on Health Services Information: A Report on the Collection and Use of Financial Information in the NHS. (Sixth Report) (Körner), HMSO, London
———— (1984e) Steering Group on Health Services Information: A Further Report on the Collection and Use of Information about Activity in Hospitals and in the Community in the NHS. (Fourth Report) (Körner). HMSO, London
Nurses, Midwives and Health Visitors Act 1979 (1979) (Chapter 36) HMSO, London
Nurses, Midwives and Health Visitors Rules Approved Order (1983) No. 873, HMSO, London
Olsen, M. E. (1978) *The Process of Social Organization: Power in Social Systems*. Holt, Rinehart and Winston, New York
Revans, R. W. (1964) *Standards for Morale: Cause and Effect in Hospitals*. Oxford University Press, Oxford
———— (1971) *Developing Effective Managers* Longman, London
Rogers, E. M. (1961) *Educational Revolution in Nursing*. Macmillan, New York
———— (1972) Change agents, clients and change. in G. Zaltman *et al.* (eds) *Creating*

Social Change. Holt, Rinehart and Winston, New York
——— and Shoemaker, E.F. (1971) *Communication of Innovation: A Cross-cultural Approach*. Free Press of Glencoe, New York
Royal College of Nursing (1943) Nursing Reconstruction Committee (Horder), RCN, London
——— (1964) A Reform of Nurse Education (Platt). RCN, London
——— (1981) Towards Standards (A Discussion Document). RCN, London
——— (1984) A Report on the Effects of the Financial and Manpower Cuts in the NHS. (Nurse Alert). RCN London
——— (1985) The Education of Nurses: A New Dispensation (Commission on Nursing Education). RCN, London
Scottish Home and Health Dept (1981) Continuing Education for the Nursing Profession in Scotland. (Report of a Working Party on Continuing Education and Professional Development for Nurses, Midwives and Health Visitors). SH&HD
Ullrich, R. A. and Wieland, G. P. (1980) *Organisation Theory and Design*. Richard D. Irwin Inc., Homewood, Illinois

Advised Further Reading

Duncan, W. J. (1978) *Essentials of Management*. Dryden Press
Fulmer, R. M. (1983) *The New Management*, 3rd edn. Macmillan, New York
Kramer, M. (1974) *Reality Shock*. C. V. Mosby, St Louis
Mauksch, I. G. (1981) *Implementing Change in Nursing*. C. V. Mosby, St Louis
Morrish, I. (1976) *Aspects of Educational Change*. Allen and Unwin, London
Rowbottom, R. *et al.* (1973) *Hospital Organization*. Heinemann, London
Zaltmann, G. *et al.* (1973) *Innovations and Organizations*. Wiley, New York

2 THE NATIONAL HEALTH SERVICE: THE CONTINUING SEARCH FOR BETTER MANAGEMENT

Aims

The aims of this chapter are:

1. To examine the concept of management in the context of
   (a) The National Health Service and
   (b) Nursing.
2. To explore problems which are central to the health care service

Learning Objectives

The purpose of this chapter is to enable the reader to:

1. Understand the concept of management within the context of
   (1) The national health service and
   (2) Nursing.
2. Appreciate problems which are central to the health care service

Background

The NHS, in Governmental terms, differs from the usual model of Government administration where the Minister heads a line command system down to local level, in so far as there are authorities such as RHAs and DHAs. Also, the NHS does not fit the model established in the nationalised industries where the Boards have delegated powers and are accountable to Ministers for achieving precise targets — financial and other. In industry members' roles are, in the main, clearly defined in terms of function. Regrettably there is a vagueness in the case of lay and professional NHS authorities, in this respect, as underlined by Griffiths: 'There is a lack of clearly defined management function throughout the NHS.' (DHSS, 1983, Para.4, p.11). There is, in essence, a confusion regarding the possession of legitimacy of authority (Regan and Stewart, 1982). Also, in the main, NHS staff loyalties are to the service itself while civil servants' actions tend to be primarily aimed at the support of their political heads. 'This division may on occasions promote inefficiencies in the NHS, not the least of which stem from a lack of proper leadership from the 'top' of the structure.' (Taylor, 1984).

Nurses, doctors and other health care professionals are aware of the problems and difficulties that confront them, e.g. lack of information, lack of involvement in decision making, unrealistic demands on their level of professional training and development, inadequate motivation, guidance and support, inefficient and/or inadequate resources and poor leadership. This information is well documented and much discussed.

There is little dispute among health care professionals on the need for a wise, effective and efficient management structure which would provide a better deal for patients, clients and staff. The central point being, that whatever organising systems are used they are not used for their own sake; but are used for 'delivering services to people' (DHSS, 1983, para.3, p.10).

Blight: The Facts

The structure of the NHS continues to be blighted in securing its primary objective, namely, the effective and efficient delivery of care to patients and clients. The recent management inquiry into the NHS (DHSS, 1983), one of two major investigations and reshuffles since 1974, highlights the weakness that continues to bedevil the management of the enterprise and which acts as an impediment to securing a quality service. However, are the shortcomings of the NHS frequently voiced by health care professionals largely unfounded, as stated in a recent report? (Taylor, 1984). Or, are they founded, as underlined by RCN evidence? (1978, 1984) and by Griffiths (DHSS, 1983)?

What are the facts?

The NHS is a large and complex organisation. It will spend around £17,000 m. in the UK in 1984. It employs more than 1.2 million full-time and part-time staff and it utilises around 6 per cent of the country's gross national product and a similar proportion of its manpower resources.

The challenges to the Service are many. For example, the last four decades have brought new challenges including the ageing of the population which has required more energies to be focused on the health problems associated with chronic, disabling diseases of later life. In addition, the emergence of a more individualistic social environment has meant that health care consumers have become less tolerant of inconvenient and/or inadequate patterns of service than they were when the NHS was first introduced. More important, the trends and tensions associated with the NHS industrial disputes of the 1970s and early 1980s together with the structural reorganisations of 1974 and 1982, with yet another due to take place in 1985, led to a belief that the NHS has reached a crisis point.

The central problem is, how can a health care system which is based on the ideal of universal welfare, incorporating values of equality, rationality and efficiency (Klein, 1983) and which was initially built on assumptions about the nature of medical authority, most efficiently achieve its aims in the present — and in the future?

To address this problem effectively, in the hope of finding some clues, attention must be focused on the health service, in its complexity organisationally, together with the nature and the purpose of health service management.

Problems and Complexities

What is unique about the NHS, and hospitals where patients are cared for? Does the NHS — and its contained professions — differ substantially from industry in terms of its general goals, activities and procedures? Clearly, the Griffiths view is, No (DHSS, 1983, paras. 1/2, p. 10).

Professor Revans, who, in the past, devoted considerable time to identifying and analysing the problems of some health care professions, says hospitals are 'institutions cradled in anxiety'. In this respect, patients are anxious about their health and about their families. Nurses, especially nursing students, are anxious about the difficulties of learning and the fear that they may be inadequate, in the care of their patients. Trained nurses, especially sisters, are often anxious about the good order of their wards and units; also their relationships with their superiors and the medical consultants. And doctors, especially the more senior ones — Registrars and Consultants — are anxious because they are often taking important decisions — sometimes on incomplete information. In fact, in Revans' (1964) view, the only persons 'who seem permanently secure in hospital are the cleaners'.

Despite the evident insecurity of staff, it is paramount to patients' recovery that they must have confidence in those who treat and care for them. Therefore, all health care professionals, particularly nurses, who are in constant touch with patients, providing round-the-clock care, must always feel assured and secure. This security is substantially enabled through effective communication. In Revans' view, 'anxiety is enhanced by uncertainity and uncertainty is magnified by communication failure'.

The difficulties of communicating and of being communicated with are highlighted by such factors as unclear or unrealistic ideas of one's role, knowledge and status — particularly in respect of authority, responsibility, and autonomy. These problems, even though highlighted in Revans' research some two decades ago, continue to be central to the nursing situation today (RCN, 1984).

The Search for Improved Management: Evolution

Management: Concept

Before discussing the many and complex variables in the search for improved management, it is appropriate to say what is meant by management.

Essentially, management is about solving problems and making decisions. Also, it is about reshaping the behaviour of staff to get them to work towards defined and agreed goals. Management includes the important functions of establishing an authority (organisational) structure which enables and enhances (or limits) organisation functions, together with those of planning — establishing agreed objectives through investigation, research and analysis; directing — which includes motivating and leading; co-ordinating — externally with allied bodies appropriate to the functioning and viability of the organisation, and internally relating the various parts and functions of the organisation; as well as communicating (which includes ensuring feedback) and controlling the activities of the enterprise. But, most importantly, it includes coping with (managing) conflict, establishing relationships and providing supportive services (i.e. counselling, appraisal and staff development) to ensure the self-actualisation of staff and to preserve the integrity of the organisation.

The search for better, improved and/or successful management in the NHS as a whole as well as in individual health care professions has continued , unceasing, since the mid 1960s. For example, the Salmon (1966) and Mayston (1969) reports led to substantial and important professional restructuring in nursing. Likewise, the Cogwheel reports (DHSS 1967, 1972 and 1974) led to a rethink in the organisation of hospital doctors' working relationships. Unfortunately, the positive philosophy displayed in these reports has not been fully, if at all, exploited.

Regrettably, as with nurses, doctors also seem to demonstrate a non-commitment to the management process. They are, of course, unlike nurses, ably supported and 'covered' in this respect, through the agency of 'clinical freedom'.

Many important initiatives designed to enhance NHS management have been adopted, and in this respect those that are paramount include, the Rayner Scrutinies, (90-day scrutinies in regions by officials reporting to Regional Chairmen, on matters such as the collection of payments to Health Authorities resulting from road accidents and catering costs); the Körner Steering Group on Health Service Information (the NHS/DHSS Steering Group on Health Service Information Systems was set up in 1980 with the remit to agree and implement the principles and procedures appropriate to guiding the development of the NHS information gathering, as well as to review existing arrangements and change them if necessary); Regional Reviews and Performance Indicators (in January 1982 the Secretary of State announced that Annual Review meetings between Ministers, RHA Chairmen and Regional Officers would be organised to help ensure the efficient use of NHS resources within Government's priorities); and Management Advisory Service which grew from a suggestion made in the 1979 Consultative Document, *Patients First* (DHSS, 1979).

Some of these initiatives, even though realistic in their aims to secure improved management, have been questioned as to their validity, practicality and reasonableness. For example, the Rayner Scrutiny into NHS accommodation, the intention to sell large amounts of NHS housing stock was seen as 'devastating', 'ignoring human cost' and having 'serious implications for nurses', by the RCN (*Nursing Standard*, Aug. Sept. Oct., 1984).

Change in the NHS: Restructuring

In Chapter 1 we discussed the concept, and the difficulties of introducing and of coping with change. In the context of change in the NHS and in nursing, which has been frequent, especially during the past two decades, one would assume (wrongly) that the experience of health care professionals of coping with change would render them immune to its effects. Regrettably, the dislocation and emotional trauma caused by repeated change continues to have devastating effects on the more vulnerable health care professionals, as evidenced currently by the introduction of some of the Griffiths' recommendations, notably the appointment of general managers.

The dislocation of the service during and following major change, and its subsequent effects on health care professionals, has many roots, e.g. fear of the unknown, loss of job, new bosses; but, most important, a new role must be learned as well as an unlearning of the old-existing role. The problem lies in the fact that one's former role will have provided a stable set of role expectations with related knowledge, skills and attitudes: this is disrupted to a greater or lesser extent by change. In this context, Smith (1971) discusses ways of reducing the emotional stress thus encountered by staff which include, 'preparation for the anticipated changes', essentially this approach entails 'making aware of the problems associated with role changes'; 'providing emotional support' by providing opportunities for discussion of the issues thus enabling staff 'to express their feelings'; and by providing them with a 'role model of the new role which they can emulate', particularly one that is 'integrated and makes sense in terms of training, skills and function'.

The 1974 Reorganisation

The 1974 reorganisation of the NHS was an attempt to correct the anomalies of the organisational problems which were inherent in the organisation created by the 1946 Act; but having corrected some, e.g. the tripartite structure was dissolved, regrettably, it created many other structural problems. In this context, the consultative paper, *Patients First* (DHSS, 1979) makes the following points: 'The structure and management arrangements of the service introduced in 1974 do not provide the best framework for the effective delivery to care of patients' (para.1, p.1). Also, there has been widespread criticism of the 1974 changes which the Royal Commission on the NHS (1979) summed up as: 'too many tiers; too many administrators in all disciplines; failure to take quick decisions; and money wasted' (para.3, p.4).

The 1974 Reorganisation: Precipitating Factors (Figure 2.1)
The important facets of the reorganisation were: the creation of Regions and Areas as Executive Authorities; the preservation of the Executive Council System; the establishment of the new boundaries of the FPCs to relate to those of the Areas; the introduction of teams of managers at District, Area and Regional levels; the integration of Training Hospitals into the unified structure; the nomination of Community Health Councils; the establishment of a comprehensive new planning system to equip the NHS to identify and pursue priorities; and an emphasis on the need to balance accountability upwards by delegation downwards. (The latter is important to note as with the advent of the Griffiths' philosophy, particularly with the appointment of general managers, the trend would seem to be to 'limit' downward delegation.)

Figure 2.1: The NHS in England in 1974

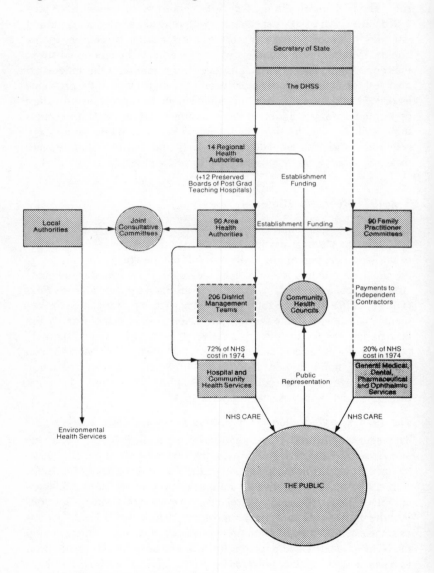

Source: Office of Health Economics.

The control of infectious diseases together with the plight of the elderly and the chronic sick led a number of professional groups to underline the inadequacy (reduced and/or inhibited co-ordination) of the tripartite division between the then local authority, executive council and hospital services. In addition, other factors which prompted the 1974 structural reorganisation of the health service included, 'the dominance of hospital-based attitudes and values throughout the NHS; poor liason between staff working in the community services and those in the hospitals which led to imbalance in standards of care; and the success of medicine since 1948' (OHE, 1974). The proposals for the 1974 reorganisation were embodied in the National Health Service Act 1972.

Aims and Objectives

The objective in reorganising the service was to enable health care to be improved. The principal aims underlying the reorganisation were to provide a fully integrated health service in which every aspect of care could be provided by the health care professions and that this care should be provided so far as possible locally and with regard to the health needs of the community as a whole. Within these aims, the specific objectives to be promoted by management included, the co-ordination of the planning and provision of all personal health services; planning of services in relation to the needs of the population; the effective working of professional practitioners; and effecting more uniform standards of care (DHSS, 1972, para.1.4, pp.9–10).

To implement these aims and objectives, health services were integrated locally, within areas, on a district basis, to ensure effective operational units, together with adopting a more patient-centred approach, in which all professionals would engage in management. Clinicians were particularly encouraged to do so (DHSS, 1972, para.4.6, p.68). Multi-disciplinary management teams were formed at each level to plan and co-ordinate health services jointly. Implicit in the patient-centred approach was the greatest possible decentralisation of decision-making and delegation from the Secretary of State down the line, i.e. an interactive planning process in which the management control exercised by one level over the level below (DHSS over RHA, RHA over AHA and AHA over District) would enable a continuous dialogue on policies and plans. This, sadly, did not occur. In this way it was hoped that there would be less delegation downwards — accompanied by accountability upwards. However, 'Accountability in the health service is not easily determined, because consultants and general practitioners are primarily accountable to their patients.' (DHSS, 1972, para.1.28, p.17).

Regrettably, the 1974 reorganisation failed to provide a satisfactory deal for patients and provided little in the way of job-satisfaction for staff. This is noted in the Consultative Paper on the Structure and Management of the NHS (DHSS, 1979) which states: 'The structure and management arrangements of the Service introduced in 1974 do not provide the best framework for the effective delivery of care to patients.' (para.1, p.1). The Paper goes on to unfold the reasons for the inappropriateness of the service to patients, underlining that the needs of patients were not regarded as paramount and that decisions affecting patients were taken at remote levels of the organisation. In this context, the paper says, 'the needs of patients must be paramount', and 'the closer decisions are taken to those who work with patients, the more likely it is that the patients' needs will be their prime objective' (para.3, p.1). It emphasises that to achieve better services to patients, management arrangements should be strengthened at local level coupled with greater delegation of responsibility, and there should be simplification of structure, i.e. removal of the area tier; simplification of the professional structure to give improved voice to professionals; and simplification of the planning system particularly to ensure that regional plans are sensitive to district needs.

The re-examination of the NHS was precipitated due to dissatisfaction with the organisation and services of the 1974 structure, and began as early as 1975. The Government of the day had reservations regarding the new arrangements evidenced by the introduction of the Consultative Paper — *Democracy in the National Health Service*, May 1974, which made provision for the inclusion of Local Government representatives on the RHAs; an increase in their numbers on AHAs together with additional powers to Community Health Councils regarding the approval of hospital closures.

It became obvious, that the earlier reorganisation had resulted in an over-centralised service, with decisions being taken too far from the point of delivery of services and that the bureaucracy had increased disproportionately as a result. These beliefs were borne out by the findings of The Royal Commission on the NHS which reported in June 1979. It was the structure of the service which was considered to be unsatisfactory. Proposals for a radical change in the management structure were issued in December 1979 in the consultation paper *Patients First* (DHSS, 1979). The strategy proposed received general support and the proposals were embodied in the *Health Services Act* 1980. This Act enabled a new structure to be established, with effect from April 1982 having the overall aim to increase the effectiveness and efficiency of the NHS whilst causing least disruption for those directly engaged in patient care.

The 1982 Reorganisation

The 1982 reorganisation was advanced following the recognition in the 'Royal Commission on the NHS' and *Patients First* of 'the heavy price in terms of personal stress and service disruption imposed by the 1974 reorganisation' (Taylor, 1984). Therefore, the search for better management in the NHS continued, ultimately heralding the 1982 reorganisation. An analysis of the events which are thought to have precipitated the 1982 reorganisation include, the Conservative Government's election pledge to reduce, where possible, the level of public spending; the Rayner scrutinies; the establishment of the Körner Working Party on Health Service Information; the introduction of accountability reviews; and the development of performance indicators (Taylor, 1984).

The 1982 structural reorganisation reflected an earnest and continuing quest for better management, 'to ensure the care and comfort of patients, central to which was the efficient use of resources and the morale of workers' (Merrison, HMSO, 1979, para.1.7, p.2).

The theme underlying the reorganisation was that of simplification of structure by the removal of the area tier. Also, the intention was to alter the planning and professional procedures which would give professionals the right to give advice on, and be consulted on, matters concerning them directly. To effect this, the number of committees was reduced together with the strengthening of unit level management thereby hopefully ensuring greater managerial efficiency together with greater accountability of the service to Parliament.

The philosophy underlying the 1982 reorganisation was that change should be effected in an evolutionary way coupled with less central guidance allowing more local freedom to effect precise arrangements. The Government's aim was that all structural changes should have taken effect by the end of 1983. Within this period RHAs would be free to make progress at whatever pace was appropriate to their circumstances (Merrison, para.29, p.15).

In reality the main effect of the 1980 Act was to reduce the many tiers of management which were deemed to be duplicative as well as inhibiting communication and decision making within the NHS. Thus the 90 Area Health Authorities (with their 208 districts) were superseded by 192 District Health Authorities which were generally smaller than AHAs and closer to the communities they serve. As a consequence, therefore, it was hoped the new structure would be more receptive to local issues and needs. Within districts, adminstrative sectors were abolished while simultaneously strengthening the units of management.

Figure 2.2: Structure of the NHS (1982)

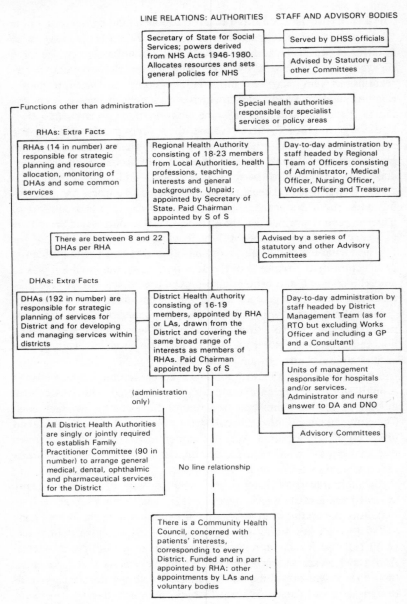

LINE RELATIONS: AUTHORITIES   STAFF AND ADVISORY BODIES

Secretary of State for Social Services; powers derived from NHS Acts 1946-1980. Allocates resources and sets general policies for NHS

Served by DHSS officials

Advised by Statutory and other Committees

Functions other than administration

Special health authorities responsible for specialist services or policy areas

RHAs: Extra Facts

RHAs (14 in number) are responsible for strategic planning and resource allocation, monitoring of DHAs and some common services

Regional Health Authority consisting of 18-23 members from Local Authorities, health professions, teaching interests and general backgrounds. Unpaid; appointed by Secretary of State. Paid Chairman appointed by S of S

Day-to-day administration by staff headed by Regional Team of Officers consisting of Administrator, Medical Officer, Nursing Officer, Works Officer and Treasurer

There are between 8 and 22 DHAs per RHA

Advised by a series of statutory and other Advisory Committees

DHAs: Extra Facts

DHAs (192 in number) are responsible for strategic planning of services for District and for developing and managing services within districts

District Health Authority consisting of 16-19 members, appointed by RHA or LAs, drawn from the District and covering the same broad range of interests as members of RHAs. Paid Chairman appointed by S of S

Day-to-day administration by staff headed by District Management Team (as for RTO but excluding Works Officer and including a GP and a Consultant)

Units of management responsible for hospitals and/or services. Administrator and nurse answer to DA and DNO

(administration only)

All District Health Authorities are singly or jointly required to establish Family Practitioner Committee (90 in number) to arrange general medical, dental, ophthalmic and pharmaceutical services for the District

Advisory Committees

No line relationship

There is a Community Health Council, concerned with patients' interests, corresponding to every District. Funded and in part appointed by RHA: other appointments by LAs and voluntary bodies

Source: DHSS.

This reorganisation led to the NHS in England being managed by 14 Regional Health Authorities (RHAs) and 192 District Health Authorities (DHAs). Each RHA comprises from 8 to 22 DHAs (Figure 2.2). The constitution of each RHA consists of 18 to 23 members from local authorities, health professions, teaching and members of general backgrounds. Each authority has a paid chairman appointed by the Secretary of State. The RHAs are responsible principally for strategic planning and resource allocation as well as monitoring DHAs. They are advised by a series of statutory and other advisory committees.

Each DHA consists of 16 to 19 members. The members are appointed by RHAs or Local Authorities and are drawn from the district and cover the same broad range of interests as members of RHAs. The chairman is appointed by the Secretary of State.

The DHAs are responsible for the day-to-day administration by staff, headed by the district management team. DHAs have responsibility for strategic planning of services for the district and for developing and managing services within districts. All DHAs are singly or jointly required to establish a Family Practitioner Committee (FPC). Currently these committees number 90 and have the responsibility for arranging general medical, dental, ophthalmic and pharmaceutical services for the district.

Units of management responsible for hospitals are headed by a Director of Nursing Services, Administrator and Senior Consultant, and are answerable to the DNO, DA and DMO.

Also, there is a Community Health Council (which has no line relationship) and which is wholly concerned with patients' interests. There is one CHC for every district. It is funded, and in part appointed by the RHA with other appointments being made by LAs and voluntary bodies.

The 1982 reorganisation was initiated to decentralise decision making, in effect to reduce central 'control' (DHSS) and to provide more local freedom to decide on precise arrangements. Did this decentralisation really happen? What changes, if any, in real terms resulted from this re-shaping of the NHS authority structure?

According to Taylor (1984) since the 1982 reorganisation, the emphasis of policy has moved towards the need to ensure the NHS upward accountability to Parliament. Also the power of the professional monopolies in the Health Service has been challenged in a number of ways. The relevant events which underlie this shift of emphasis and challenges are seen to include industrial action involving groups including nurses and ancillary workers, which accentuated and increased NHS waiting lists to unacceptable levels, together with Government expenditure adjustments of 1983 which resulted in a loss to the hospital services equivalent to £140m. To compound the problem, there was dispute over Norman Fowler's direct attempts to reduce the NHS manpower levels and, most important, there was the report of the 1983 NHS Management Inquiry (DHSS, 1983).

Clearly, in the light of much evidence the changes envisaged, and intended by repeated and sometimes extensive reorganisation, did not fully materialise, as evidenced by the findings of the Griffiths Inquiry (DHSS, 1983). And so, the search for an improved authority structure — a suitable framework — which would ensure the delivery of quality care to patients and clients and afford the staff a measure of job satisfaction, continued.

The Griffiths Inquiry (DHSS, 1983)

In 1983, Norman Fowler announced the establishment of an inquiry into NHS management practices in England. The team responsible for conducting this exercise was headed by Roy Griffiths. The inquiry focused on the need to create a new managerial structure.

The philosophy of the report is simply stated: 'The National Health Service is about delivering services to patients.' 'All that we recommend is the desire to secure the best possible services for the patient' (DHSS, 1983, paras. 3/4/30, pp.10/11/21).

In view of the potential importance of the Griffiths report, particularly in hopefully providing a future effective and appropriate framework for the management of the NHS, a detailed analysis of its philosophy, observations and recommendations, together with the comment and observations of professionals, follows.

Critique of the Present Service

The Griffiths report is critical of NHS management at all levels, particularly in such vital areas as, 'the lack of identifiable individuals to accept personal responsibility for planning and implementing objectives'. In addition, the report emphasises 'lack of a clearly defined general management function' throughout the NHS and, not surprisingly, there is no real continuous evaluation of its performance against criteria such as levels of service, quality of product, meeting budgets, cost improvement, productivity and motivating and rewarding staff. The report emphasises that central, isolated instances should disappear and that, given an effective management process, the same levels of care could be delivered more efficiently at lower cost, or a superior service given at the same cost. Also, the report emphasises the importance of units of management (particularly the major hospitals) which provide the bedrock for the whole NHS management process. It is noted that many hospitals do not yet have budgets and that urgent management action is required, if units are to fulfil their role and provide the most effective management of their resources. This, the report says, particularly affects the doctors as 'their decisions largely dictate the use of all resources and they must accept the management's responsibility which goes with clinical freedom'.

General management defined as 'the responsibility drawn together in one person, at different levels of the organisation, for planning, implementation and control of performance' is disturbingly lacking. 'At no level', says the report, 'is the general management role clearly being performed by an identifiable individual and, as a result, there is no driving force seeking and accepting direct and personal responsibility for developing management plans, securing their implementation and monitoring actual achievements'. In addition, the process of devolution of responsibility is far too slow and units and the authorities are being swamped with directives without being given direction. Following from this appraisal, the report advocates establishing a general management process to provide the necessary leadership to capitalise on the existing high levels of dedication and expertise, to stimulate initiative, urgency and vitality, to bring about a constant search for major change and cost improvement and to secure proper motivation of staff.

Recommended Changes

The report recommends changes that are radical and which have major implications (some of which are already clear, i.e. the removal of chief nursing officers from post) for all health care professionals. In this context, the report sees as paramount to a successful and productive service, the appointment of a Health Services Supervisory Board, chaired by the Secretary of State together with any NHS Management Board chaired by the General Manager. The function of these Boards is to ensure that statutorily appointed Authorities engage in day-to-day management at all levels; and, that the central objective is securing quality of care and delivery of services at local level.

The report recommends the appointment of a general manager who should be identified on the criteria of general management skills and experience, from within the existing team (already the managers have been appointed from outside the existing team), the exceptions to the rule being the Chairman of the NHS Management Board and the Personnel Director. The reasons given for this approach are: 'the people concerned would require to have considerable experience and skill in effecting change in a large, service orientated organisation as well as having credibility in establishing the new management style'.

The purpose of appointing General Managers is to 'sharpen up the process on decision taking where there is disagreement, and, on implementation, by identifying personal responsibility to ensure that speedy action is taken and that the effectiveness and efficiency of such action is under constant review'. In support of this, the report says that consensus management can lead to 'lowest common denominator decisions and to long delays in the management process'.

It is proposed that the role of RHAs be strengthened — they will need to ensure that districts, hospitals and units are liberated to manage the service and be held to proper account for performance and achievement. Each authority will have to clarify its own role together with the general management function.

The Griffiths inquiry established that the 1982 reorganisation had not resulted in the devolution of real decision making to unit and hospital level; stressing that hospitals do not have budgets. Some observers support (Evans, 1983) the approach advocated by Griffiths, in so far as it intends 'to promote the control change in a much more positive manner; it is about transforming the NHS into a managed rather than a merely administered service'.

Comment

How have nurses and other health care professionals reacted to the findings and recommendations of the Griffith Inquiry?

The proposals (depending on whether they suit or do not suit professionals) have been interpreted in different ways. The key questions being asked include: In what way, if at all, will designating one member of each regional health authority, district health authority or unit, as a general manager (with the power to reduce time on consultative procedures as well as to over-rule dissenting members) affect the health service? Is it envisaged that general managers at district level, would act as team co-ordinators without altering functional command lines, e.g. between district nursing officers and their nurse managers? Can there be true democracy and efficiency in the management of health care where doctors continue to retain medical autonomy — despite a deliberate intention to emasculate them? Currently, doctors continue, due to their power and authority of prescription, to make major demands on NHS resources. Will this situation change? Will the general management function emerge intact, and effective?

Observations by Professionals

The General Secretary of the RCN, Trevor Clay, made a number of observations on the report. For example: 'The report's recommendations for what amount to yet another reorganisation of the Health Service, are illtimed and disturbing'; 'these proposals will have a shattering effect on personnel in the Health Service'. More recently Mr Clay has become more optimistic. Following the publication of the DHSS Circular (HC(84)13, DHSS, 1984), he said: 'As a profession nurses are strong and powerful and will seek to extend the leadership they have built up into the new structure for the benefit of patients and society as a whole.' (*Nursing Standard*, Oct./Nov.1983/June 1984). Sadly, this optimism was short-lived following virtual insurrection by chief nursing officers (rightly) as they saw their very necessary expertise being despised and their role apparently (sometimes actually) becoming redundant.

The President of the RCN, Miss Sheila Quinn, was also equally concerned about some of the effects of Griffiths on the nursing profession; 'The report brought into question the whole issue of leadership in nursing in a way that would not be beneficial to all concerned.' (*Nursing Mirror*, Nov.1983), and 'the report threatened to stop nurses of the right to manage patient services'. (*Nursing Standard*, Nov.1983). More recently Miss Quinn had this to say: 'The Griffiths' report was discredited in the eyes of professionals because of its misplaced emphasis on "productivity".' (*Senior Nurse*, May 1984).

Administrators were initially hostile to the idea of the appointment of Chief Executives, understandably seeing their own jobs under threat through appointments other than from the ranks of administration. More recently (presumably sensing that they would become the 'leaders'), this hostility had turned to euphoria, as indicated by the first General Manager to be appointed as Regional General Manager for the North West Thames RHA (as administrator) who said, 'The new style management should help the nursing service.' (*Nursing Standard*, July 1984). The way in which this new management could help nurses, was not qualified. Treasurers feel that the issue of consultants' freedom has been imperfectly grasped by Griffiths in so far as he rightly emphasises the importance of clinicians' decisions in all matters with consequent management modifications; but he has not tied them down by insisting that they should be employees of the Authority.

The doctors' enthusiastic welcome for Griffiths is not, one suspects, for the concept of accountable management it embraces but more cynically perhaps because they see the NHS being broken down into units through which they can give rein to their own views. Also, doctors' initial disquiet at the introduction of Griffiths has been allayed, presumably because of the carrot offered in the form of financial allowance for additional managerial responsibilities as well as ensuring a high proportion of top management posts filled by doctors.

What about Griffiths' personal views and those of his team as to the validity and efficacy of their philosophy?

In an interview with the *Daily Telegraph* (Nov.1983) Roy Griffiths made the following points: 'The General Manager is going to be the person best suited to the job, regardless of profession, and it can quite easily be a nurse. Nurses exhibit very strong potential for general management in many cases; the proposals don't threaten them at all.' He also emphasised that the role of the general manager is to ensure that decisions are taken and that problems are addressed. In addition, they are intended to fill the 'vacuum of authority' left by the present NHS system of consensus management. He saw the problem with consensus management as leading to the 'lowest common denominator' approach — the level at which managers easily get agreement, so that the really contentious issues don't get on to the table or, if they do, are not decided.

In the light of the exhaustive debate on the report, are the many comments about Griffiths justified, particularly in the light of the publication of the DHSS circular 'Implementation of the NHS Management Inquiry Report (HC(84)13) (DHSS, 1984)? Are the 'off-the-cuff' comments of health care professionals valid and realistic? Are the fears expressed by some health care professionals justified? In short, despite inevitable bias, is the future viability of the NHS assured by adopting this 'new' approach to management?

The main areas of concern expressed by nurses on publication of the DHSS circular (HC(84)13) relate to the function of general management (para.4, p. ii). In this context, the circular underlines: 'direct accountability to the authority, or in the case of units to the District General Manager, for the general management function' (para.4.1, p. ii). And, 'Professional Chief Officers, on matters relating to the fulfilment of the general manager's responsibility, will be accountable to the general manager for the day-to-day performance of their management functions.' (para.5, p.iii). The view apparently being expressed by nurses is that they do not wish, for reasons undisclosed, to be accountable to somebody other than a nurse. In recent months, regrettably, their worst fears have been realised with the removal from post of some chief nursing officers, following the appointment of a general manager.

The alleged improvements in NHS management since the introduction of the Griffiths recommendations are catalogued in the DHSS circular (HC(84)13) and include: the establishment of DHAs which now serve smaller populations; greater responsibility being devolved to hospital and community services at unit level; the strengthening of accountability with the introduction of annual reviews of performance against agreed objectives; more effective monitoring of manpower nurses; and the introduction of the Rayner Scrutiny technique. This list (which is only part of a long catalogue of alleged improvements) is disputed in a recent publication (Davidmann, 1984).

Davidmann (1984) is scathing of the Griffiths report insofar as he says that the recommendations of the report 'should be rejected'. The author makes this uncompromising conclusion, despite his difficulty in evaluating the report, because of its 'brevity and the absence from the document of back-up material supporting the proposals'. He rationalises his decision on such key issues pertaining to the report as:

> management (executives) are apparently to provide patients and the community with what management think is good for them instead of reacting to their needs; the potential reduction in functional management, consultation and teamwork together with the associated move of decision making to the top; judging the extent of a manager's performance by the extent to which he accepts the new style of management and by the extent to which he can persuade his subordinates to accept the new style of management and its objectives; that functional managers are to be responsible first to the newly appointed executives instead of to their functional managers; and, that changes for functional chief officers and managers amount to demotion and its consequent effects e.g. reduced chances of promotion and consequently reduced chances of better pay for functional managers such as doctors and nurses.

Recent information on the potential effects of the Griffiths recommendations on the position of the ward sister/charge nurse indicates that this significant and vital role may be taken over by a ward manager! If this is to be the model for the future of nursing one must seriously question the centrality of caring to nursing and indeed wonder if the words of Professor Revans (1962) on humanising the system have gone wholly unheeded.

Impact of Griffiths' key question of course cannot be answered directly: Will the service to patients be improved if the service is manned by managers rather than by civil servants as at present?

Taylor (1984) says that the impact of the Griffiths' recommendations will ultimately depend on detailed arrangements finally agreed; but the combination of a strong NHS Management Board head, together with significant delegation of existing DHSS powers into the NHS if realised, could free the upper echelons of the organisation of excessive and unnecessary involvement in the day-to-day working of the service thus enabling those officers to concentrate on making the more fundamental decisions about health policy

In the final analysis, the acid test of an improved NHS will be the provision of a more humane, caring and personal service to patients and clients by managers and professionals who collectively pool and use their skills and knowledge in providing the highest standard of care.

References

Davidmann, D. (1984) Reorganising the National Health Service. An Evaluation of the Griffiths Report. Social Organisation Ltd., Middlesex

DHSS (1972) Management Arrangements for the Reorganised National Health Service (Grey Book). HMSO, London

────── (1972, 1974) Reports of the Joint Working Party on the Organisation of Medical Work in Hospitals (Cogwheel). HMSO, London

────── (1979) Patients First (Consultative Paper on Structure and Management of the National Health Service). DHSS

────── (1982) Health Service Development: Professional Advisory Machinery, HC(83)1. DHSS, London

────── (1982) Health Service Development, HC(82)2, HC(FP)(82)1, LAC(82)2. DHSS, London

────── (1983) NHS Management Inquiry (Griffiths). DHSS, London

────── (1984) Implementation of the NHS Management Inquiry, HC(84)13. DHSS, London

Draper, P. (1971) Changes within the National Health Service. *Community Health, 3,* 51–5

Evans, T (1983) Griffiths — The Right Prescription? Transcript of Paper Delivered to CIPFA-ASHT Conference, Nov.1983

HMSO (1979) Royal Commission on the National Health Service (Merrison). Cmnd, no.7615. HMSO, London

Klein, R. (1983) *The Politics of the National Health Service.* Longman, London

Office of Health Economics (1974) *The NHS Reorganisation.* OHE, London

Regan, D.E. and Stewart, J. (1982) An essay on the government of health: The case for Local Authority control. *Journal of Social Policy and Adminstration, 16,* 19–43

Revans, R.W. (1964) The morale and effectiveness of general hospitals, in G. McLachlan (ed.) *Problems and Progress in Medical Care.* Oxford University Press, Oxford

Royal College of Nursing (1978) An Assessment of the State of Nursing in the National Health Service. RCN, London

────── (1984) A Report on the Effects of the Financial and Manpower Cuts in the NHS (Nurse Alert). RCN, London

Smith, R.L. (1971) Management of change, in R.C.Jelinek *et al.* (eds.) *Service Unit Management: An Organizational Approach to Improved Patient Care*. W.Kellog Foundation, Battle Creek, MI, pp.57–78
Taylor, D. (ed.) (1984) *Understanding the NHS in the 1980s*. OHE, London

Further Advised Reading

Brown, R.G.S. (1978) *The Changing NHS*. 2nd Edn. Library of Social Policy and Administrators, London
———— (1979) *Reorganisation of the National Health Service*. A Case Study of Administrative Change. Blackwell and Mott Ltd., London
Brown, W. (1974) *Organisation*. Pelican, London
DHSS (1980) Patients First — Summary of Contents Received on the Consultative Paper. DHSS
———— (1980) Health Service Development: Structured Management HC(80)8, LAC (80)3, DHSS, London
———— (1981) Priorities for the New District Health Authorities (81/252), DHSS, London
———— (1981) Determination of Regions (S.1.1981/No.1836). DHSS, London
———— (1981) Determination of Districts (S.1.1981/No.1837). DHSS, London
———— (1981) Constitution of DHAs (S.1.1981/No.1838) DHSS, London
Draper, P. (1973) Value judgements in health service planning. *Community Medicine, 23*
Draper, P. and Smart, T. (1972) *The Future of Our Health Care*. Dept of Community Medicine, Guy's Hospital, London
Drucker, P.F. (1974) *The Practice of Management*. Harper and Row, New York
Evans, T. and Maxwell, R. (1984) Griffiths: Challenge and Response. (Evidence to the Select Committee on Social Services) Unpublished. King Edward's Hospital Fund, London
Handy, C.B. (1976) *Understanding Organizations*. Penguin, Harmondsworth
Heirs, B. (1982) *Organisations, Management, Decision-Making*. Harper and Row, New York
Klein, R. (1983) *The Politics of the National Health Service*. Longman, London
Levitt, R. and Wall, A. (1985) *The Reorganised National Health Service* 3rd edn. Croom Helm, London
McLachlan, G. (ed.) (1964) *Problems and Progress in Medical Care*. Oxford University Press, Oxford
March, J.G. and Simon, H.A. (1958) *Organizations*. Wiley, New York
Taylor, D. (ed.) (1984) *Understanding of the NHS in the 1980s*. Office of Health Economics, London

3 NURSING: STRUCTURE AND FUNCTIONS

Aims

The aims of this chapter are:

1. To examine the concept of nursing.
2. To discuss the organisation of nursing.
3. To explore the problems which are central to nursing.

Learning Objectives

The purpose of this chapter is to enable the reader to:

1. Understand the concept, structure and functions of nursing in the context of the largest health care profession.
2. Appreciate the problems which are central to nursing.

Delivery of Care: Health Care System

One of the most important current issues facing health service managers in general and nurse managers in particular is how to preserve the integrity of their organisation whether at national, regional, district or hospital level, in a constantly changing and increasingly more complex and demanding environment, while at the same time attempting to develop and encourage their staff to secure the highest standard and quality of care. Central to this ideal is the acknowledgment of the patient as a person which is realised, as far as practicable, through individualised patient care.

Currently, the delivery of patient care takes place within an organisational framework that is in essence, hierarchical (a succession of superior-subordinate relationships). This applies to the NHS as a whole and to the health care professions in particular.

Central to the nursing organisation, is that nursing service and nursing care should be as effective and efficient as possible. This encompasses the notion of productivity, i.e. the effectiveness of care relates to its quality and the efficiency of care relates to the use of resources in the most effective way (DHSS, 1983, para.1, p.10).

This framework for 'productivity' of the nursing organisation includes nursing inputs — nurses, equipment, information, together with everything that is required in providing a service to patients; transformation — technology, the nursing process, the medical process and the para medical process, i.e. methods of changing inputs into desirable output; and output — an improved and/or rehabilitated patient together with happy and satisfied staff. Two additional but vital aspects of the health care system include those of evaluation of the services given and feedback to ensure its adjustment and regulation.

The open system is in continual interaction with its environment and achieves a state of dynamic equilibrium — homeostasis. The survival of the system is dependent on the input, transformation and output.

Nursing, medicine, the paramedical professions together with other supportive disciplines, e.g. catering, pharmacy, administration and accounting, form the main components of the health care system — the National Health Service. Each of these professions can be regarded as a lesser system — a subsystem within the total system. In this complex arrangement of interrelated subsystems, any alteration in one subsystem inevitably affects the whole system, to a greater or lesser extent, e.g. if there is a dysfunction of the pharmacy, catering or domestic supportive service (subsystem) this can have an adverse effect immediately or ultimately — minimally or optimally (depending on the extent of the dysfunction), on the care and wellbeing of the patient within the total system.

Some twenty years ago a special paper examined the hospital as a human system (Revans, 1962). In his paper, Professor Revans discusses the concept and relevance of communication within the health care system. He depicts a situation in a hospital ward where, if there is rigidity of the communication system — communication is poor, information is lacking — decisions are bad and the students become afraid and discouraged. And, that 'certain identifiable human attitudes are transmitted between the organisational layers of the hospital system'. In a sample of 350 ward sisters he found:

> The attitudes that they feel they perceive in those from whom they receive instructions are the attitudes they exhibit to those to whom they transmit them. There is a statistically significant association between the attitudes that the ward sisters detect in their superiors and those which they themselves display towards their subordinates.

Human Purpose

The hospital is a system built around a set of human purposes, within which patients undergo treatment and receive care (Revans, 1962).

In general terms the open system depicts the hospital as an organisation in which there is a constant inflow of patients together with an input of staff and other resources; the processing (transformation) of those resources takes place through the agency of the nursing process and the medical process and eventually an output is produced of patients who are rehabilitated to a greater or lesser extent. In productive terms (the Griffiths philosophy highlights this aspect), the hospital can be viewed (rather inhumanely) as a people — patients processing institution. In essence, the organisation of the hospital (system) consists of many interlocking subsystems, i.e. nursing, medical, paramedical, pastoral, educational and administrative, each having their own specific functions, but contributing to the general aims of the hospital — the reception, care, treatment, comfort and rehabilitation of the patient.

Concept of Nursing

Many definitions of nursing exist (WHO, 1966; EEC, 1977; Henderson and Nite, 1978; RCN, 1981). However, as yet, there is no internationally agreed definition. Negative images of the nurse continue to linger and nurses are often portrayed in the media as 'angels of mercy', 'handmaidens', 'sex symbols' and 'battleaxes'. Such stereotypes even though apparently innocent, may have positive adverse effects on the quality of the nursing service, e.g. the negative image may affect recruitment of nursing students as well as discouraging trained nurses from continuing in practice. Also, the image portrayed can (I am convinced does) affect the status and authority of the nurse particularly in relation to decision making, the renumeration (only in recent years taken seriously by government), and most important the bargaining power of nurses to secure the necessary resources to maintain a satisfactory service to patients and clients. These, according to a recent observer, are a 'substantial impurity that needs to be filtered from nursing if its maximum quality is to be achieved' (Bennett, 1984).

The arguments as to whether nursing is a science or an art have continued over the years without any final agreeement. Some official views include:

Nursing is concerned with helping the patient with his daily pattern of living or with those activities that he normally performs without assistance i.e. eating, drinking, sleeping, moving. And to provide for those activities that make life more than a vegetable process — namely, social intercourse, recreational and productive occupations. In other words, the nurse helps the patient to maintain or to create a health regime that, if he were fit and well, he would carry out himself. (WHO, 1966, para.3.1, p.10).

In the context of providing a nursing service, Professor Baroness McFarlane (1983) said:

If one looks at the cost of the nursing service, the nursing needed to give a basic level of care and to maintain the demands of technological support to the medical function, it is unrealistic to expect the nursing service also to support informed personalised care. If it is unrealistic then we should cease to call nursing 'nursing'. Our new name should denote the role of technical aids and our training should reflect the objectives of competencies in tasks rather than role.

And:

In nursing there is an inherent conflict between scientific or competency values and moral values: the tension between competency and caring provides one of the ethical dilemmas of nursing and is only resolved when we regard scientific stringency as a way of achieving excellence in care. *(Nursing Mirror,* June 1983).

The principal objectives of the training of nurses include: the ability to identify, formulate and put into practice methods of satisfying the various health needs of patients and clients; ability to guide student nurses and other groups involved in the care of patients and clients; ability to plan, organise, implement and evaluate nursing services; ability to be involved in nursing research; ability to contribute to the promotion of an efficient health policy; ability to accept professional responsibility; and a willingness to carry on further education in nursing.

The training of nurses results from the inter-relationship of theoretical instruction, i.e. that part of nursing training where students acquire the knowledge, understanding and professional skills to plan, provide and assess total nursing care and clinical instruction on the basis of their acquired knowledge and skills.

Nursing involves a specific and individual responsibility towards the patient/client and the family, and, in this context, has as its focus the identification of the needs of individuals and groups together with the promotion of health including health education, the prevention of illness. Also, nursing must include the provision of measures to assist — both with physical, psychological, social and ethical aspects in hospital and in the community. The process of nursing must include the proper training and education of student nurses (and trained nurses) to effect the satisfactory delivery of care by nurses and auxiliary staff and the ability to guide other health personnel and to promote and maintain the necessary teamwork with health care staff. Most important, the nurse must contribute to basic and applied research in nursing, and utilise research findings and scientific techniques in the care of patients and clients (EEC.111/D/76/6/80-EN, 1981).

Even though nurses may have difficulty in defining what nursing is, there seems to be little difficulty in saying what nursing is not. Miss Nightingale underlined her views on 'non-nursing' duties by stating that nurses should not be expected to do 'scrubbing and scouring' (1859).

In 1949 the General Nursing Council for England and Wales made it clear that student nurses should not undertake what they regarded to be 'non-nursing' duties. These duties included domestic work, i.e. cleaning and dusting of wards. Also it has been emphasised over the years, by statutory and professional bodies, that nurses should not be engaged as messengers and porters and that the clerical work undertaken by them should be reduced.

The Salmon Committee (HMSO, 1966) underlined the many tasks of which ward sisters could be relieved which included administrative work and the supervision of domestic staff 'to enable them give more direct care to the patient' (para.4.22, p.34). Regrettably, despite continued effort to free nurses of non-nursing duties, tradition dies slowly, and even today some nurses seem to get 'security' from engaging in these activities — perhaps an escape from the real pressures of patient care, thus limiting the time for direct nursing care. However, as a matter of fact it is well known that in 'emergency' situations nurses continue to have non-nursing duties thrust upon them, sometimes I suspect because of sheer exploitation by other groups. And so, does an examination of what is 'non-nursing' give some clues as to what nursing really is? Obviously there is little dispute over the centrality of nursing — the care of the patients and clients by meeting their needs together with enabling their rehabilitation.

The problems of definition of nursing relate particularly to boundary issues, i.e. the problems, the conflict, and lack of clarity that are associated with the extended — specialist-practitioner — role of the nurse and its incumbent degree of authority, responsibility, accountability and autonomy, particularly in the context of attempting to define nursing's boundaries with medical and paramedical professionals. It is clear, however, that nursing practice must, of necessity, extend beyond the boundaries of other health care professions. The management and care of patients/clients is by its very nature, a team approach. This concept acknowledges the inter-dependence of health care professionals. During the past decade particularly with the emergence of the 'nursing process', the nursing situation has become complicated, largely with the development of the role of nurse practitioner and its implicit 'prescribing' role (nursing care) together with its implied and/or actual autonomy for making nursing decisions, which is frequently misinterpreted by other health care professionals, notably doctors, as signifying the total autonomy of the nurse for patient care and, as a consequence, having potentially major implications for the medical role. This point has been highlighted by some doctors who clearly feel threatened by a nursing 'take-over'. However, in this situation, there is a salutory lesson to be learned by nurses, who, in their demand for autonomy must not become so rigid in their practice as to isolate themselves from other health care professionals thereby having the effect of further reducing the quality of service provided to patients and clients. In addition, this rigidity could substantially reduce the capability of the nursing profession to respond promptly and realistically to constant changes in technology, education, and legislation and most important meeting the ever-increasing demands of an educated and knowledgeable clientele.

So, are we any nearer to knowing what nursing is? Does the 'nursing process' shed light on what nursing is, or what nurses do?

The nursing process will be discussed fully (Chapter 4), but, in the interest of clarifying what 'nursing' is, it may help to look at its accepted concept, i.e. an approach by nurses to organise the care of their patients — nursing practice, on the basis of a system which is logical, rational, includes patient/family participation and which has central to it, a problem-solving approach. Unfortunately, the concept has become clouded by mystique through the use of terminology which has become unnecessarily confusing. The process is further complicated by an apparent lack of a team approach where it is being used, an alleged increase in the clerical work (records) involved and the problems of 'breaching' role boundaries particularly with the medical profession have compounded the situation. It appears that nurses in attempting to define nursing have caused some problems (which need to be corrected promptly in the interest of sound patient care), by highlighting their move towards independence — autonomy of role — at the expense (either consciously or otherwise) of underplaying the vital and indispensible inter-professional relationship. The subsequent conflict which has arisen between nurses and doctors is substantially a communication problem: the inability of nurses to state, in unambiguous terms, that it is now a planned and systematic process, whereas in the past it was very often unsystematic, unplanned, and delivered on demand as the situation dictated. In essence, nursing was carried out in an *ad hoc* way, substantially unrecorded and with the emphasis on the nurse and procedures rather than on the patient as an individual.

Nursing and medicine can operate to a degree in parallel, i.e. nursing decisions can be made and taken by doctors; but, it is important for both professions to work in concert, to pursue the same objectives in relating to ensuring the total care, management and rehabilitation of the patient.

The problems of being decisive about what nursing is, are many, and relate to such central issues as role, functions, education and training of nurses. This indecisiveness is largely due to the complexity and lack of definition of nurses' work as stated by the EEC Nursing Directives (Nursing Directive 77/452/EEC) and by the ICN (1965). The concept expressed embodies supplying a most responsible service for the promotion of health, the prevention of illness, and the care of the sick. These requirements are as complex and demanding as they are vague, and require an extensive knowledge and skill base as well as the use of professional judgement. According to Bennett (1984) 'it is this area of subtle interaction between the nurse, patient and family, that lies at the centre of nursing, the actual caring role'. She continues, 'this area (fulfilling the preventive role) remains largely undercover. Yet, it is an integral part of the art of nursing'.

Before proceeding to discuss the management of care, let us first examine the concept and philosophy of care.

Nursing Care: A Philosophy

Caring is viewed as a discipline and is described as: 'A process, a way of relating to someone that involves development through mutual trust, a deepening and qualitative transformation of the relationship'. This discipline has eight elements, knowledge, alternating rhythms, patience, honesty, trust, humility, hope and courage (Mayeroff, 1971).

In caring, one experiences what is cared for as 'having a dignity and worth in its own right with potentialities and need for growth'.

Relevance of Mayeroff's Components of Caring as Epitomised in the Nursing Process

1. Knowledge: General and specific. This includes the possession and use of general knowledge and skills, e.g. knowledge and skills of interviewing: specific knowledge and skills, e.g. those of nursing knowledge, management and clinical knowledge and skills.
2. Alternating rhythms: Understanding and acknowledging the physical, emotional, social and spiritual needs of the patient; realising that these are ever-changing therefore requiring intentional acknowledgement and appropriate modification of nurses' approach to care (care plan).
3. Patience: Adapting to patients'/clients' pace.
4. Honesty: Open, self-critical approach to oneself, one's practice, one's profession and to patients, clients, colleagues and other professionals.
5. Trust: Respecting the independence of others: valuing one's ability, competency and judgement to take informed nursing decisions.
6. Humility: Accepting one's limitations in terms of knowledge and skills — and taking appropriate measures to reduce those limitations — knowledge gaps, through improved and continuous education and updating.
7. Hope: Being aware and acknowledging situations which merit encouragement — commitment.
8. Courage: Taking informed nursing decisions: limiting risks by knowledge and trust in one's own ability.

Despite a philosophy of care together with the availability of guidelines, in the form of the Code of Professional Conduct for Nurses and required nursing competencies, nursing continues to be tradition based where the emphasis continues to be on experience and expository methods of education rather than being problem-solving (Gestalt) based (McFarlane, *Nursing Mirror*, June 1983; Chapman, *Nursing Standard,* Nov.1982). In addition, despite many research reports and research findings which could benefit nursing education, nursing management and nursing practice, it is debateable how much, if any use is made of this information by nurse educators, nurse managers and nurse practitioners, even though nurses in practice remain accountable round-the-clock.

The performance of nursing depends on a complex interaction of many variables which embrace the person — their capability, preparations, motivation, interest and commitment; the nature and demands of the job;

and the nature of the environment in which the job is done. The successful interaction of these variables determine how well the nurse performs. Obviously if the nurse is not of the right personality, does not have the right aptitude, attitude and ability, no amount of education and training will ensure success and satisfaction when coping with the demands of nursing. In addition, if the demands of nursing outstrip the level of readiness of the nurse to take responsibility; or if education and training is inadequate or insufficient to allow the nurse to deal effectively with current problems and demands, job performance will be reduced or ineffective; and, if the environment in which nursing takes place lacks the necessary resources — human and non-human — emotional and educational support and suitable social relationships, then problems may arise.

The Role of the Nurse

Nurses have to promote their own workforce; but they have to do it within a context of professional responsibility (Bosanquet, *Nursing Times*, 1981).

The nursing care of the patient today makes great demands on nurses' knowledge and skills, especially if the care given is to be competent, efficient and effective. For example, the assessment of patients' needs together with the planning, implementing, monitoring and evaluating of the care plan, according to an RCN report (1981), 'demands a greater degree of knowledge than does the application of procedures and rules. Also, the improvement of nursing standards requires a major investment in staff development and in continuing professional education.' Such an investment must involve 'the willingness of nurse practitioners to update their knowledge, the agreement of nursing managers to provide the resources, facilities and opportunities, and the ability of nurse educators to provide the new knowledge required.' I would add that senior nurses must adopt the role of educators-enablers: they must enable nurses to acquire the skills of learning and motivate them into using their skills. In addition, the successful implementation of educational policies depends substantially on the ability of senior clinical nurses and nurse managers to interpret and meet the educational and training needs of the nursing service. But, does this really happen? Some observers think not, and state that; 'Nursing practice is still based on tradition and more credence is given to experience than to logical argument and rational problem solving.' (*Nursing Standard*, November, 1982)

A structure for the development of the nurse in education and clinical practice has already been discussed. However, defining a model or framework is one thing, putting it into practice — operationalising it through the reality of the nurse's role — can be quite different and fraught with problems.

The role of the senior nurse is very demanding, detailed and complex; but is the role occupant given the necessary recognition, authority, autonomy and preparation — initially and on-going — to ensure meeting the obligations of responsibility and accountability to practice their role in enabling and maintaining the requisite quality care?

The changing role of the nurse — particularly the front-line nurse, has been a topic of extended discussion in recent years. This change in role has its roots in the reports of Salmon and Briggs together with the guidelines developed by professional bodies. For example, the RCN considers it essential that the nurse practitioner should be able to progress to a post of consultant/specialist in a particular branch of nursing, being recognised as an expert on specialist nursing care, and being consulted by nursing colleagues and other health care professionals. In addition, Merrison (HMSO, 1979) recommends that:

> Examination should be given to the possiblility of extending the role of the nurse and enabling them to undertake tasks traditionally the province of the medical staff. Nurses should be enabled and encouraged to prescribe nursing care programmes, including the mobilisation of other services such as physiotherapy and occupational therapy. (Para. 13.16/13.17, pp. 190–191).

The Briggs report (1972) underlines the 'consultancy' function of the ward sister (para. 541, p. 164).

The problem of interpretation of role is to some extent related to the tradition, education and training of the nurse, together with the attitudes developed by senior nurses during those formative years. Where serious thought is given to effective and major change in the existing role, then there must be an effective re-education of nurses — at basic and post-basic levels, in their knowledge, skills and attitudes. Nurses must tread cautiously, in their own interest — avoiding litigation; and in the interest of the patient — ensuring optimum and safe care. This is not happening to any extent (Bowman 1980).

The lack of clarity of role gives rise to feelings of insecurity, uncertainty, lack of recognition and direction in nurses' work. Central to this uncertainty is lack of, unclear, or uncertain authority, responsibility and autonomy of trained nurses which produce unclear boundaries in relation to their work. Also the inadequacy of definition, perception and interpretation of the nursing role poses special problems for the development of a suitable curricula.

Before becoming preoccupied with the extended/expanded role, the Merrison report makes clear what is the nature and criteria of the clinical role of the nurse.

A conference (RCN, 1982) identified the different types of senior clinical role as 'senior sister/clinical leader and clinical specialist' (para.2, p.2). And stated that, 'the criteria for the nurse exercising advanced clinical skills would include: evidence of innovative initiative; clinical teaching — peer groups, multidisciplinary groups, staff in designated training areas, involvement in nursing research, consultancy — the credibility and expertise of the nurse is such that they are acknowledged and used as a source of nursing advice by colleagues, and exceptional leadership characteristics.' (para.1, p.4).

Research carried out at Brunel University (Cang *et al.*, 1981) on the role of the ward sister in general hospitals, underlines five main responsibilities which include: ensuring that patients are made physically, psychologically and socially comfortable, ensuring that special procedures required for individual patients are carrried out, ensuring that doctors' prescriptions for individual patients are carried out, the management and control of the ward environment and of the ward's relationships with the hospital and external world, and teaching and training.

A seminar (RCN, 1982) indicated its 'concern' over the extent to which the ward sister's role has been eroded and proposed that 'accountability should be matched by the necessary authority to control the environment for patient care'.

There is growing concern and urgency among nurses which is particularly demonstrated by professional and statutory bodies, to clarify the role of the nurse, particularly nurses' 'responsibility', 'accountability', 'authority' and 'autonomy', in the context of the delivery of quality care. Before examining these concepts together with identifying their interrelationships and applicability to nursing, certain questions are prompted. For example: How can nurses argue with conviction for increased authority, and autonomy? Has their responsibility, authority and accountability increased? What is the relevance of these elements in relation to the exercise of the nurse's role in the management of patient care and in the professionalisation of nursing? Is the situation right legally, educationally and skill-wise for nurses to cope effectively with — and to accept the consequences of — autonomy of role in relation to clinical decision making, together with coming to terms with the incumbent responsibility and accountability? Are nurses ready to be judged/assessed on their competency in relation to nursing standards by peers and/or other criteria? Have nurses, in fact, the necessary motivation and expertise to secure, and maintain, an extension of their role? What are the problems — educationally, professionally, emotionally and legally — associated with the exercise of an extended role?

Problems and Dilemmas: The Real Issues

If nurses are to be regarded as professionals then it follows that important issues relating to their responsibility, authority, accountability and autonomy must be acknowledged, not only in their practice, but also, most importantly, priority must be given to their training and development to fit them for, and safeguard them in the decisions they are obliged to make in the proper execution of their job, in setting and maintaining standards of care.

The principal dilemmas for senior nurses and nurse managers relate to maintaining an effective nursing service in an environment which presents vagueness of the role, functions and professional parameters of key nurses, not knowing the area of legitimate clinical freedom and practice. It follows that nurses must exercise caution, particularly in the areas of the 'extended' role and/or 'practitioner' role, as the carrying out of procedures or the conduct of activity, for which nurses are not trained, should an accident occur, may lead to a situation where they are charged with negligence. In this situation there is a need to define operational policy particularly related to indemnity insurance requirements, i.e. the vicarious liability of the employer needs to be clarified.

A major problem is that the authority, responsibility, accountability and autonomy and development of senior nurses do not match their role functions and expectations and negate against nurses meeting the needs and demands of their patients/clients. In essence, their imprecise role is unproductive and unmeaningful to the demands placed upon them and to their own security and job-satisfaction.

How do Nurses see their Role? The Real Issues

Research shows that sisters see their role 'as being founded on and related to their professional as opposed to their managerial activities'. (Williams, 1969; Bowman, 1980). The ward sister's role was seen by Williams to be made up of a kernel of professional-clinical activity which is surrounded by responsibilities that are both clinical and administrative in nature and around these tasks are activities which are managerial in nature. Bowman found that front-line nurses saw their role mainly as 'nurse';

but identified their functions as 'managerial'.

The role of the nurse is influenced by many factors including social change, new technology and medical progress — all of which affect nurses' approach to patient management. Because of these changes the role of the nurse can never be static (even though it must be accepted that it contains a substantial nursing element), but be constantly review- ed, updated and extended — within the framework of education and agreed legislation, to permit safe practice.

Therefore, does the role of the nurse embody those vital elements which enable them to do their job with confidence and competence? In essence, to enable them to perform at a professional level, how relevant is the research to identifying the true perspective of nurses' role?

Nurses, through encouragement from their professional bodies as well as through the trigger of various Government reports, notably Salmon (1966), Briggs (HMSO, 1972) and Merrison (1979), have in recent years focused on the much discussed 'extended' role together with its elements of responsibility, accountability, authority and autonomy. In this con- text there are important implications that need to be considered. For ex- ample, any increased responsibility inevitably brings with it increased accountability. The further transfer of authority through increased autonomy for decision making on matters relating to the nursing care of the patient and/or through the adoption of a 'practitioner' role (prescribing nursing care) which is central to the nursing process, brings in its wake problems which relate to other health care professionals, as exemplified by the 'offence' taken and resistance offered by some doctors to the introduction of the nursing process. These problems would seem to have their roots in tradition, fear and faulty communication between professionals. I would venture to say that this resistance could be reduc- ed or obviated by improved communication together with improved con- fidence by professionals in the professional integrity of their colleagues.

In addition to these problems there are also educational issues that need to be examined, i.e. the acquisition of new knowledge and skills to cope with the new and/or additional cognitive, effective and psychomotor problems which may be encountered by the potential role occupant. In effect, nurses must be prepared educationally, skill-wise and emotionally to enable them cope effectively with their new role.

Most important, there are potential legal problems arising from the increased authority, responsibility and autonomy of the nurse. In the legal context 'change the ground rules and take on additional functions and the next few years will unquestionably see more nurses being named as defendants in negligence actions'. And, 'the standard of care required of nurses is based on the level of skill and competence that might reasonably be found in adequately trained members of the profession. It is here that any widening of the nurse's role could lead to trouble' (Martin, 1982).

In this respect, in any action by a patient/client for damages, which involves a nursing decision, a nurse may be held legally liable if it can be shown either that she has failed to exercise the skills properly expected of her, or that she has undertaken tasks she was not competent to perform.

Delegation of Tasks

The doctor may be held to be guilty of negligent delegation if it can be shown that he conferred authority on nurses to perform tasks which were either outside the scope of the duties they were normally expected to perform, or for which they had no special qualification. Tasks which have hitherto been carried out by doctors before they were delegated to nurses should only be undertaken if: nurses have been specifically and adequately trained for the performance of the new tasks; the training needed for the efficient execution of the task has been recognised as satisfactory by the employing authority; nurses agree to undertake the new tasks; the tasks have been recognised by the respective professions and by the employing authority as tasks which may be properly delegated to nurses; and the delegating doctor has been assured of the competence of the individual nurse concerned.

Effects of Vagueness of Role on Practice and Professionalism

What are the effects on nurses and their patients, of working in an environment which remains 'grey' on the chief elements of nurses' role, i.e. responsibility, actual or implied, an indecisiveness of authority and lack of autonomy to make nursing decisions, but still major accountability for ensuring safe practice?

The absence of a clearly defined role makes it increasingly difficult for nurses to maintain standards of care let alone improve the quality of care. Because of this inability to maintain standards of care nurses' morale is reduced and stress is accentuated. This is substantiated by research which shows: 'Failure to live up to unrealistic standards set by themselves and others is placing many nurses under stress.' Also, the inability of the nurse to know when she has done a job well — an inherent problem of the nursing profession — was blamed on, 'the nature of the job and the nature of the profession' (Hingley, 1984).

The essence of nursing is ensuring care of patients. To enable this requires the requisite authority to make decisions on patient care. This can only be effective if appropriate autonomy for making clinical decisions is incumbent in the role of the senior nurse. 'The sister should decide the standards of care to be given, within resource limits and be answerable for the performance of all staff who nurse on the ward' (Cang *et al.*, 1981). Also, excessive work demands cause the nurse to suffer tension and frustration which may lead to aggression and aggravate existing difficulties in interpersonal and intraprofessional relationships leading to conflict. Conflict may also be caused because of differences between the roles — nurses', doctors' and managers'. Essentially, the orientation of nurses' and doctors' role is professional while the manager's is efficiency seeking (Wieland, 1981).

The implications for nurses and nursing of an unclear role is that of increased stress for nurses and inefficient and ineffective care for the patient. In addition, as already mentioned, lawyers have commented on the legal problems of moving prematurely into the 'extended role' now much discussed.

Research by Cang and his colleagues on the future emerging role of ward sisters proposes: 'The Sister role requires to be pitched at a higher level of work than is the case at present.' The implications of this they see as being 'substantial for recruitment, career development, relationships with medical and other staff, including senior roles'. They say in this situation, 'much more could be expected to be decided at ward level, by Sister, than is now possible'; the ward would become an organisationally more significant part of the overall service. And, in the absence of this role the envisaged, potential, consequences for patient care are serious and include:

> Priorities cannot be properly set; policies also will not be set as they should be set, with the proper involvement by the nursing staff; unrealistic resource levels may be set, leading to an unreliable service to Sister, and in turn to an effective undermining of her position of responsibility, leaving patients unduly exposed.

To date, regrettably, nursing has tended to focus on non-nursing activities rather than on what nursing is about — the activities of nursing, or what nurses do. In this respect, the role of the nurse, which is central to sound education, development, practice and management, remains unclear and ambiguous.

Generally there is little dispute among senior nurses on the central caring role. The problem relates particularly to the operation of nursing — to defining the boundaries, i.e. the parameters of nursing practice (Barnard, 1984). For example, the expanded role of the nurse, central to which is a practitioner function, is seen by doctors to intrude into the domain of medicine (Mitchell, 1984). However, in the final analysis the nurse's role must remain flexible to enable the profession to respond readily to changes in society, to meet the ever-increasing demands of patients and clients and to help nurses to cope with the introduction and effects of new technology.

Nursing Organisation and Structure: Evolution

The nursing organisation can be viewed as a three-tiered structure. The front level is the interface between the patient/client and the rest of the organisation. This level, the operational level, is of particular importance as the nurses are in immediate contact with the patients, clients and the public. Major decisions on nursing policy taken by managers at the 'top' level of nursing management are put into effect on the ward and in the community.

The second level, that of middle management, is essentially concerned with the day-to-day operations of the organisation. Decision making and monitoring are central functions of this level.

Top level management is primarily concerned with general organisation and planning, together with monitoring of the lower levels of management.

Nurse Education

The organisation of the Nurse Education Department School of Nursing may vary slightly for each district, but substantially consists of the following: Director of Nurse Education (DNE); in line relationship with the DNE may be two or more Assistant Directors with particular responsibility for basic and post-basic education; next in line are the Senior Nurse Tutors (SNTs) with particular responsibility for day-to-day educational activities and specialisms, i.e. the basic curricula in general nursing, psychiatry, paediatrics, and post-basic curricula, e.g. ENB courses and continuing education.

The front-line teachers include Nurse Teachers (NTs) and Clinical Teachers (CTs) who are particularly charged with the implementing of the main educational programme theoretically as well as in the clinical setting.

The development of nurses in the skills and knowledge of nursing, has, over the years, made the standard of nursing and the image of British nursing to be rated highly internationally. Yet, despite the emphasis on the caring aspect, little in the way of training for the management content of the job took place before the advent of the Salmon (1966) and Mayston (1969) reports. Even today, there is much debate, and rightly so, on how to make best use of the skills, knowledge and other attributes of nurses at basic and post-basic levels to ensure the improved care of patients. (Continuing education will be discussed in Chapter 11).

Nursing Structure: Future Trends

Nursing is a practice discipline and as such relies substantially on society's support. Therefore, in return, nursing must endeavour to meet society's needs by ensuring it keeps pace with changes in technology and public opinion. These needs are not static. This clearly means that nurses and the profession of nursing, to fulfil these requirements, must be able to respond positively and effectively to change, while simultaneously nurses must act as change agents.

Even though the challenges, demands and opportunities for nurses are many and great, regrettably, the structure of the profession and the many constraints placed on nurses, central to which is the ineptness and inadequacy of their education, minimises their ability to meet the changes, needs and demands which confront them. The evidence for this is great and will be unfolded as the text progresses. (Education will be discussed in Chapter 11.)

Essentially, the philosophy and structure in which nursing is taught and practised and on which nursing is managed, at least is inept and at most, is impotent. The reasons for this are many with their roots in tradition and nursing culture. However, increasing pressure for improved career prospects in nursing education, clinical nursing and nursing management (the latter presently being somewhat blighted through uncertainty as to the future of chief nursing officers in the wake of the Griffiths' Inquiry), together with the many changes over recent years in the management strucure of the health service, have given impetus to the need to establish the way in which the education, management and clinical nursing function should be clarified, substantiated and developed. The seed for a new, a more logical, rational and career-satisfying, nursing structure which would enable the development of staff and utilise their skills and abilities to the full, in essence their self-actualisation, was sown at a DHSS seminar (DHSS, 1981). The objective of the seminar was to develop initiatives which would reinforce and develop the clinical nursing function and to define a strategy for their achievement. The principles underlying the recommendations of seminar syndicates included, 'commitment to the idea of professional development as a continuous educational process and acceptance of the principle of accreditation'. (The appointment to clinical posts at any level must be in accordance with specified criteria which indicate that the person appointed is suitably qualified in terms of formal qualification, experience and other relevant attainment.)

The recommendations for a clinical career pattern acknowledge that immediately following registration nurses should have a required period for professional consolidation and development. Also, the post of staff nurse should no longer have automatic progression from student to staff nurse. In addition, there should be a 'clinical leader' role, e.g. head of ward or leader of community team, which is regarded as a senior designated post. Most important, there should be progress to advanced clinical grades which could be based on participation in research, published articles, peer group reviews together with teaching expertise.

In the wake of the DHSS seminar, a second seminar was arranged (RCN, 1982), the intention being to continue the work of the previous seminar. The principles endorsed by the seminar participants included:

that every registered nurse is responsible and accountable for their own nursing actions; every post designated 'clinical' would have a specified clinical (geographical) base; the concept of an 'advanced clinical role' should be developed by establishing clinical career progression with 'senior clinical posts'.

In the quest for securing a structure for nursing, in an attempt to facilitate the highest standard of care, a discussion document was prepared and published (RCN, 1981). This document was prepared 'in response to the frustration and dissatisfaction voiced within the nursing profession' which were echoed in the RCN Council's emergency resolution to its representative body (1980).

In July 1980 the RCN Council agreed to the setting up of a working group 'to examine and made recommendations on a professional structure for nursing and midwifery staff'. The working group subsequently published a discussion document — *A Structure for Nursing* (RCN, 1981). This document contained proposals for a new professional nursing structure for clinical nurses, nurse managers and nurse educationists.

Clinical and Managerial Structure

1. Clinical Structure (Figure 3.1)

In the context of the clinical structure, the qualified nurse is defined as, 'the holder of a statutory nursing qualification who has been prepared to assess, plan, implement and evaluate nursing care and who is professionally accountable for the care he/she gives'. All qualified nurses should hold the title of 'Staff Nurse'. At this basic level of experience it is advised that the provision of care should be directed and guided by the 'Primary' nurse, who is identified as the leader of the care team, by virtue of experience and expertise and who has total responsibility for planning and implementation of care for a specific group of patients or client group.

'Sister II' is a grade which is intended to encompass the qualified experienced nurse who is in the process of undertaking or has undertaken an appropriate post-basic qualification and/or recognised training within the specialty in which he/she is practising and who is responsible for the total provision of nursing care to a specific group of patients or clients.

Advanced clinical roles include 'Sister I', the designated leader of the clinical team for a defined clinical area who has appropriate post-basic qualifications and/or substantial experience in the clinical area for which he/she is responsible and who has total responsibility for the overall provision of care. The Working Group also envisaged the role of 'Sister I' as clinical specialist providing advice across the range of a unit or district.

2. Management Structure (Figure 3.1)

The management structure presented includes 'Director of Nursing Services' whose functions are envisaged to include assistance with and control of district nursing policies; control, co-ordination and development of nursing staff within the unit; initiation and implementation of unit nursing policies; management of the unit budget; service planning; and the provision of current nursing advice to the Chief Nurse. The 'Assistant Director of Nursing Services' would provide support and advise the DNS probably in relation to personnel and clinical practice as well as assuming line management control over other members of the clinical team. The 'Chief Nurse' would be accountable to the authority for the provision of a nursing service within the district. The functions of the Chief Nurse would include the formulation, allocation and control of the nursing budget; advising the authority on all matters relating to the nursing service; overall control and co-ordination of all nursing staff; and responsibility for the education and training of all nursing staff. 'Nurse Advisors' as envisaged in the structure, could provide advice to the Chief

Nurse and/or DNSs on matters such as service planning, personnel and research.

Education Structure (Figure 3.2)

The envisaged education structure is depicted to include the role of 'Nurse Teacher'; a qualified nurse who also has attained an advanced professional qualification, e.g. Diploma in Nursing, Advanced Diploma in Midwifery, who has undertaken a common course of preparation as a Nurse Teacher and who is responsible for the preparation, provision and assessment of theoretical and practical education and training programmes for nursing staff. The Working Group also envisage the role of 'Senior Lecturer', being a qualified nurse teacher who undertakes direct responsibility for a defined functional area within nursing education or who, by virtue of additional expertise in areas such as research or published works can demonstrate a contribution to the education centre. The role of 'Vice Principal' is seen as a staff post with a qualified Nurse Teacher assuming one or more of the functions of the 'Principal'. The role of Principal is that of a qualified, experienced Nurse Teacher who has undertaken managerial training and who is responsible for the provision of basic, post-basic and in-service education for all nursing personnel, who is head of the nurse training school and whose functions include the implementation of agreed nursing education policies, budget control of all nursing education costs, liason with statutory and non-statutory educational bodies, control and co-ordination of all staff within the Education Division and advising the Chief Nursing Officer and the authority on all matters pertaining to nursing education.

The proposed grades of Senior Lecturer, Vice Principal and Principal were probably based on the assumption that Colleges of Nursing and Midwifery would be established. An assumption that no longer seems soundly based. The present situation indicates the likelihood of nurse education being centred (if not wholly, at least in part) in institutes of higher education. No doubt if the present pilot studies are successful, ultimately a decision will be made to site the more formal aspects of basic nursing education in polytechnics or universities (which is currently happening to a minor extent), and using parent hospitals and the community for the acquisition of clinical skills and expertise.

Following the publication of the discussion document (RCN, 1981), a report of the Working Group on a 'Professional Nursing Structure for the NHS' was published by the RCN (1983). The Working Group in

Figure 3.1: Organisation: Clinical and Managerial

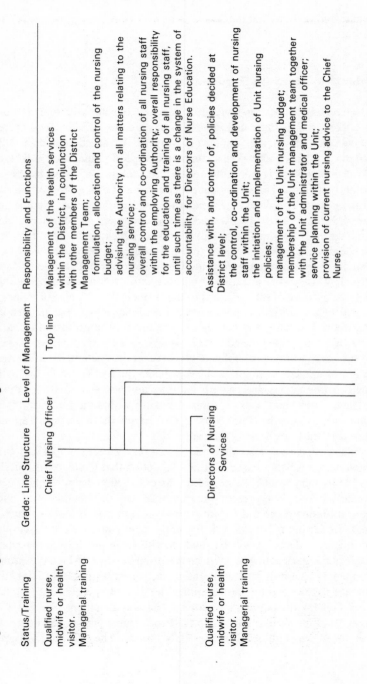

Qualifications	Title	Level	Functions
Qualified experienced nurse. Managerial training. Specialist skills and knowledge	Asst. Dirs. of Nursing / Night duty / Clinical / Capital planning / Personnel	Middle	Night duty co-ordination; continuing education; management of clinical specialties, e.g. paediatrics, geriatrics; occupational health/counselling/support; service planning and development; recruitment, advertising, personnel development.
Qualified experienced nurse. Advanced clinical skills. Expertise and qualifications.	Sen. Sisters / General Admin. Asst.	Front-line	Leader of the clinical nursing team for a defined care area or client group — in hospital or in the community. Clinical specialist with responsibility for a specific patient or client group.
Qualified experienced nurse: Post-basic training in specialty, DIP. in nursing	Sisters		Organisation and total provision of nursing care for specific groups of patients or clients.
Qualified nurse	Sen. Staff nurses / Clerical Staff	Front-line	Leader of a care team in a ward. By virtue of her experience and expertise, she has total responsibility for the assessment, planning and implementation of care for a specific group of patients or clients.
Qualified nurse: Primarily a period of further experience	Staff Nurses		Responsibilities would involve planning, implementing and assessing the nursing care of a group of patients.
	Nursing Students		Increasing responsibility: no accountability.

Figure 3.2: Organisation of Nursing Education

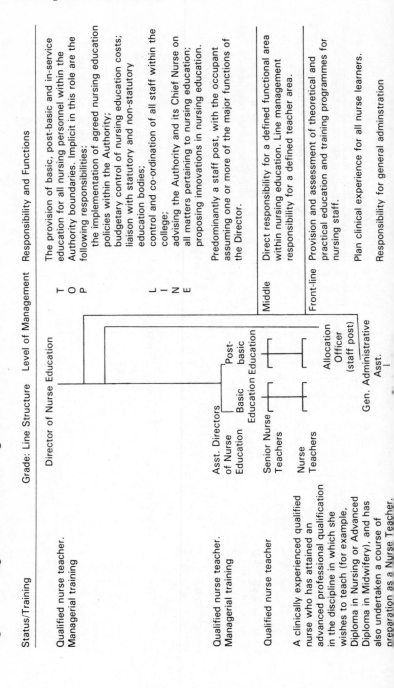

Status/Training	Grade: Line Structure	Level of Management	Responsibility and Functions
Qualified nurse teacher. Managerial training	Director of Nurse Education	TOP	The provision of basic, post-basic and in-service education for all nursing personnel within the Authority boundaries. Implicit in this role are the following responsibilities: the implementation of agreed nursing education policies within the Authority; budgetary control of nursing education costs; liaison with statutory and non-statutory education bodies; control and co-ordination of all staff within the college; advising the Authority and its Chief Nurse on all matters pertaining to nursing education; proposing innovations in nursing education.
Qualified nurse teacher. Managerial training	Asst. Directors of Nurse Education — Basic Education / Post-basic Education	LINE	Predominantly a staff post, with the occupant assuming one or more of the major functions of the Director.
Qualified nurse teacher	Senior Nurse Teachers	Middle	Direct responsibility for a defined functional area within nursing education. Line management responsibility for a defined teacher area.
A clinically experienced qualified nurse who has attained an advanced professional qualification in the discipline in which she wishes to teach (for example, Diploma in Nursing or Advanced Diploma in Midwifery), and has also undertaken a course of preparation as a Nurse Teacher.	Nurse Teachers; Allocation Officer (staff post); Gen. Administrative Asst.	Front-line	Provision and assessment of theoretical and practical education and training programmes for nursing staff. Plan clinical experience for all nurse learners. Responsibility for general adminstration

its opening statement underlines: 'The group wishes to emphasise that flexibility is desirable, because the same structure may not be appropriate for every situation'. The proposals were published as a 'general framework for consideration and development within the profession'.

On the clinical structure, the titles 'Staff Nurse' and 'Senior Staff Nurse' are used: the latter title being equated with that of 'Primary Nurse'. Their functions, as stated in the original discussion document substantially remains unaltered. The main difference being that, 'the clinical managerial responsibility with its leadership functions places the 'Senior Staff Nurse' on a qualitatively different level'. Also, the titles of 'Sister' and 'Senior Sister' replace the original titles. Their functions remain unaltered.

The management structure substantially remains as set out in the discussion document.

The education structure also remains as originally described with the exception of the titles used: instead of the use of the previously mentioned titles, those of 'Nurse Teacher', Senior Nurse Teacher', 'Assistant Director of Nurse Education' and 'Director of Nurse Education', are used.

One of the major problems which confronts nurse managers, nurse educators and nurse researchers is that of establishing how better management (knowledge and skills) and improved education and training can contribute to improving the environment in which patients are nursed, and, overall, enhance their quality of care and life while simultaneously improving the job satisfaction of staff.

Miss Nightingale (1860) concluded that wards are healthy or unhealthy, according to the knowledge or ignorance of the nurse (Notes on Nursing, p.134).

The Briggs Committee (HMSO, 1972) saw nursing and midwifery as 'the major caring profession' (para.38, p.11). The report referred to 'the unique caring role' of the nurse (paras.39/41, pp.11/12), and emphasised the skills of observation, assessment, planning and responsibility, as well as having a legal duty for comprehensive patient care. In the latter context, nurses are required to exercise the degree of knowledge and skill which could reasonably be expected of one trained in their particular profession. If they fall below this standard and the patient is harmed they will be regarded as negligent and will be legally liable for the damage resulting from their negligence.

Disabling Impediments

In endeavouring to maintain a quality service to the patient, the nurse has to contend with impediments which tend to negate against smooth and effective practice. These are many and include economic difficulties and their effects on public expenditure restraint, particularly on staffing and other resources, together with changing roles and relationships of professionals, including the increasing use of industrial action which inevitably accompanies the increasing encouragement, and influence, of nurses in decisions about the management of services and the care of patients. Also, stress arising from the reorganisation of the NHS affects nurses in many ways particularly in the context of an unclear role, and, most important, the uncertainty which tends to be generated through repeated change. Public criticism of the NHS, even though warranted, additionally tends to undermine the morale of staff, particularly their confidence in what they are doing. In addition, the urgent move towards professionalism in nursing, even though fundamentally good, generates problems for nurse practitioners and nurse managers of using staff flexibly, as skills become increasingly narrow and specialised. The various branches and specialties in nursing are largely separated, in reality, by obviating and/or limiting the interchangeability of nurses. Specialist training has developed in a range of nursing fields clearly benefiting the service to patients from the increased skills and knowledge of nurses, but, paradoxically, ensuring that the total nursing manpower available is less interchangeable and becomes impossible to re-deploy without further training.

Nursing is substantially dependent on unqualified and/or untrained staff. About 25 per cent of all nursing staff in the UK are nursing auxiliaries and 25 per cent are nurse learners (Merrison, paras. 12.36/13.39, pp. 170/195). In view of the development of specialised units, and their requirement for qualified nurses, this can result in units becoming more dependent upon unqualified and/or untrained staff.

Current problems which face nurse managers and nurse educationists, in selecting, training, educating and developing nurses, are many. The central problems are those of selecting candidates for nursing who have the right education, motivation and physical and emotional make up to cope with the demands of the profession — in the absence and/or non-use of effective personality screening tests this important function is done with the minimum of information and guidelines. Having selected nurses, managers and educationists must do everything possible to ensure that the nursing students are prepared, nurtured and developed, educationally, socially and emotionally, to enable them to cope with new technology and its effects on them (stress) and on patient care ensuring that the needs of patients are understood and met in a sensitive and proper manner. But, can this be realistically accomplished in the present environment which lacks proper expertise and resources? The training of nurses does not enable them to acquire the necessary social, behavioural and educational skills to master the problems of co-operation between professionals thereby helping them as well as coping with new technology and new trends in education and practice. The approach to the learning of nurses with the emphasis on expository learning rather than insight (Gestalt) learning, poses special problems for nurses in the clinical setting, particularly as this approach may limit their understanding — and their success in nursing decision making.

Central to nurses' problems is the inheritance of tradition in the nurses' culture which can, to a great extent, be identified as a formidable drag on doing what needs to be done in nursing education, nursing management and nursing practice. Some of this tradition is good, useful and has obvious benefits for patients and clients, particularly the nursing ethic of service which puts patient/client interest before self. Regrettably, however, some tradition is also disabling to the profession, notably the substantial reliance of the health service on unqualified and/or untrained staff to provide a 'satisfactory' service for patients and clients. The continuing debate on the status of learners, even though clarified by the recent legislation (1979), remains unresolved: there is still disagreement as to whether the learners should be regarded as 'nursing students' and thereby coming under the major influence and control of nurse educationists or whether they should be afforded 'protected employee' status, thereby potentially enabling the employing authority to have a major say in their employment. The lack of a clear role poses problems for nurse educationists, particularly limiting their scope to develop realistic and appropriate curricula to meet nurses' needs at basic and post-basic levels.

A problem of major proportions has resulted over the past two decades due to; 'a noticeable increase in the complexity of the work carried out by nurses as well as a decrease in the number of trained nurses available to do the work' (RCN, 1984). This anomaly produces in its wake a situation whereby nurses are overworked and in a hurry, to the extent that they spend only the minimum of time with patients and clients — sometimes even to the neglect of their nursing duties — with the results that some patients at most may feel at peril and at least are uncomfortable' (Merrison, para.13.5, p.185). As a direct result of this neglect, communication with patients is diminished and the value of the nurse-patient relationship is reduced. Relating to this, research carried out two decades showed that patients who could not get their questions answered, or their troubles aired, took longer to recover. The difference lay in 'the quality of communication maintained throughout the hospital hierarchy' (Revans, 1964).

The problem of better use of nurses' time continues. There is no generally accepted estimate of the proper number of nurses to care for a given number of patients: in practice the number needed is usually the number that can be found. The daily workload is found to vary widely from ward to ward. Today, demands on the nurse are greatly accentuated because of increasing technology together with the now common use of complex medical and surgical interventions, which demand highly skilled and time-consuming nursing for their success. This necessitates a rational preparation, direction and use of nursing manpower to ensure the satisfaction and success of nurses in their search for the improved care of their patients and clients. (This will be discussed more fully in Chapters 4–9.)

The NHS and Nursing: Links between Management and Care

Nurses, as professionals, are obliged to provide a service to their patients and clients which in essence means ensuring safe practice by maintaining the quality and standard of care. This, in turn, implies securing, and using, the knowledge and the skills which nurses have acquired (or ought to have acquired) at basic and post-basic levels of training, to enable the satisfactory care of their patients and clients.

A publication by the RCN (1980) underlines the necessity for the nurse as a professional to acquire and keep up to date with new techniques and knowledge in helping patients to attain their health potential and independence. Implicit in this is the responsibility of management education, the specific role of management in achieving and maintaining the highest standards of care. The report says: 'Nurses as managers have primary and secondary responsibilities connected with standards of care.' The primary duties include such vital factors as, 'ensuring resources' as well as 'enabling nursing policies democratically within the enterprise'. The secondary duties relate to 'monitoring the clinical environment and its activities' (para.79, p.18).

How do these views match what is happening in relation to the proper preparation of nurses, at all levels, in professional and managerial skills and knowledge?

In the late 1960s there was a rapid growth of activity and interest in management education for nurses. This growth has its roots and guidelines in the Salmon (1966), Powell (1966) and Mayston (1969) reports.

The Salmon Committee recommended: 'For successful performance of the job, vocational training is necessary; this can be practical — given 'on-the-job' or theoretical — through formal instruction.' (para.9.11, pp.93–94). Following from this and inspired by the wisdom and industry of the National Staff Committee for Nurses and Midwives, during the next five years or so, a great number of nurses throughout the UK undertook management courses. (No official record of numbers undertaking management courses is available.) From 1970 onwards there was much questioning of the value of management training, particularly 'off-the-job' training. Also, doubts were expressed by senior nurse managers and employing authorities as to the 'value-for-money' for the substantial investments of time and money on such training. Some critics questioned the nature of these management courses where the subject content was often varied, profuse and apparently irrelevant and/or unrelated to the needs of nurses (Haywood, 1968, Williams, 1969, Bowman, 1980).

Even though evident progress was made, through the agency of the philosophy and structure which followed the publication of the Salmon and Mayston reports, the need for development in management skills and knowledge was again highlighted in the *Grey Book* (DHSS, 1972) which stated: 'If the proposed management organisation is to be effective in its ultimate aim of securing improvements to health care for patients, highly skilled and experienced managers will be needed at all levels of the organisation in many functions.' (para.3.62, p.64).

Also, the Briggs report (1972) highlights the link between nursing care and management by emphasising: 'Just as every qualified nurse must be in some sense an educator, so every qualified nurse must be in some sense a manager.' And, 'Good management is a precondition of good care.' (paras. 54/55, p.15). The report leaves nurses in no doubt about the importance and relevance of their professional experience and its impact on care.

> Nurses, with professional experience at their command, will be in a position at every level — beginning at the level of the clinical team, to explain what the acceptable minimum of nursing care is, what in any given situation is the best pattern of care, and how external restraints on money, manpower and hospital resources will affect its provision. (para.55, p.15)

The present hierarchical structure of power is seen by some observers as being inappropriate to the requirements of the Health Service in so much as it tends to become rule-bound, inflexible, and insensitive to the needs and changes in the world around them (Draper and Smart, 1972; Draper, 1973). Also, from the mouthpiece of the DHSS, it is stated that there is inherent difficulty with advisory machinery in a profession that is hierarchically structured and has a clearly defined role for nurse managers (DHSS Circular HC(82)1). The general hierarchial management of the Service has meant that decisions are taken at inappropriate levels (*Patients First — Summary of Comments* (DHSS, 1980) para.19). And, most important, this form of management leads to communication problems in nursing (Revans, 1964, 1972; Briggs, 1972, paras.67–69, 107, 594).

Patients First states: 'The structure and management arrangements of the Service introduced in 1974 do not provide the best framework for the effective delivery of care to patients.' 'The service must be managed in a way that enables those with prime responsibility for providing the services to patients to get on with the job.' And, 'Our approach stems from the profound belief that the needs of patients must be paramount. Whichever structure and management arrangements are devised must be responsive to those needs.' (paras.1,3,5, pp.1,5).

Griffiths (DHSS, 1983) is critical of the NHS as a whole, especially of the way it is managed, underlining the lack of a clearly defined general management function through the NHS, particularly in relation to developing management plans, effecting their implementation, monitoring achievement, devolving responsibility, lack of leadership together with the motivation of staff: and, most important, swamping units and authorities with Directives — without direction (paras.4,5,6,9,29, pp. 6, 11, 12, 13, 21).

In view of the depressing catalogue of evidence, can the service be improved — managed more effectively and efficiently?

Guidelines for Better Management in the NHS and Nursing

Pertinent questions arise from the variety and extent of reports underlining major problems and advising ways to improve the lot of patient, clients and staff. For example, have the quantities of guidelines and advice designed to foster better management been heeded? Will the organisation and management of the NHS and nursing, following the many re-shuffles, be enhanced, become more humane and acceptable to patients and clients? Have the messages in the litany of reports, documents and memoranda been understood, accepted and implemented? Has decentralisation of decision making which is taking place in the NHS and in nursing, and consensus management highlighted in the *Grey Book* (DHSS, 1972) worked both in the NHS and in nursing? Has the early investment of time and money provided nurses with a greater influence on the management and control (nursing) of the environment in which patients are nursed?

Answers? Outcomes?

The answers to these questions reside to a considerable extent in the revelations of Merrison (1979), *Patients First* (DHSS, 1979), Griffiths (DHSS, 1983) and *Nurse Alert* (RCN, 1984) which, without doubt reflect the real and intolerable environment and structure in which care is given.

On standards of care Merrison (1979) said: 'We received much evidence expressing concern about declining standards of care which was often attributed to the structural changes arising from the Salmon and Mayston Committees' recommendations.' (para.13.5, p.185). Merrison also emphasises problems associated with 'consensus management' once much applauded, but clearly also having its inherent limitations such as, 'clashes of personality'; domination by an individual; the need to reach compromises; prompting members to ignore a difficult problem or to present a united view — when what is needed is to present health authorities with options for decision; and delay in decision making (para.20.14, p.314).

The challenge of establishing, and maintaining, efficient and effective management in the NHS as a whole and ensuring that all available resources are focused upon reducing ill health, even though clearly desirable, raises many questions and poses many problems, especially in the context of control of available resources while simultaneously attempting to raise 'productivity' as indicated by Griffiths. Additional challenges relate to the real role of the general manager, in the proposed new structure. Will it be that of co-ordinator? Facilitator? Will it alter functional command lines? If so, what will be the consequences for professionals together with their patients and clients?

What will be the future for nurse managers? Present discussion and views indicate that some feel threatened and uneasy about the proposed management changes. This initial unease was precipitated by the regrettable initial omission of the Chief Nursing Officer on the new Supervisory Board (now corrected). More recently, a press headline read: 'Griffiths causing Major Upheaval in NHS' (*Nursing Standard*, March,

1985). Will the current fuctional management position — management of nurses by nurses — be altered? Is there bias against nurses? Or, is this mythical? Roy Griffiths is optimistic about the future of nurse managers (*Daily Telegraph*, Nov. 1983). Clearly there are problems associated with the organisational structure within which patients are nursed, as evidenced in recent reports.

What about the role of doctors in the envisaged NHS? Clearly doctors continue to have substantial membership on management teams (three doctors out of a total of six members of the DMT). Also the preservation of autonomy, 'clinical freedom' for doctors in the proposed management structure, continues to be a bone of contention in decision making — their major stake together with the prescription and use of resources; yet their accountability remains unclear, medical influence remaining paramount. When discussing the participation by clinicians in management the *Grey Book* (DHSS, 1972) emphasised: 'To do their work properly, consultants and general practitioners must have clinical autonomy. It follows that these doctors' and dentists' work are each others' equals and that they are their own managers.' (para.1.18, p.13). In this context, Taylor (1984) asks: 'How, given the reality of medical power and the essential desirability of local freedom of action for individual clinicians, can the NHS management effectively influence medical action?' Griffiths in answering this says:

> Urgent management action is required, if Units are to fulfil their role and provide the most effective management of their resouces. This particularly affects the doctors. Their decisions largely dictate the use of all resources and they must accept the management responsibility which goes with clinical freedom. (para.19, p.18).

And, 'Clinicians must participate fully in decisions about priorities in the use of resources.' (para.8.2, p.6). 'Doctors must accept the management responsibility that goes with clinical freedom.' (para.19, p.18).

What about the use of incentives — rewards and sanctions — to motivate professionals? Will the revision of Whiteley Council system (para.9.1, p.7) for determining NHS pay levels together with such practices as redeployment of non-efficient personnel trigger improved performance? (para.(c), (d), (e), pp.13, 14) (DHSS, 1976). Briggs (1972) referring to an outstanding deficiency of nursing and midwifery manpower policy said: 'At present there are no financial incentives to the "manager" to utilise manpower more efficiently, the primary incentive for the nurse manager being the care of the patients.' (para.491, p.149).

Can nurses be encouraged into greater 'productivity' by a system of rewards and incentives?

Despite much advice, in the absence of effective education, training and development of staff together with the inadequate provision of resources, the chances of maintaining present levels of care, let alone improving standards, remain but a pious hope.

In the next chapter we shall examine the issues which are paramount in meeting patients'/clients' needs in the delivery of care.

References

Barnard, K. (1984) Social policy statement: Implications for nursing. in M.J. Kim *et al.* (eds.) *Classification of Nursing Diagnoses.* C.V. Mosby, St Louis

Bennett, M. (1984) Quality of Nursing — Strained or Thrice Blessed.? Paper given at Royal Melbourne Hospital Oration.

Bowman, M.P. (1980) The Management Education and Training Needs of First-line Nursing Officers. Unpublished MEd thesis, University of Newcastle upon Tyne.

Cang, S. *et al.* (1981) An Emerging Model for Ward Sister Roles in General Hospitals. Health Services Organistion Research Unit, Brunel University

Chapman, C. (1982) The paradox of nursing, *Nursing Standard*, 270

DHSS (1969) Report of the Working Party on Mnagement Structure in the Local Authority Nursing Services (Mayston). HMSO, London

—— (1972) Management Arrangements for the Reorganised National Health Service (Grey Book). HMSO, London

—— (1972, 1974) Reports of the Joint Working Party on the Organisation of Medical Work in Hospitals (Cogwheel). HMSO, London

—— (1976) Making Whitley Work. (A Review of the Operation of the National Health Service Whitley Council System by Lord McCarthy). HMSO, London

—— (1980) Patients First — Summary of Comments. DHSS, London

—— (1981) Seminar: Professional Development in Clinical Nursing — The 1980s. DHSS, London

—— (1983) NHS Management Inquiry (Griffiths). DHSS, London

—— (1984) Implementation of the NHS Management Inquiry. HC(84)13. DHSS, London

EEC (Commission of the European Community) (1977) Legislation. *Official Journal of the European Communities, 20*, no.L176.

—— (1981) The EEC Advisory Committee on Training in Nursing (Report on the Training of Nurses Responsible for General Care in Particular on the Balance to be found between Theoretical and Clinical Instruction for this Category of Nurse). EEC 111/D/76/6/80-EN 1981. EEC

Draper, P. and Smart, T. (1972) *The Future of Our Health Care.* Dept of Community Medicine, Guy's Hospital, London

Haywood, S.C. (1968) The unwilling managers. *British Hospital Journal and Social Services Review. LXXVIII*, 297–8

Henderson, V. and Nite, G. (1978) *Principles and Practice of Nursing*, 6th edn. Macmillan, New York

Hingley, P. (1984) Stress: A Report of the King Edward Hospitals Fund.*Nursing Standard, 352*, 3

International Council of Nurses (1965) Special and Committee Reports Presented to the ICN Board of Directors and Grand Council Meetings, Frankfurt. June

McFarlane, Baroness (1983) 'Mirror mirror on the wall', Nursing Mirror Lecture 1983. *Nursing Mirror*, 8 June, pp. 17–20

Martin, A. (1981) Easy does it! *Nursing Mirror, 152*, 30

Mayeroff, M. (1971) *On Caring*. Harper and Row, New York

Mitchell, J.R.A. (1984) Is nursing any business of doctors? A simple guide to the 'Nursing Process'. *British Medical Journal, 288*, 216–19

Ministry of Health Central Health Services Council (1966) The Post-Certificate Training and Education of Nurses (Powell). HMSO, London

———— (1966) Report of the Committee on Senior Nursing Staff Structure (Salmon). HMSO, London

Nightingale, F. (1960) *Notes on Nursing: What it is and what it is not*. Dover Publications. (Unabridged republication of First American Edition, 1860). London

Revans, R.W. (1962) The hospital as a human system. *Journal of Physics in Medicine and Biology, 7*(12), 147

———— (1964) The morale and effectiveness of general hospitals. in G. McLachlan (ed.) *Problems and Progress in Medical Care*. Oxford University Press, Oxford

———— (1972) *Hospitals: Communication, Choice and Change*. Tavistock, London

———— (1976) *Action Learning in Hospitals: Diagnosis and Therapy*. McGraw-Hill, New York

RCN (1980) Standards of Nursing Care. RCN

———— (1981) Towards Standards (Discussion Document). RCN

———— (1982) Seminar on Advanced Clinical Roles. RCN

———— (1983) Towards a New Professional Structure for Nursing. RCN

———— (1984) A Report on the Financial and Manpower Cuts in the NHS (Nurse Alert). RCN

Taylor, D. (1984) *Understanding the NHS in the 1980s*. Office of Health Economics

WHO (1966) WHO Expert Committee on Nursing (Fifth Report). WHO, Geneva

Wieland, G. (ed.) (1981) *Improving Health Care Management: Organization Development and Organization Change*. Health Administration Press, Ann Arbor, MI

Williams, D. (1969) The administrative contribution of the nursing sister. *Public Administration, XLVIII*, 307–328

Advised Further Reading

Clarke, C.C. (1977) Reframing. *American Journal of Nursing, 77*, 840–1

DHSS (1982) Health Service Development, HC(FP)(82)1, HC(82)2, LAC(82)2, DHSS, London

———— (1983) NHS Management Inquiry (Griffiths). DHSS, London

———— (1984) Implementation of the NHS Management Inquiry HC(84)13. DHSS, London

Grusky, O. and Miller, G.A. (1970) *The Sociology of Organizations*. Free Press, New York

HMSO (1942) Social Insurance and Allied Services (Beveridge), Cmnd 6404, HMSO, London

McLachlan, G. (ed.) (1964) *Problems and Progress in Medical Care*. Oxford University Press, Oxford

Maloney, M.M. (1979) *Leadership in Nursing: Theory, Strategies, Action*. C.V. Mosby, St Louis

Revans, R.W. (1972) *Hospitals: Communication, Choice and Change*. Tavistock

RCN (1984) A Report on the Financial and Manpower Cuts in the NHS. RCN, London

Williams, D. (1969) The administrative contribution of the nursing sister. *Public Administration, XLVIII*, 307–28

4 PATIENTS AND THEIR NEEDS

Aims

The aims of this chapter are:
1. To discuss the patient and his needs.
2. To examine the role of the nurse in meeting patient needs.

Learning Objectives

The purpose of this chapter is to enable the reader to:

1. Understand the needs of patients in hospital.
2. Appreciate some of the major issues surrounding the role of the nurse.
3. Apply management stategies and management techniques in the delivery of care.

Background

'The NHS is about delivering a service to people. It is not about organising systems for their own use.' (DHSS, 1983). Nursing is about meeting individual patients' nursing needs; it is about caring — enabling and ensuring optimum standards and quality of care.

Health care is organised and delivered within a large, complex, hierarchical structure — The National Health Service. The NHS is probably the nation's largest institution. It employs more than 1.2 million full-time and part-time staff. Its budget for the UK in 1984 is in the order of £17,000m.

There are about 2750 hospitals in the NHS. The number of hospital beds is about 480,000 of which 80 per cent are occupied on any one day. Out-patient and accident and emergency departments serve some 100,000 patients daily. Hospital services account for 70 per cent of total NHS expenditure (Merrison, para.102, p.125).

Any organisation of this magnitude, which employs and utilises such sizeable resources — 6 per cent of the country's gross national product and a similar proportion of its manpower resources — cannot avoid its central responsibility, the effective and efficient use of its resources (Taylor, 1984).

When people have to use hospital services, either as out-patients or in-patients, they are invariably at their most vulnerable, removed from the security of the home, their relatives, and their friends. Most important, they are dependent on others, professional and ancillary staff, for meeting their needs, the success of which, is central to ensuring their successful treatment and care.

When discussing needs in the context of patients and clients, it becomes necessary to use a psychological framework of reference so as to focus on their relationships and functions in the context of patient/client care, treatment and rehabilitation together with their relevance to the self-actualisation of staff.

In any care situation, patients are at a disadvantage to a greater or lesser degree — physically, socially and emotionally — because of the effects of their illness, separation from family and friends (if hospitalised), and the foreign and traumatic environment of the hospital. Therefore, it is imperative that all staff responsible for their care fully understand and acknowledge this disadvantage, and ensure that they and their relatives are comforted, reassured and shown kindness and sensitivity.

At the best of times, hospitals tend to be charged with drama, emotion and anxiety because of the nature of the work. Patients may feel emotionally threatened, anxious and insecure; an insecurity that may be compounded by inadequate, infrequent or incomplete communication; problems that have been highlighted by many researchers.

Because of the stress which is inevitably associated with illness and hospitalisation, it is imperative that all staff ensure that the experience of the patient is as happy and tolerable as can be provided within the complex environment in which care takes place. Staff must be sensitive to the stresses and the needs of their patients and do everything possible by their attitudes and in their work to treat them in a personal and humane way and reduce their stress through reassurance, improved communication, establishing a satisfactory relationship and be comforting and caring for them.

The aim of nurse managers, at all levels of the organisation is to ensure quality of care. This aim can be difficult to achieve for many reasons, central to which is the magnitude of the task in getting different groups, i.e. nurses, doctors and paramedicals, together with administrators, and ancillary workers, to blend, to integrate and direct their energies towards securing the main needs of patients, i.e. information, comfort, security, care, treatment and rehabilitation.

Needs: Concept

Patients have needs arising from their own unique makeup i.e. the

physical, psychological, social and spiritual components of their personality. Essentially, a need is that which is necessary, or desirable to
maintain homeostasis. Human needs, when met satisfactorily, help to
maintain physical, social and emotional homeostasis.

The satisfaction of needs requires interaction among the components
of the person — and between the person and the environment. Needs
are the triggers for behaviour. They may be met consciously or un-
consciously.

Physical needs can be divided into two groups, survival and stimulation (Kalish, 1973). Survival needs include the need for food, water,
bodily protection, rest, and avoidance and relief of pain. Stimulation
needs include those for activity, exploration and stimulation. Emotional
needs include those to love and be loved, self-esteem, self-sufficiency,
to be wanted, adequacy, ability to meet physical needs, and creativity.
Social needs include the need to belong (the family, social groups), and
to learn, and spiritual needs arise out of the person's search for the meaning of life.

These needs are never static, but vary according to individual patients,
medical and technical advances and developments such as a unified nursing service (Briggs, (HMSO, 1972), para.13, p.3). In this respect, Mayeroff (1971) says: 'To care for someone I must know what his needs are.'

Patients must have their innate needs as well as those that are
specifically related to their clinical condition, recognised and met, to
ensure their full and speedy recovery. In this context, communicating
with patients and reducing their level of fear and anxiety accelerates their
recovery (Revans, 1964).

Motivation links needs and motives: in essence it is an energised state
of the person. Motivated behaviour has many characteristics. Primarily
it is directed at correcting a deficit within the person arising from an
unsatisfied need and/or some incentive external to the person; 'the
behaviour is focused on or away from something. Also, the behaviour
is selective in so far as achieving a practical goal: when the goal is attained, the behaviour alters.' (Strongman, 1979).

Motivation is important to the nurse and to the patient, enabling the
achievement of their respective goals, i.e. patients in their striving for
recovery and nurses in their drive to achieve and maintain standards and
quality of care as well as getting the most and best from their patients
and clients to ensure their full recovery. Motivating high levels of performance in staff must incorporate standards and quality. Therefore,
'when defining standards the goal should be both to offer a challenge
and to encourage high levels of performance' (Smith, 1982).

A knowledge of needs is important to the nurse as a prerequisite to understanding human behaviour which is motivated through the basic needs: behaviour represents an effort to satisfy those needs. The person/patient is motivated through their needs and, in this respect, nurses need to differentiate between needs and problems of their patients and clients. Needs are requirements for the maintenance of wellbeing, therefore the person unable to have his needs gratified experiences a problem (Wolfe *et al.*, 1979).

Needs' Fulfilment Theory

Maslow's (1954) work on animal behaviour demonstrated not only that behaviour varied in accordance with experimentally induced needs but also that needs seemed to have a hierarchy of importance. From these observations he developed a framework in which man's needs are organised in a series of levels: a hierarchy of importance. In this framework he suggests that the fundamental motivational tendencies which he calls 'needs', are organised in a hierarchy. At the bottom are the physiological needs; then safety, love, self-esteem and the esteem of others, and, at the summit, self-actualisation — the effort to realise the maximum fulfilment of all the person's potentialities and abilities, including that of creativity. Needs develop as a person grows; the higher needs become evident only when the lower are reasonably satisfied. The expression of the higher level needs leads to continued activity and the search for new and higher goals, though satisfaction may be more readily postponed than in the case of the lower needs. 'The lower needs, those below the level of consciousness as long as they are reasonably well satisfied, may emerge and dominate behaviour in conditions of deprivation or frustration.' (Vernon, 1971).

In practice, the needs' levels are both interdependent and overlapping. The hierarchy indicates an order of priority of satisfaction; for most people, a higher satisfaction at the lower than the higher need levels. People are said to possess drives towards the satisfaction of certain needs, e.g. the need for food and shelter, security, interpersonal activity, ego and self-actualisation, in their lives: Maslow suggests that these needs can be arranged in descending order of basic importance to the individual, and descending order of approach to the most developed stage of self-actualisation.

Maslow's need-fulfilment theory of human motivation is widely accepted. He argues that humans are born with a set of needs that not only energise but direct behaviour: these needs are organised in a hierarchical fashion whereby needs lowest in the hierarchy must be satisfied first. He depicts the need hierarchy as a pyramid where the needs, such as hunger and thirst, dominate the person's attention until satisfied. When these basic needs have been satisfied, the next set of needs in the hierarchy come to exert their influence. This framework helps the understanding of the strength of certain needs, i.e. a hierarchy of needs. When one group of needs becomes partially satisfied other levels of needs dominate the behaviour of the person, and so on up the hierarchy.

He believes that a person strives for self-fulfilment — to become everything he is capable of becoming. He suggests that until lower level needs, i.e. physiological, are met (at least in part), upper level needs, i.e. self-actualisation, will not be met. In this way when physiological needs (they tend to have the highest strength until they begin to be satisfied) begin to be fulfilled other levels of needs, e.g. safety, social esteem, self-actualisation up the hierarchy, become dominant until satisfied. Essentially, there tends to be greater satisfaction of physiological needs (99 per cent) and safety needs (80 per cent) and less satisfaction at the social (60 per cent), ego (esteem) (30 per cent) and self-actualisation (5 per cent) levels.

Maslow's needs' model is intended to demonstrate a pattern of activity that operates most of the time.

Relevance of Theory to Nurses and Patients

Nursing involves a total specific and individual responsibility towards the patient/client and family, which as an inseparable part of the provision of nursing care and all this entails (i.e. promotion of health — including health education) must ensure, by observation and communication with the patient/client, the identification and acknowledgement of their needs: physical, emotional, social and spiritual. Outstanding in patients'/clients' needs are those of emotion — the need for support, reassurance and security; communication — the need for information and personal recognition; and dehospitalisation — the need to maintain independence (EEC 111/D/76/6/80-EN, 1981).

Therefore, central to any nursing care plan is the identification and gratification (as practicable) of patient/client needs.

The 'needs-reduction model' is one partial attempt to explain how human behaviour is determined. This theory assumes an individual's behaviour, at any moment, is presumed to be directed towards satisfying what he considers to be the most pressing of his needs, at that time. Having in mind this assumption, in relation to satisfying human needs, if nursing management has provided for the physiological and safety needs of its employees, substantially in doing so it will cause motivation to move to the social and ego needs and, unless it provides opportunities for satisfying these needs, staff may feel deprivation which may be reflected in their behaviour in striving to their fulfilment.

A recent publication underlines the link between the responsibility to assess and meet patient needs and that of managing and co-ordinating resources and services (RCN, 1980, para.64, p.16).

In the nursing context, the needs' model lends itself to particular use within the context of nursing care in general, and the nursing process in particular. In general nursing a patient may present with an emergency clinical condition, e.g. cardiac arrest, in which many physiological needs present and between which the nurse must differentiate and decide their priority. For example, there will be pain, discomfort and difficulty in breathing, which demand prompt action in the interest of patient resuscitation and survival.

'The aim of nursing is to define goals with, and for, the patient towards the achievement of these activities of daily living which ensure the patient's maximum independence' (RCN, 1981). And, in this way nursing care is concerned with helping the patient with his daily pattern of living or with those activities that he normally performs without assistance, that is, breathing, eating, drinking, eliminating, resting, sleeping and moving, cleaning the body, and keeping it warm and properly clothed. 'Nursing helps to provide the patient with those activities that make life more than a vegetative process, i.e. social intercourse, recreational activity and other productive rehabilitating occupations' (WHO, 1966).

The care of the patient is personified in the nursing process which is a system of planned nursing care and which includes determining and assessing patients' needs, constructing a nursing care plan on the basis of the assessment, and implementing and evaluating the nursing care, and using the results of intentional monitoring and evaluation to perfect the process. In practical terms the nursing process (discussed in Chapter 2) is structured to identify the patient's clinical problems and is intended to support patients' efforts to satisfy their needs. It is a problem-solving approach which is based on individual patients' needs.

Central to effecting nursing care is the nurse-patient relationship, the basis of which is interaction between the nurse and the patient and the nurse and other health care professionals, i.e. doctor, physiotherapist, etc. The implementation of the nursing care plan embraces a relationship in which the nurse helps the patient to achieve the goals set — goals which have arisen out of the patient's needs. The goals of nursing care are defined co-operatively with colleagues and the patient, in terms of the patient's needs, e.g. improving and increasing the patient's independence together with their general physical and social wellbeing. This helping, co-operative relationship is central to the nursing care.

The function of nursing management is to match necessary and available resources to patient needs. The needs of patients are never static, but vary according to individual patients, therefore the provision of nursing services and nursing care must always be directly related to meeting those needs. In this way, nursing becomes a patient-centred approach which is must usefully effected through the agency of the nursing process whose usefulness is high-lighted in a survey conducted by the Briggs Committee, which found: that over half those nurses interviewed agreed that a system of patient allocation was more efficient in meeting the patient's needs, as opposed to a system of task allocation (para.124, p.41).

Patients who are nursed in ICUs, who are critically ill, need constant, individual, skilled nursing, which entails frequent personal attention together with the use of special equipment and facilities. Conversely, there are patients who are ready for going home and need little or no nursing care. Intermediate to these two groups are those patients who form the bulk of patients requiring 'intermediate' care: this group of patients give scope to front-line nurses, particularly the ward sisters and staff nurses to deploy their staff creatively and imaginatively marrying their nursing skills with the needs of their patients, using particularly their skills of developing, motivating and leading the nursing team while simultaneously optimising their resources in meeting patients' needs.

In Chapter 5 we shall discuss what meeting patients'/clients' needs mean in the context of the management of care.

References

DHSS (1983) NHS Management Inquiry (Griffiths). DHSS, London

EEC (1981) Advisory Committee on Training in Nursing (Report on the Training of Nurses Responsible for General Care, in Particular on the Balance to be found Between Theoretical and Clinical Instruction for this Category of Nurse). EEC, 111/D/76/6/80-EN 1981. EEC

HMSO (1972) Report of the Committee on Nursing (Briggs), Cmnd 5115. HMSO, London
———— (1979) Royal Commission on the National Health Service (Merrison). HMSO, London

Kalish, R. (1973) *The Psychology of Human Behaviour*, 3rd edn. Brooks/Cole

Maslow, A.H. (1954) *Motivation and Personality*, Harper and Row, New York

Mayeroff, M (1971) *On Caring*. Harper and Row, New York
RCN (1980) Standards of Nursing Care (Discussion Document). RCN, London
———— (1981) Towards Standards (A Discussion Document). RCN, London
Revans, R.W. (1964) The morale and effectiveness of general hospitals. In G McLachlan (ed.) *Problems and Progress in Medical Care*. Oxford University Press, Oxford
Smith, J. (1982) Managing employee performance. *Nursing Management, 13*, 14–16
Stongman, K.T. (1979) *Psychology for the Paramedical Profession*, Croom Helm, London
Vernon, M.D. (1971) *Human Motivation*. Cambridge University Press, Cambridge
Wolfe, L. *et al.* (1974) *Fundamentals of Nursing*. J.B. Lippincott Co., Philadelphia
WHO (1966) WHO Expert Committee on Nursing (Fifth Report). WHO, Geneva
———— (1976) The Nursing Process (Report on the First Meeting of the Technical Advisory Group, ICP/HMP 049(1). WHO, Geneva

Advised Further Reading

Altman, J. (1966) *Organic Foundations of Animal Behaviour*. Holt, Rinehart and Winston, New York
Cole, G.A. (1982) *Management: Theory and Practice*. D.P. Publications, Eastleigh, Hants
Diekelman, N. *et al.* (1980) *Fundamentals of Nursing*. McGraw-Hill, New York
Drucker, P.F. (1974) *Management: Tasks, Responsibilities, Practices*. Harper and Row, New York
Fayol, H. (1938) *The Functions of the Executive*. Harvard University Press
Franken, R.E. (1982) *Human Motivation*. Brooks/Cole Publishing, Monterey, California
Fulmer, R.M. (1983) *The New Management,* 3rd edn. Macmillan, New York
Gregory, J. (1978) Patient's Attitudes to the Hospital Service. Royal Commission on the National Health Service (Research Paper no. 5). HMSO, London
Hersey, P. and Blanchard, K.H. (1982) *Management of Organisational Behaviour: Utilising Human Resources*. Prentice-Hall, New Jersey
Herzberg, F. (1959) *The Motivation to Work*. 2nd edn. Wiley, New York
Strongman, K.T. (1979) *Psychology for the Paramedical Professions*. Croom Helm, London
Taylor, F.W. (1947) *The Principles of Scientific Management*. Harper and Row, New York
Vernon, M.D. (1971) *Human Motivation,* Cambridge University Press, Cambridge
Wong, R. (1976) *Motivation: A Biobehavioural Analysis of Consumatory Activities*. Macmillan, New York

5 THE MANAGEMENT OF CARE: MEETING PATIENTS' NEEDS

Aims

The aims of this chapter are:

1. To discuss the concept of management.
2. To examine the role and functions of management in enabling the care of patients.

Learning Objectives

The purpose of this chapter is to enable the reader to:

1. Appreciate the nature of management.
2. Relate and apply the principles of management to enabling the care and wellbeing of patients.

The functions of the manager were described by Fayol (1916), who identified planning, co-ordinating, organising, staffing, directing and budgeting as being the key elements for effective management. Also, one must include six more vital functions: leadership, motivation, forecasting, monitoring, assessing and appraising.

The planning process, he concluded, includes establishing goals — setting targets; deciding policy — strategic and long-term; organising tactical action — setting short-term objectives; and appraising and evaluating outcomes. Co-ordinating means establishing links with other departments through discussion and final agreement on a coherent, fulfilling and appropriate policy. Organising includes what Fayol refers to as the 'scalar chain' — the span of control, i.e. the number of subordinates reporting to one manager: for effective management, Fayol suggests this number should not exceed seven or eight. Staffing means ensuring through recruitment, interviewing, and selection that staff appointed are suitable to the job — and to the organisation. Directing includes complex processes such as communicating, relating counselling, motivating and appraising staff to ensure that the goals of the organisation are fulfilled as well as enabling the advancement and fulfilment of the person. Budgeting is essentially the expression of targets in financial terms.

Reporting is the analysis of information, data processing to provide essential feedback to front-line and senior managers.

Fayol's original thesis on the functions of the executive lists no fewer than fourteen principles of management, i.e. division of work, authority, discipline, unity of command, unity of direction, subordination of individual interests to the general interest, remuneration, centralisation, scalar chain — line authority, order, equity, stability of tenure of personnel, initiative and esprit de corps.

In addition to the ideas of Fayol, the theories of McGregor (1960) have important things to say about certain aspects of management, particularly that which is concerned with motivation.

In McGregor's view one of the major tasks of management is 'to organise human effort in the service of the objectives of the enterprise'. He also suggests that: 'Successful management depends not alone, but significantly upon the ability to predict and control human behaviour'. It is his belief that underlying the method of influence used in organisations to achieve its objectives are certain assumptions (held by managers) about the nature of man, his attitudes to work, and his needs and their satisfaction. He suggests that behind every managerial decision or action are assumptions about human behaviour, which he refers to as 'Theory X' and 'Theory Y'.

Theory 'X' assumes that:

> the average human being has an inherent dislike of work and will avoid it if he can and because of this, people must be coerced, controlled and directed to get them to put forth adequate effort towards the achievement of organisational objectives; and, the average human being prefers to be directed, wishes to avoid responsibility, has relatively little ambition, and wants security above all.

Among the assumptions of Theory 'Y' are that: staff will exercise self-direction and self-control in the service of objectives to which they are committed; and that commitment to objectives is a function of rewards associated with their achievement. However, he also emphasises that 'perfect integration of organisational requirements and individual goals and needs is not a realistic objective'.

Herzberg's (1959) theory assumes 'a hygiene environment prevents discontent with a job, but, cannot lead the individual beyond a minimal adjustment consisting of the absence of dissatisfaction'. He emphasises that a positive ''happiness'' seems to require some attainment of psychological growth'. In this respect, the hygiene factors fail to provide for positive satisfaction because they cannot lead to this psychological growth. To feel that one has grown psychologically, depends upon achievement in tasks that have meaning for the individual and since the hygiene factors do not relate to the task they are powerless to give such meaning for the individual. The message for managers is that roles, where necessary, must be re-defined to build in psychological factors — to improve output.

A satisfied need is no longer a motivator: it does not influence behaviour, therefore what satisfies that need is no longer an incentive. Herzberg says that 'unless the basic needs are satisfied, nothing higher in the hierarchy of needs will be right'.

Fulfilment of needs at the highest level is achieved by such things as recognition of abilities, acceptance of the individual and allocation of responsibility, according to the potential of that individual, together with establishing a relationship which involves a high level of trust.

Herzberg's hygiene factors surround a job, but are not directly concerned with its operation. They relate to organisation, policy, and administration — the way the organisation is run; the nature of the supervision; the climate of interpersonal relations — how people relate to each other; and to the working conditions and salary.

Work, responsibility and advancement are the major factors involved in producing high job attitudes. Conversely, the policy of the organisation, its administration, supervision (both technical and interpersonal relationships), and working conditions represent the major job dissatisfiers.

Herzberg says that, 'any organisation can expect trouble of some kind from its employees if the above factors are not satisfactory, and that however good they are, they do not motivate people.'

Having examined some theories which relate to management and workers, how do the views and ideas expressed relate to the reality of nursing — to the role and functions of nursing management?

In the context of nursing management many questions arise. Some dilemmas are presented. For example, what should be the main concern of nurse managers — their staff, patients/clients or, as recently mentioned (DHSS, 1983) and since much debated, 'productivity'? Are there links between effective nursing care and the use of management skills and knowledge? How should nurses be prepared in the skills and theory of management? These are questions and issues which, in part will be entertained in this section, and a more thorough discussion will take place in Chapter 11.

Role and Functions of Nursing Management: Is the Preparation of Nurses Realistic? Adequate?

Having discussed patients, clients and their needs, we now examine the role of nurses at different levels of nursing, in meeting those needs by applying management skills and management knowledge to their professional (nursing) activities: in essence, the management of care.

The essence of management education is to enable nurses, at all levels of nursing, to gain an understanding of the philosophy, aims and objectives of the organisation and, by applying the skills and knowledge of management to their professional practice, to provide an acceptable standard of care.

Concerns of the Manager

'Management must always be conceived of in the right way as the effective development of the full potential of precious human resources.' (Briggs (HMSO, 1972), para.728, p.211).

The manager is essentially concerned with the problems of the organisation: he is a problem-solver — decision-maker. This is underlined by Revans (1971) who writes: 'The manager's principal perception is not of objectives nor of resources, nor of good, nor of means, but of problems.' Drucker (1974) makes the point: 'Whatever a manager does he does through making decisions.'

An integral part of the decision-making activity of managers is deciding what needs to be done within their area of responsibility and inducing others, usually subordinates, to implement their decisions as well as controlling the implementation of these decisions and observing, evaluating and amending them as deemed necessary. Ultimately, they must accept responsibility for their decisions and the consequences of their implementation.

Managing the Clinical Environment: Links between Education, Service and Management

Following the 1974 reorganisation of the NHS, in each district the nursing service was managed by a DNO (District Nursing Officer) who was a member of the DMT (District Management Team) and directly accountable to the AHA. The DNO had functional co-ordinating responsibility within the DMT. Under the DNO the nursing service was organised in 'divisions' each under a divisional nursing officer. The nursing divisions comprised two or more hospital nursing divisions together with a community nursing division. Essentially, functional nursing divisions aligned, to some extent, with 'health care groups' e.g. a general nursing division, a midwifery division, a psychiatry division and a community care division. Each division was managed by a divisional nursing officer accountable to the DNO.

The aim of these arrangements for nursing was to provide for integrated community and hospital nursing services within districts and co-ordination with other disciplines at each level of management to facilitate effective, efficient and optimal patient/client care.

Nursing is one of the principal professions in the NHS, committed to the care and management of patients.

Nurse managers have the central responsibility of enabling standards of care by ensuring that the environment in which patients are nursed is appropriate to meeting their needs and enabling staff needs, in so far as resources are readily available and used and that the ward climate, in terms of the sensitivity, relationships, attitudes, aspirations and goals of staff are in harmony with ensuring patient care satisfaction. It is numerically the largest profession. Paradoxically, because of its innate weaknesses due to the negative image of nursing that is projected, together with its associated lack of real authority and autonomy and negotiating ability, it is probably the most powerful of the health care professions. Contributing to this lack of real power is the fact that its peer professions, especially medicine, are unwilling to relinquish even a proportion of its power. Clearly, for one group of professionals to 'gain' power another group must relinquish some. The power struggle, to me, is exemplified in the present conflict between nurses and doctors in the context of the nursing process.

The emergence of new knowledge, technology and legislation together with the development of associated policies and frequent change in the NHS and in the professions makes the continuing development (career-long) and updating of nurses, at all levels of nursing, a prerequisite to ensuring competent practice, i.e. maintaining quality of service. In this context, the central duty of nurse managers is to maintain and to improve the care provided for patients/clients by optimising human resources — the skills, knowledge and expertise of nurses — and by providing a suitable environment for the practice of care.

Even though primarily management is the concern of the explicit appointed managers, the practice of management is an important aspect of the jobs of all those concerned with the running of hospitals. It is not the special concern of administrators, nor is it the special concern of senior managers. Therefore, if nurses are going to accept fully their emerging role as highly trained nursing managers, how should they be educated to do their job? What are the things they must be able to do?

To establish the rightful place and role of management knowledge and management skills in nursing, it may help the reader first to examine the views and the guidelines suggested for the management preparation of nurses, in some major reports, in an effort to establish the general philosophy and the links between the practice of nursing, the achievement of quality care, and the use of a management methodology.

Management education is about informing and enabling nurses, at different levels of the NHS and/or nursing, to recognise, understand and cope effectively with situations which relate to the organisation and delivery of health care, as well as helping them to understand the inherent philosophy aims and activities of the organisation in which care is delivered to patients, i.e. its aims, objectives and fuctions, together with the required interrelationships and behaviour of professionals and the effects of this on the patient.

Many reports during the past two decades highlight the management role and functions of nurse and relate them to sound nursing practice and the realisation of effective and efficient standards and quality of care.

The Platt report (RCN, 1964) indicated 'the difficulty of meeting demands for skilled nursing care within the context of a rapidly developing and increasingly complex service'. Also a report by Revans (1964) underlined 'dissatisfaction expressed by nurses is centred around conditions of employment, which include matters such as staffing, pay, hours, training, promotion and job-satisfaction, communication, social relations and personal security'.

The management function of the nurse was discussed in the reports of Salmon (1966) and Mayston (DHSS, 1969) which established the framework for, and underlined the importance of, management education in securing sound nursing practice. This message from the 1960s has subsequently been reflected in the philosophy of many reports and legislation.

The link between good nursing and management is also emphasised in the Briggs report which states: 'Good management is a precondition of good care' (para.55, p.15). Also, the Briggs guidelines highlighted anaomalies in nursing education, some of which were discussed by the Platt Committee, paramount to which was the inadequacy of the existing pattern of nursing education and the difficulty of meeting demands for skilled nursing care.

The report, *Management Arrangements for the Reorganised National Health Service* (DHSS, 1972) which prompted the integration of the NHS, attempted to provide a more effective working of professional practitioners through the provision of a structure and systems that would support them both educationally and administratively. The education and training of staff was seen to be central to producing 'the best health care' (para.1.4, p.10).

The Merrison report and the Consultative Paper *Patients First* (DHSS, 1979) said that the structure and management arrangements introduced in 1974, were an inappropriate framework for the effective delivery of care. And the Griffiths report (DHSS, 1983) said: 'The NHS demands top class management' (para.4, p.11).

These reports, either explicitly or implicitly, underline the centrality of the relationship between Education, Service and Management in providing and delivering health care to patients and clients.

The EEC Nursing Directives (1977) together with the *Nurses, Midwives and Health Visitors Act* 1979 are most important developments in the advancement of nursing philosophy and nurses' aims, through improved education, training and development, to realising their own professional aspirations — in essence, their self-actualisation — and through this, successfully determining and maintaining nursing standards.

A report on 'Foundation Management Training' (National Staff Committee, 1980) said:

> The prime purpose of nurse managers is to maintain and improve the standard of care provided for patients and their families through the effective use of availiable resources: Management Education and Training and its integration with Clinical Training is essential to enable nurses to provide an acceptable standard of care, to gain an understanding of the real purpose of the organisation and to act as a basis upon which to build further training. (para.2, p.3)

In 1981 the NSC published a report on 'The Organisation and Provision of Continuing In-Service Education and Training' which emphasises the link between the emergence of new knowledge and technology and continuing social change and staff development, 'to maintain and improve competency in practice' (para.1.2, p.5). Also in 1981, a DHSS seminar on 'Professional Development in Clinical Nursing', among its proposals endorsed 'the need for professional updating on a regular basis if a high standard of nursing care is to be maintained throughout a nurse's whole career' (para.8, p.4). In addition an RCN Discussion Document, *Towards Standards* (1981), on discussing the management of change in the context of 'individualised care' underlined, 'innovation of this sort requires skilled management if it is to be successfully achieved' (para.1, p.9).

In 1983, a report published by the RCN, *Toward a New Professional Structure for Nursing*, said:

> The possession of clinical skills and expertise alone cannot ensure that high standards of clinical care are maintained: they must be accompanied by the authority to manage the clinical environment. The role of the ward sister implies extensive clinical expertise and preparation for clinical management. (paras. 2.5/2.6, p.6)

In managing the clinical environment, two things are paramount, namely, the authority to act and having the knowledge, skills and confidence to act.

So, do trained nurses have the necessary authority to manage the clinical environment? Do nurses have autonomy to make decisions about nursing care? And, most important, is the preparation for clinical management adequate? And what of the clinical expertise? Are the basic nine competencies (these will be discussed later in the chapter) hopefully acquired during basic nursing training, refined, developed and updated to allow the trained nurse to practice with assurance and confidence?

Preparation of Nurses for Management: Role of Education and Training

The Salmon and Mayston reports, among their many useful effects and some criticism, gave the nursing profession the opportunity to scrutinise the management of the nursing services together with the personnel, training and education arrangements required.

The Briggs Committee indicated their unease about sharp distinctions in nursing, between clinical and managerial responsibilities in so far as there are managerial elements in the role of all nurses who have finished their training, e.g. assessing, planning, co-ordinating, monitoring, evaluating, the care of patients, as well as communicating, motivating and leading the ward team. More important, the Committee advised that senior nurse managers and teachers should have substantial clinical experience particularly at middle management level, to enable them to 'continue to exercise clinical judgement' (para.538, p.163). In this respect, the Committee concluded: 'Management and care are not conflicting conceptions, good management is a precondition of good care.' (para.55, p.15).

The ultimate aim of the management of the NHS and nursing is to secure improvements to health care for patients. In this respect, highly skilled, experienced and competent managers, of all professions, of which nursing is central (because of the size of its workforce and its close and continuous relationship with the patients), are needed at all levels of the organisation, but particularly at the front line, the ward/community level, where nurses afford round-the-clock nursing care and where prompt and accurate decision making is required by health care professionals in the interest of the integrity of care.

Hypothetical Qualities

The hypothetical qualities of the effective manager include: command of the basic facts of a situation; relevant professional understanding; continuing sensitivity to events; analytical and problem-solving skills; social skills and abilities; emotional resilience; inclination to respond purposefully to events; balanced learning habits and skills; mental agility; and creativity (Burgoyne and Stuart, 1976).

In reality, are these qualities purely hypothetical, whose only value is academic, or are they qualities of significance to every nurse manager? If they can be accepted as being relevant to enabling nurse managers to perform their role with efficiency, at what stage should these qualities, aptitudes, abilities, knowledge and skills, be developed?

The preparation of the nurse in management theory and management practice begins at the level of the nursing student. The basic training of nurses is particularly concerned with the professional (nursing) aspects of the job; but there should also be learnt on-the-job some of the basic managerial skills which are important to the operational manager in managing the ward or community which include those of co-ordination of services, supervision and counselling (staff, patients, clients and relatives), communication, decision-making and leadership. This is necessary to enable nurses to utilise their professional (nursing) knowledge and skills optimally in the care and management of the patient (NSC Report, 1980, para.2, p.3).

Senior nurses at ward and community level have substantial managerial and clinical commitment, i.e. setting of work objectives, planning, the co-ordination of the work of nurses and other professionals and non-professionals working in the wards. Nurses of higher and specialised clinical skills additionally may be required to exercise advisory functions to nurses and other professionals — the 'consultancy' function (Briggs 1972).

If the theory of management, management knowledge, is to play an effective part in the total development of the nurse in so far as enabling nurses to improve the quality of nursing care, then ways of linking theory with practice must be found and used. In effecting these links three factors need to be considered; nurses, the hospital/ward/community environment, and the situational opportunities.

Nurses need to have their practice supervised and in this respect they need to be supported, counselled and, most important, need to be motivated and allowed to participate in the activities of the service, through examining real problems. The environment in which practice takes place needs to be sound, to contain the necessary resources and be devoid of conflict, if possible. And use must be made of situational opportunities by ensuring more on-the-job training as well as effecting an 'action learning' approach, to maximise the learning experience of the nurse. However, despite the enthusiasm and desire of nurse managers to effect the latter, a major problem that may present is the absence of, or the inadequacy of, numbers of suitably trained and developed staff who are capable of adequately supervising and guiding nurses to optimise on-the-job and problem-solving learning. Therefore, nurses at operational level must be helped to develop skills which will enable them to co-ordinate services; to teach and supervise; to counsel staff, patients, clients and relatives; to understand their legal responsibilities and to lead their nursing team in such a way to enable nurses to utilise and to apply their clinical and professional skills to their full advantage for the benefit of patient.

The Salmon Committee (1966) emphasised as being central to the managerial role the 'quality or type of the decisions to be taken' (para.3.35, p.25) i.e. whether they are appropriate to top management — assisting in the formation of policy and applying it to the sphere controlled; middle management — programming, formulating procedures for applying policy; or first-line management — executive, seeing that the work programme is carried out. This means that the formulation of policy should be done by nurses in top management, decisions on its detailed application should be made by nurses in middle management and decisions on its execution should be taken by nurses in first-line management.

The job of nurse managers, at different levels, is likely to involve them in playing several roles. It will also enable them to bring to the job their characteristic set of attitudes which will mould the way in which they fulfill their roles. The effectiveness with which they do the job will depend on the various skills and knowledge, e.g. behavioural — communication, leadership, interviewing; organisational — policies and procedures, managing, industrial relations, finance; and legislative — health and safety, industrial relations, disciplinary and grievance procedures, which they have acquired. The role of the front-line nurse manager includes information gatherer, listener, counsellor — helping others to solve problems; consultant — advising on procedure; director — telling people to do something; co-ordinator — bringing resources together; standard-setter; teacher; and ward-team representative.

They must (in the philosophy of Fayol) plan — decide what to do and how to do it; control — see that the plans have been achieved; co-ordinate — make provision for all necessary resources in the right place at the right time. They must also motivate, encourage their staff to develop their own drive towards achieving the aims of the ward within the aims of the NHS.

Deciding what has to be done is called planning; it involves making oneself quite familiar with all that is involved in a given situation and deciding in reasonable detail how it should be tackled. Also, it includes understanding the techniques of nursing, professional ethics, and understanding the broad plans of top management.

Deciding how to do the job is another aspect of policy. Nurse managers must explain and interpret hospital/district policy to their staff in terms which they can understand and put into action. They must organise and co-ordinate the operation. Having communicated their plans and checked that they have been understood, they must ensure that there are enough nurses to do the job.

In addition to their responsibilities to patients and clients, nurses have a personal responsibility, that of ensuring their own professional educational development to enable them to make informed judgements and to maintain safe and competent practice. This is underlined by the UKCC in its Code of Professional Conduct (1984) and in The Nurses, Midwives and Health Visitors Rules Approval Order, 1983 (EEC, 1983).

These responsibilities are deemed to be vital prerequisites of successful patient care, yet in the current industrial and social climate, are difficult to realise. The main impediments to their realisation being the uncertainties of the nurse's role, manpower and other resource constraints; rapid and continuous technological and social change; lack of research into nursing problems and/or failure of nursing to use the results of proven research; and the preoccupation of nurses with the ideal of professionalisation of nursing.

The task of management education and training resides substantially at the workplace rather than in the formal situation of the classroom (Revans, 1971). The success or failure in the transfer of this learning into improved managerial performance on the job, is the collective responsibility of nurses, their immediate superiors and senior management. Progress in performance is substantially dependent upon the attitudes and aspirations of nurses, the nature of their working environment together with the attitudes of their colleagues and superiors. However, for progress to be made, management knowledge needs constant application, management skills need regular use. The keynote is practice: to focus on getting right one aspect of performance at a time, rather than identifying several aspects. In addition, feedback is important to get the views of others on how effective performance is. Also, if skills are to be acquired and/or developed, time must be made available for practice and discussion. Essentially getting this right, or management action, is about securing the best deal for patients and the community within available resources and the best motivation for staff (DHSS, 1983, para.3, p.11).

Management education viewed in the context of clinical training and practice, has a three-fold function: 'To enable nurses to provide an acceptable standard of care and, for nursing students to gain an understanding of the real purpose of the organisation — the effective and efficient care of the patient as well as to act as a basis for further training.' (NSC, 1980). A DHSS (1973) document states: 'The purpose of management education and training is to help to improve the quality of management and thus to contribute to better health care'. It continues, 'In the absence of appropriate training opportunities (this will be discussed in Chapter 11) there is a great risk of bad management, with its attendant isolation of the health care professions, continuance of out-dated practices and, inevitably, poor organisation of patient care services.' (para.2, p.1).

The purpose of management education and training is similar to any form of education and training: it has to do with developing knowledge and skills, usually specific to one's job, and providing the requisite information and abilities to effect development — fulfilment of the person. In nursing this development is directly related to enabling the comfort, security and well-being of patients, thus ensuring their proper care, in terms of the standard and quality provided, and ultimately contributing to their rehabilitation.

Management is good and useful only in so far as it leads to greater efficiency in enabling the care of the patient. How is this enabled? What is the official view? What are the hallmarks of the effective management, and of effective and efficient management?

To be effective, management education should build on and relate to the underlying professional education of the nurse. In this respect, ensuring the proper development and realisation of the management potential of their subordinates is a responsibility of senior nurse managers. Apart from the use of management developmental devices as staff training, staff apraisal procedures and career guidance, ability to plan the nurse's career is a corollary of management education and a vital prerequisite for developing nurse managers. How can this best be achieved? One approach to developing management potential, which is currently being used in the NHS, is that of role-based training.

Role-based Training

In recent years role-based training has been considered as a means of developing nurse managers. In this situation, management development centres help individual nurses to function more effectively in the role they currently occupy by providing them with an opportunity to gain greater understanding of that role together with the skills and knowledge needed for its successful occupancy. Essentially the approach is three pronged, namely: direct focus on the nurse's current work programme; professionally led training — senior nurse managers act as educators and have continuous involvement in the planning and implementation of the programme as well as linking with nurses' managers; and diagnostic — a phase designed to determine and agree individual training needs which are met during the subsequent training phase.

In role-based training members have control over the training content and are able to make a significant contribution to their own training and development. Also, the ambiguity/confusion of role is less of a problem in so far as there is increased understanding together with the provision of appropriate skills thus enabling the job to be done more effectively. There is also a broadening of horizons enabling nurses to think more clearly and plan improvements in the delivery of patient care (NSC, 1983).

Despite sound management education and training, impediments may present, which in practice negate against or limit its use. Therefore, such factors as uncertainty about role, lack of guidance and support from superiors together with frequent changes to the organisational structure within which health care is practised, i.e. district, hospital, ward or community, may adversely affect nurses' approach to their work. In addition the preoccupation of nurses with the more personal and professional issues of nursing including inadequate status and recognition, industrial relations, ethical issues and the professionalisation of nursing, even though important and relevant, may affect nurses' morale, causing them to lack belief in what they are doing resulting in inadequte or sub-standard care for patients and clients.

This situation, in the words of Merrison, can cause patients to lose out on care, 'if those caring for patients are more concerned with their own status and problems, than the patients' health and well-being then the patients will be the losers.' (para.12.30, p.169).

Regrettably, even if the existing organisational and educational climate is in favour of encouraging the managerial potential of nurses, there continues to be a lack of the necessary authority and autonomy to enable them to fulfil their professional responsibilities: this overall is due to 'the absence of an appropriate educational system which gives them insufficient knowledge, skills and values from which to discharge their responsibility' (McFarlane, 1983).

Clearly, in the present disquieting situation, nurses cannot fulfil their professional obligations to their patients and clients. Also, in the absence of clearly defined role criteria it becomes impossible for nurse educationists to prepare nurses to meet the demands of their nursing role. Currently discussions and seminars are being held to establish the feasibility of advanced clinical roles, central to which is that of establishing clinical career progression with senior clinical posts. This is laudable and long overdue; but, before progressing to this stage, a vital prerequisite is that of establishing unequivocally the basic role of the trained nurse.

And so, in the final analysis, have the many attempts over the past two decades to reshape the NHS in the search for better management, proved to be successful? Some observers, notably Williams (1969) conclude:

> There is the tendency for each main professional group in the NHS to produce and associate itself with its own set of proposals for training and structural change. Also, there is the deference that some of these policy statements show to the idea that there are certain 'principles of management' that can be used to increase the efficiency with which hospitals are managed. And the willingness of some parties to advocate major structural changes with basing their recommendations on a searching analysis of what hospital members do and how they see their jobs.

He also highlights some contradictions in the reports of Salmon (1966), Godber (1967) and Howard (King Edward Hospitals Fund, 1967) and says that these contradictions are understandable if the reports are viewed as 'delineations of desirable occupational spheres of influence and power as well as attempts to prescribe managerial solutions to organization problems'.

Williams argues that the concern of the Salmon report was almost wholly with the administrative functions of nurses together with the means of preparing them for their responsibilities. This approach, intentionally or otherwise, disregards professional interrelationships and interdependence in the total care of the patient.

The Godber report underlined that: 'practically every clinical decision affects the administrative running of the hospital'. Despite this, doctors continue to remain impervious to administrative 'interference' even in a remote way, over clinical decision making, despite the guidelines of the *Grey Book* (DHSS, 1972) and Merrison and the more positive approach of Griffiths (DHSS, 1983). The Godber report makes it clear that, 'the greatest benefit to participants and to the service is most likely to be derived from a multi-disciplinary approach'.

This practice was acknowledged by the *Grey Book* and the Merrison report which favoured a consensus approach to decision making; now in some disfavour with Griffiths.

The 1967 report on hospital management called for structural changes which had their foundations in the idea that professional services must be managed by trained managers. It said: 'No hospital or group can be successfully administered by a triumvirate of equal and independent senior officers. Someone must be in charge.' A philosophy now overtaken by the ideas inherent in Griffiths. In fact, to date, there has been the appointment of two general managers from outside the NHS. The quest to find a secure management framework for the NHS and nursing continues, albeit unsuccessfully, as evidenced by the 1972 and 1982 NHS reorganisation, and much documentation.

So, at the end of 1985 (the deadline for implementing the new Griffiths structure) the search for effective management which hopefully, though belatedly, will meet the needs of patients, clients and staff, will start to be tested. Will this new structure provide the right approach (organisationally) to the management of care? Clearly, only time will tell. Perhaps the time is now right to privatise the Service and aim for the motive of 'productivity', underlined by Griffiths.

References

Burgoyne, J.G.. and Stuart, R. (1976) The nature, use and acquisition of managerial skills and other attributes. *Personnel Review, 5*, 19–29

DHSS (1969) Report of Working Party on Management Structure in the Local Authority Nursing Service (Mayston). HMSO, London

———— (1972) Management Arrangements for the Reorganised National Health Service (Grey Book). DHSS, London

———— (1973) Personnel Management in the National Health Service Management and Training (No.1). DHSS, London

———— (1979) Patients First (Consultative Paper on the Structure and Management of the NHS). DHSS, London

———— (1981) Seminar: Professional Development in Clinical Nursing — the 1980s. DHSS, London

———— (1983) Report of the Inquiry into the National Health Service (Griffiths), DHSS, London

Drucker, P.F. (1974) *Management: Tasks, Responsibilities and Practices*. Harper and Row, New York

———— (1975) *The Practice of Management*. Heinemann, London

EEC (Commission of the European Communities) (1977) Legislation. *Official Journal of the European Communities, 20*, no. L176

———— (1983) *Nurses, Midwives and Health Visitors Rules Approval Order*. HMSO, London

Fayol, H. (1916) *General and Industrial Management*. Translation by Constance Storr, 1949. Pitman, London

Herzberg, F. (1959) *The Motivation to Work*, 2nd edn. Wiley, New York

HMSO (1972) Report of the Committee on Nursing (Briggs). Cmnd no. 5115. HMSO, London

———— (1979) Royal Commission on the National Health Service (Merrison). Cmnd no. 7615. HMSO, London

King Edward Hospitals Fund (1967) The Shape of Hospital Mangement in 1980? (Howard). King Edward Hospital Fund, London

McFarlane, Baroness (1983) 'Mirror, mirror on the wall', Nursing Mirror Lecture, 1983. *Nursing Mirror, 156*, 17–20

McGregor, D. (1960) *The Human Side of Enterprise*. McGraw-Hill, New York

Ministry of Health, Scottish Home and Health Dept (1966) Report of the Committee on Senior Nursing Staff Structure (Salmon). HMSO, London

———— (1967) First Report of the Joint Working Party on the Organisation of Medical Work in Hospitals (Godber). HMSO, London

National Staff Committee (N&M) (1980) Foundation Management Training. NSC

———— (1981) The Organisation of Continuing Education. In-service Education and Training. NSC

———— (1983) Role Based Training as a Means of Developing Nurse Managers. NSC

Nurses, Midwives and Health Visitors Act 1979 (Chapter 36). HMSO, London

Revans, R.W. (1964) *Standards for Morale: Cause and Effect in Hospitals*. Oxford University Press, Oxford

———— (1971) in G.F. Wieland and H. Leigh (eds.) *Changing Hospitals: A Report on the Internal Communication Project*. Tavistock, London

RCN (1964) A Reform of Nurse Education (Platt). RCN

———— (1981) Towards Standards (Discussion Document). RCN

———— (1983) Towards a New Professional Structure for Nursing. RCN

Williams, D. (1969) The administrative contribution of the nursing sister. *Journal of Public Administration, XLVII*, 307–28

Advised Further Reading

Bennett, M. (1984) Quality of Nursing — Strained or Thrice Blessed? Paper given at Royal Melbourne Hospital Oration, October

Block, D. (1977) Criteria, Standards, Norms. *Journal of Nursing Administration*, Sept., pp. 20–30

Bowman, M.P. (1980) The Education and Training Needs of First-line Nurses. Unpublished

MEd Thesis, University of Newcastle upon Tyne

Carlson, D. (1982) *Modern Management: Principles and Practices*. Macmillan, New York

Carson, S. (1981) What every Head Nurse should Know about Management. *Health Services Manager, 14*(3), 11–12

Clark, C.C. and Shea, C.A. (1979) *Management in Nursing: A Vital Link in the Health Care System*. McGraw-Hill, New York

Colavecchio, R. (1982) Direct patient care: a viable career choice? *Journal of Nursing Administration, 12*(8), 17–22

Crosby, P.B. (1982) *The Art of Getting Your Own Sweet Way*. 2nd end. McGraw-Hill, New York

Davis, C.K. *et al.* (1982) Leadership for expanding influence on health policy. *Journal of Nursing Administration, 12,* 12–21

Degreene, K.B. (1982) *The Adaptive Organisation: Anticipation and Management Crisis*. Wiley, New York

EEC (Commission of the European Communities) (1981) Advisory Committee on Training in Nursing. Report on the Training of Nurses Responsible for General Care. (lll/D/5). EEC

——— (1981) Legislation. *Official Journal of the European Communities*, 24, no. L385

Gordon, G.K. (1982) Motivating staff: a look at the assumptions. *Journal of Nursing Administration, 12,* 27–8

Fayol, H (1938) *The Functions of the Executive*. Harvard University Press

Fulmer, R. (1982) *Supervision: Principles of Professional Management*, 2nd edn. Macmillan, New York

General Nursing Council for England and Wales (1980/1) Annual Report. GNC, London

Henderson, V. and Nite, G. (1978) *Principles and Practice of Nursing*, 6th edn. Macmillan, New York

International Council of Nurses (1965) Special and Committee Reports presented to the ICN Board of Directors and Grand Council Meetings, Frankfurt, June 1965, ICN

Kramer, M. (1974) *Reality Shock*. C.V. Mosby, St Louis

MacGuire, J.M. (1980) *The Expanded Role of the Nurse*. King Edwards Hospital Fund for London

Mayeroff, M. (1971) *On Caring*. Harper and Row, New York

McCarthy, M. (1983) A management say in NHS pay. *Personnel Management (UK), 15,* 26–9

Nightingale, F. (1980) *Notes on Nursing: What it is and what it is not*. Originally published in London, Hainson, 1859. Includes: Notes on Nursing: The Science and the Art. By Skeet, M. Churchill Livingstone, Edinburgh

Rowbottom, R. *et al.* (1973) *Hospital Organisation*. Heineman, London

RCN (1943) Nursing Reconstruction Committee (Horder). RCN

——— (1978) An Assessment of the State of Nursing in the National Health Service. RCN

——— (1979) Working Committee on Standards of Nursing Care and Related Matters (England and Wales). RCN

——— (1982) Seminar on Advanced Clinical Roles. RCN

——— (1984) Nurse Alert, RCN

Schweiger, J.L. (1980) *The Nurse as Manager*. Wiley, New York

Wieland, G. (ed.) (1981) *Improving Health Care Management: Organization Development and Organization Change*. Health Administration Press, Ann Arbor, MI

Williams, D. (1969) The administrative contribution of the nursing sister. *Public Administration, XLVII,* 307–28

Wolff, L. *et al.* (1974) *Fundamentals of Nursing*. J.B. Lippincott Co., Philadelphia

6 PROFESSIONALISM IN HEALTH CARE AND NURSING

Aims

The aims of this chapter are:

1. To discuss the concept of professionalism.
2. To examine the criteria of professionalism in the context of providing quality care.

Learning Objectives

The purpose of this chapter is to enable the reader to:

1. Understand the nature of professionalism.
2. Appreciate the relevance of the nursing competencies to the nurse.
3. Understand the place of the code of professional conduct in nursing.

Concept of Professionalism

'Nurses must develop a professional identity and promote an image of nursing which will cause doctors to regard them as colleagues and no longer as subservient handmaidens or a threat to their own practice' (McFarlane, 1984).

Special competence, implying complex formal education, is central to most definitions of the professional. As the need for education increases 'amateurs' may be edged out (O'Connor and Meadows, 1976).

The evolution of professional criteria includes a move from:

service provided by the individual to a team approach; knowledge from a single discipline to knowledge from diverse fields; altruism — selfless service limited to increased opportunity for selfless service; restricted colleague/peer evaluation of work to increased opportunity for colleague/peer evaluation; and from relative privacy in the client — professional relationship to decreased privacy. (Goodlad, 1984)

A UKCC Paper (1982) in defining the 'professional nurse' says:

'Members of a profession are characterised by an attitude of service to clients.' (Section 2, p.5).

Professionalism is regarded by some observers to consist of a body of knowledge which is applicable; exclusive competence in so much as others are unable or are prevented (legally and professionally) because of this exclusive competence, to assume professional status and to practice; responsibility for the development and the transmission of knowledge; primary ethic of service; and controlled entry and exit to the profession (Rowbottom *et al.*, 1973).

Nursing, in the concept of a profession, is assumed to be unique, distinct and different, by virtue of its exclusiveness through its standard of entry, the education, training and development of its members code of professional conduct, ethic of service, nursing competencies, together with the responsibility, authority and autonomy of trained nurses to perform the nursing function and to make decisions about nursing care.

To provide a service at a professional level, implicit in which is enabling and ensuring an acceptable standard and quality of care, nursing must embody all these elements. In their absence, how can a service of professional integrity be ensured?

To ensure that the highest achievable standard of care is secured, nurses, if they are to be recognised as true professionals, must be properly educated, trained, developed and updated in knowledge and skills at all nursing levels. In doing so the educational methods used must ensure that the creative, intellectual and other abilities and skills of the nurse are developed: there must be greater emphasis on problem-solving and action-learning; expository methods of learning must give way to insight (Gestalt) and autonomous learning — where the person and the situation are focal. In addition, nurses must become more open-minded — self-critical to themselves and their practice.

In the ultimate, this approach I believe would produce increased job-satisfaction, improved patient care and greater self-actualisation of nurses (realising their full potential in terms of their abilities, skills and knowledge).

Many writers have grappled with the notion of, and criteria for, the professional. Notable names include those of Butcher and Stelling (1969), Engel (1969), Rowbottom (1973), Kramer (1974). In addition, much evidence on the elements of professionalism is available in many reports and documents, by professional and statutory bodies, e.g. WHO (1966), RCN (1981, 1983), DHSS (1981) and UKCC (1984).

The word profession can be defined in different ways. However, when used in the context of nursing it can be described as a learned calling, as distinct from a trade, whose members choose human service as a career and who share a client-centred orientation.

Do the implications which are inherent in this concept, or definition, match the criteria on professionalism discussed in the literature? Do they relate to the expectations of nurses and the practice of nursing? Are they reconciled to the image and aspirations of nurses? Is there consensus on professional criteria? More important, what is the relationship between the assumed professional role and functions of the nurse as opposed to their extant role? In effect, what is the reality of being a professional? What is the essence of professionalism?

Official View

A report published by the WHO (1966) commenting on the education development of the nurse said:

> Nurses should have a broad general education as well as nursing training which would enable them to develop their ability to provide the most skilled nursing care and their judgement to make independent decisions based on scientific, clinical and management principles: that is to say, they should provide service at a professional level. (pp.12, 13)

To provide this service, the report underlined that governments should assume the same responsibilities towards nursing as towards any other profession'; that the education of nurses, from the beginning, should adopt 'a problem-solving approach to prepare them to face a future of change'; and that their education should be 'abosrbed into the system of higher education'.

Cohen (1981) makes the point: 'Professionalism is about controlling one's own practice and making one's own decisions.'

In recent years, the concept of professionalism in nursing is being increasingly questioned for its validity and reality in the context of the framework within which the practice of nursing takes place. Vital and related issues which have been discussed in this context relate to the education, training and development of the nurse, together with the nature of the nursing role and especially nurses' associated authority, responsibility, accountability and autonomy to act.

The centrality of nursing as a profession is probably best exemplified by defining the services which it renders to patients and clients, and by the criteria which distinguish nurses as professionals: or through the absence of those allegedly valid criteria which disable nurses, reduce their status as professionals and diminish or undermine, by their absence, the service to patients and clients. Therefore, any examination of the nurse as a professional must include an analysis of such factors as: nursing, care, quality and standards of competence, methods of assessment and evaluation of the care provided, the nature of the education, training, development and appraisal of nurses; and, the nature of the role of the nurse within the context of its dispensable elements of nursing competencies together with the responsibility, authority, accountability and autonomy of the role occupant.

Personal Professional Development: The Caring Role

In the context of Cohen's observations, courses of training leading to a qualification, the successful completion of which shall enable an application to be made for admission to Part 1, 3, 5 or 8 of the Register, must provide opportunities to enable nursing students to accept responsibility for their professional development and to acquire the competencies underlined in the Nurses, Midwives and Health Visitors Rules Approval Order (1983), i.e. to:

a. advise on the promotion of health and the prevention of illness;
b. recognise situations that may be detrimental to the health and well-being of the individuals;
c. carry out those activities involved when conducting the comprehensive assessment of a person's nursing requirements;
d. recognise the significance of the observations made and use these to develop an initial nursing assessment;
e. devise a plan of nursing care based on the assessment with the co-operation of the patient, to the extent that this is possible, taking into account the medical prescription;
f. implement the planned programme of nursing care and where appropriate teach and co-ordinate other members of the caring team who may be responsible for implementing specific aspects of the nursing care;
g. review the effectiveness of the nursing care provided, and where appropriate initiate any action that may be required;
h. work in a team with other nurses, and with medical and paramedical staff and social workers;
i. undertake the management of the care of a group of patients over a period of time and organise the appropriate support services;

related to the care of the particular type of patient with whom she is likely to come in contact when registered in that Part of the register for which the student intends to qualify.

Courses leading to a qualification, the successful completion of which shall enable an application to be made for admission to Part 2, 4, 6 or 7 of the register, shall be designed to prepare nursing students to undertake nursing care under the direction of a person registered in Part 1, 3, 5 or 8 of the register and provide opportunities for the students to develop the competencies required to:

a. assist in carrying out comprehensive observation of the patient and help in assessing her care requirements;
b. develop skills to enable her to assist in the implementation of nursing care under the direction of a person registered in Part 1, 3, 5 or 8 of the register;
c. accept delegated nursing tasks;
d. assist in reviewing the effectiveness of the care provided;
e. work in a team with other nurses, and with medical and paramedical staff and social workers;

related to the care of the particular type of patient with whom she is likely to come into contact when registered in that Part of the register for which the student intends to qualify.

Caring and Care: Centrality to Professionalism

Do patients and clients need to be cared for by highly skilled people? Is the title of nurse something special — to be treasured and to be protected? If the answer to these questions is 'Yes', then they invite many supplementary questions, paramount of which are: Why is the care of patients and clients entrusted to a large workforce of unqualified (nursing students) and/or untrained (care assistants) people? And, why has it taken 65 years, since the passing of the *Nurses Act* 1919 (which legislated against the abuse of the title 'nurse') to implement effectively this aspect of the legislation?

The recent nursing legislation (*Nurses, Midwives and Health Visitors Act* 1979) has attempted, after some six decades punctuated by debates on the education of the nurse, with professionalism, role and functions of the nurse and, most important, a growing apprehension among nurses because of declining standards, to provide a sound and appropriate educational and managerial framework to enable the professionalisation of nursing strongly advised in many reports, but particularly underlined in those of Platt, Salmon, Briggs and Griffiths)?

The events which have occurred since 1919, particularly in nursing education, even though laudable have done little to enable nurses to establish a full professional role. In this respect the Platt report (RCN, 1964) despite containing sound recommendations to enable the future education of nurses was effectively shelved for reasons undisclosed, though one can assume that some of the more far-reaching recommendations of the report, e.g. 'students should not form part of the basic staff of the hospital' and 'students should receive training allowances from Exchequer funds', were 'unacceptable' to the government of the day, especially as these recommendations, if implemented, would require an increase in the workforce and cost, to enable the workload of 'students' to be expedited. Clearly, the additional funding would require government support. However, some eight years later some of the Platt recommendations formed a basis for the Briggs report (1972), notably the recommendations on the status and education of the learner together with some useful comment on the future role of the nurse. (Points also made by the Merrison Committee, 1979.) Regrettably, it took a further nine years of gathering dust before the recommendations, in part, were implemented through the agency of the *Nurses, Midwives and Health Visitors Act* 1979.

Caring and its Centrality to Professionalism

To care for patients and clients nurses must know what their patients'/clients' powers and limitations are, what their needs are and what is conducive to their growth. In addition they must know how to respond to those needs, and in the process understand their own powers and limitations.

Mayeroff (1971) describes components which are central to 'caring'. They include: general and specific knowledge, together with alternating rhythms which include attempting different approaches to care, acting with certain expectations and identifying whether what was expected was achieved and, in the light of results maintaining and/or modifying one's behaviour. The use of specific, technical professional knowledge is basic to meeting these needs. Patience, which includes participation with the patient or client and adapting to their pace, is central to the care of all patients and clients. Honesty includes actively confronting and being open with oneself and others. Trust involves acknowledging the independent existence of the patient/client and includes an element of risk and a leap into the unknown — making and taking informed decisions. Humility means that the care given by nurses is not privileged: what is important is that the nurse is able to care and has a patient/client to care for; it embodies nurses' limitations and their dependence on others — an element which seems unacknowledged in the development and practice of the 'nursing process'. Hope is hope for the realisation of the patient/client through nurses' caring: it implies that there is or could be something worthy of commitment. Courage is informed by insight from past experiences and is open and sensitive to the present. Autonomy, in Mayeroff's view, does not mean being detached and without strong ties: it does not mean being self-enclosed. Its essence is dependence on others and others' dependence on oneself. In this context the role of the nurse must explicitly acknowledge, e.g. engage, other professionals. Self-actualisation means highlighted awareness, greater responsiveness to others and oneself, and the fuller use of one's distinctive powers. This places a responsibilty on the individual nurse for developing and using to the full their potential, and on nurse managers for ensuring that potential is developed and used.

Clearly, the caring role as depicted by Mayeroff is central to the health care professions, especially nursing, and has many distinct messages particularly at a time when nurses are preoccupied with their role, the nursing process, and the underlining of nursing as a profession.

In addition to the 'caring' role, nurses must also develop a helping relationship with patients and clients, in which nurses must be aware of their own needs, feelings and sentiments (understanding of self); there should be feelings of acceptance between the nurse and the patient; patients should not be judged but encouraged to participate in their care programme; and an environment should be established where patients can be motivated to change and to cope with their problems. The helping relationship is fully described by Rogers (1974).

Professionalism: A Discipline

The responsibilities of the nurse to the patient are largely embodied in the code of professional conduct. These responsibilities are primarily the concern of senior nurse managers in providing the necessary resources and ensuring a suitable environment in which the care of the patient can be effected, and of front-line nurses whose principal responsibility is in utilising these resources in the most efficient way to ensure the care of the patient. In effect, enabling a secure environment for effective care and helping the patient to attain a rapid and uneventful recovery.

The nurse's responsibilities include ensuring that patients are cared for satisfactorily by effecting the highest standard and quality of care, ensuring patients' treatment is carried out as prescribed; acknowledging their religious beliefs, values and social customs; ensuring confidentiality of all matters and records concerning the patient; ensuring their privacy and respecting their sensitivity particularly in relation to their diagnosis, treatment, fears, apprehensions and anxieties; ensuring their general safety; understanding and meeting their needs, basic and clinical, as well as helping them to realise their aspirations for independence and rehabilitation: in essence helping them to become self-actualised.

To acknowledge the individuality of the patient, the nurse must ensure that nursing care of each patient is individually planned; the care given is systematically recorded and subsequently reviewed to see how far the goals have been reached; and the individual nurse must accept accountability for her individual nursing action (RCN, 1981, para.5, pp. 9 and 10).

Even though nurses have the responsibility and the accountability for the care of the patients, in their 'caring' and 'service' roles (often blurred by the employment of many untrained and unqualified staff who operate at ward/community level), do they have the proper authority together with the necessary autonomy of role, to make decisions on the nursing care delivered to patients? Do they operate within a framework of professionalism? Does their authority to act — to make nursing decisions — and their autonomy, in this respect, match the level of their accountability and responsibility?

Professional Elements

One of the central attributes of professions is the existence of specialist knowledge, a knowledge that can be usefully applied only by the practitioner and which it is impossible even for the most intelligent to grasp and apply in full, i.e. it is beyond the 'lay' person. As well as the existence of an exclusive body of knowledge at a scientific level the profession must itself be responsible for the transmission and development of knowledge through training and research. Members of the profession subscribe to a prime ethic of service rather than self interest and the profession controls entry and exit (Rowbottom, *et al.*, 1973). Rowbottom goes on to say that only a professional can be in full managerial relationship to another professional, since the managerial relationship implies the ability to assess the total work of the subordinate.

The criteria that constitute a profession and the process of the development of a profession — professionalisation — have been much discussed and researched. Goode (1969) says that there is considerable agreement among writers on the criteria to prove the existence of a profession. He suggests two care hallmarks, i.e. a basic body of abstract knowledge and the ideal of service. Other agreed characteristics include:

> The existence of a body of knowledge at a scientific level; the knowledge is applicable — a technology exists; there is exclusive competence — the science and technology is accepted as beyond the 'lay' group; there must be planning and research; members subscribe to a prime ethic of service rather than self interest; and there are controls of entry and exit (Rowbottom, 1973).

In practice, professional discipline relates to the individual and their profession. Nurses need to act responsibly in accordance with the code of professional practice of their profession together with their own individual conscience. At the collective level, professional discipline, allows the use of sanctions on nurses who are found guilty of professional misconduct. Therefore in view of the use of potential sanctions by the statutory body, nurses must be allowed, to a substantial degree, to control nursing practice. In this respect, they must be given the necessary authority and autonomy to complement their responsibility and accountability in ensuring patients' needs are met and standards are maintained. These issues have been highlighted by both professional and statutory bodies (RCN, 1979; UKCC, 1984).

The issues of responsibility, accountability, authority and autonomy of the senior nurse were prompted initially by statements made in the Briggs (HMSO, 1972) and Merrison (HMSO, 1979) reports. The Briggs report said: 'The "consultancy" function of ward sisters should be encouraged and should extend beyond the boundaries of the hospital.' (para.541, p.164).

The *Code of Professional Conduct* (UKCC, 1983) makes clear, in the context of delivering patient care, that nurses must be responsible and accountable for their own actions (paras.2, 8). It follows logically, if nurses are to be held responsible and accountable for nursing practice, that they must also be given the necessary authority and autonomy if they are to act effectively in the management of care, i.e. meeting the patient's needs, defining attainable goals, specifying, planning and organising appropriate resources to meet these goals, and monitoring, evaluating and adjusting the care plan as and when required.

Concepts of Responsibility, Accountability, Authority and Autonomy

To understand and answer these questions, and their implications for nurses and their patients/clients, necessitates an examination of the concepts mentioned together with their interrelationship and relevance in the context of the requirements of statutory bodies, patient care, and the professionalism of nursing.

Responsibility

The *Code of Professional Conduct* (UKCC, 1983, 1984) says: 'In fulfilment of professional responsibility and in the exercise of professional accountability the nurse, midwife or health visitor shall accept a responsibility relevant to her professional experience for assisting her peers and subordinates to develop professional competence.' Commenting on the responsibility of the nursing student, UKCC Working Group 3 (January 1982) said: 'While never being in a position of professional accountability, nevertheless is required to assume increasing responsibility for the care of his/her patient/client.'

Responsibility is 'A charge for which one is answerable. The focus is on the charge, not on how or to whom the answering would or should occur.' (Batey and Lewis, 1982). On the basis of the new legislation (1979) nurses are responsible for the delivery of nursing care to patients as well as for ensuring and maintaining the standard and quality of the care delivered. Implicit in this is the promotion and safeguarding of the physical, mental and social wellbeing, and interests of patients. It also embraces responsibility for nurses' own professional development — continuing education and updating — in the quest for standards. It is envisaged that more responsibility will be devolved to nurses, particularly front-line nurses, through the agency of the extended role of the nurse (Briggs, 1972, Merrison, 1979), as well as being an integral part of the philosophy of NHS reorganisation (1982, 1983).

Accountability

Accountability is 'the particular and concentrated responsibility of the individual for performance in keeping with the expectation of his own particular role' (Rowbottom, 1973). In can also be viewed as, 'the fulfilment of a formal obligation to disclose to others the purposes, principles, procedures, relationships, results, income, and expenditures for which one has authority. This disclosure which is systematic and periodic occurs so that decisions and evaluations can be made' (Batey and Lewis, 1982).

Nurses are accountable for their practice and must improve their knowledge and skills to sustain and improve their professional competence.

Accountability is a requirement of the members of an organisation — being answerable for work and decisions. Senior nurses are answerable for their work and the decisions they take relating to their work.

Accountability should not be viewed in punitive or in organisational control terms — although this is how it is sometimes presented and interpreted. It should be presented and acknowledged in positive terms, as a prerequisite to sound management practice (UKCC, 1983).

The accountability of clinical nurses for nursing care 'depends upon the willingness of nurse managers to push the accountability downwards, as well as on the willingness of the nurse to accept the responsibility' (RCN, 1981).

Authority

If nurses are to have confidence in themselves and in their superiors their authority to act, to make decisions, must be acknowledged, supported and become a reality.

Authority to act — to make decisions about the work for which one is responsible and accountable — is also a prerequisite of sound management practice. Authority to act is delegated. It is related to responsiblity and accountability in so much that in the absence of 'real' authority and responsibility nurses cannot make decisions — they cannot act with conviction and confidence. In essence, authority is 'the legitimate power to fulfil responsibility' (Batey and Lewis, 1982). In practice it is related to such things as position in the organisation — status, proficiency, experience, expertise, knowledge, education and training.

According to Rowbottom *et al.*, (1973):

The specification of the freedom of movement open to the role performer in carrying out functions, the right of the performer to act at his own discretion; or the range of authority in the role, generally, tends to be given little emphasis.

The Code of Professional Conduct, even though rightly highlighting the obligations of nurses in carrying out their work, ironically does not acknowledge, in any explicit way, the legitimate authority of the senior nurse. In fact authority and its importance to the role occupant, in general term seems to rate little attention.

Autonomy

Autonomy of the role of the nurse has been much discussed in nursing circles in recent years as well as being afforded much attention in national reports (Briggs, 1972; Merrison, 1979) and in statements made by professional bodies (RCN, 1979). The issues of autonomy relating to role are many, but unclear; for example, some commentators want unqualified autonomy of role.

A central question underlying autonomy of role is: Can nurses make creditable decisions about the care of their patients, in isolation? However, does a nursing authority system which tends to discourage decision making at the nursing front-line — the ward and/or community — encourage the emergence of an autonomous role for senior nurses? In fact, is autonomy of role feasible in a clinical situation which necessitates, for effective care, a multi-professional team approach to patient care and which is based (however effectively) on consensus between professionals, i.e. nurses, doctors and paramedicals?

Autonomy can be described as, 'Freedom for the professional to practice their profession in accordance with his/her professional training' (Engel, 1970). Structural autonomy is: 'When professional people are expected, in the context of their work, to use their judgement in the provision of client services'. Attitudinal autonomy 'exists for people who believe themselves to be free to exercise judgement in decision making' (Hall, 1968).

The autonomy of the clinical nurse is an issue that has been discussed with passion since the advent of the Briggs Committee. An RCN document (1979) says: 'At the very least the clinical autonomy of the nurse must involve the ability to prescribe and effect nursing care and also the responsibility of controlling the provision of care to determine standards'.

Clinical autonomy is that which arises directly out of the nature of the nurse-patient relationship. Rowbottom *et al.* (1973) see clinical autonomy in terms of 'personalised treatment'.

Batey and Lewis (1982) suggest that the principal consequence of autonomy is accountability — 'the individual is answerable for the freedom inherent in autonomy'.

Controlling Practice — Ensuring Standards: What is its Reality? How is it Achieved?

Controlling nursing practice through the prescription of nursing care, making decisions about patient care, organising nursing leadership, having a realistic knowledge base and a lack of subordination to other professions, are all vital prerequisites of the professional. And, in this way:

Nurses should be able to develop their ability to provide the most skilled nursing care in the hospital and in the community service and their judgement to make independent decisions based on scientific, clinical, and management principles: that is to say, they should provide service at a professional level. (WHO, 1966)

A standard is 'the desired or achievable level of performance corresponding with a criterion, against which actual performance is compared' (Bloch, 1977).

Nursing standards are how well an individual nurse meets an individual patient's nursing needs. Such standards depend on nurses being responsible and accountable for meeting an individual patient's needs by setting explicit goals for them. The nurse has the responsibility of specifying, planning and also of evaluating the extent to which the goals — set by herself and the patient — have been met. (RCN, 1981, para.3, p.2)

The senior nurse — ward sister, staff nurse — has a central and vital role in ensuring the organisation of the ward/special unit, and, in this way ensuring an environment, organisational framework, within which standards and quality of care are ensured.

A prerequisite to ensuring standards and quality of care, to enable nurses to discharge their responsibility effectively and efficiently, is that of recognising the problems and demands of the job, and providing appropriate back-up in the form of clinical, educational, managerial and research support. The prerequisites for the professional control of standards are also described in a RCN (1981) document as including: a philosophy of nursing; relevant knowledge and skills; the nurse's authority to act; accountability; control of resources; organisational structure and management style; the doctor-nurse relationship, and, the management of change.

Nurses, because of their unique role and function in society, which albeit they engage in freely, must always ensure that service to the patient is never eroded. In saying this, it becomes essential that society, through its government, together with nurses' statutory and professional bodies, have the over-riding responsibility to ensure that they are properly and adequately supported and acknowledged in respect of their social and economic needs, status and salary, and, most important, provide them with the requisite authority to do the job for which currently their responsibility and accountability is excessive, unrealistic and disproportionate to their real authority and autonomy. As a result, the high standards of care which most nurses strive to attain and effect, result not in the improved care and wellbeing of their patients and clients; but very often, due to this fight against the odds of inadequate training, education, support, counselling and resources, result in a decline in care and increased stress for themselves (Hingley, 1984).

The professional conduct function of the UKCC and the National Boards is a vital one. Previously, this was described as the 'disciplinary function'. Dame Catherine Hall (1983) states:

> I believe that the professional conduct function should be seen in positive terms — as one of the means through which a regulatory body, acting on behalf of the profession, honours the contract between the profession and society, by ensuring that any member of the profession who has failed to meet the trust which society has placed in him or her is not permitted to continue to practice or, if the failure has not been a serious one, is reminded of the standards which professional practitioners are expected to meet.
>
> The underlying philosophy of the professional conduct function, as perceived by the new statutory bodies, is to protect the public, to promote high standards of professional practice and conduct on the part of nurses, midwives and health visitors, to ensure that justice is done, and is seen to be done, in respect of those brought within the function and that every encouragement is given to the individual practitioner to re-establish himself or herself, if it can be demonstrated that this is not contrary to the public interest. (Hall, 1983)

The *Code of Professional Conduct* was first published in 1983 and revised in 1984. The code, which is based on ethical concepts and is central to professional practice and its many demands, requires nurses, midwives and health visitors to comply with the law of any country, state, province or territory in which they work, as well as to be accountable for their practice, and, in this respect, have regard to the customs, values and spiritual beliefs of patients/clients. They must hold in confidence any information of patients/clients and avoid abuse of the nurse-patient/client relationship, by promoting and safeguarding their wellbeing and interests. In addition, nurses must accept responsibility for their peers and subordinates to develop their professional competence and acknowledge their workload and pressures and take appropriate action if these are seen to be such as to endanger safe standards of practice, and, make known to the appropriate authority any conscientious objection they hold which may be relevant to professional practice.

As the title of the code indicates, nurses are regarded as professionals and must provide a service at professional level. This is made clear by the UKCC (1984) in the following statement:

> Each registered nurse, midwife and health visitor shall act, at all times, in such a manner as to justify public trust and confidence, to uphold and enhance the good standing and reputation of the profession, to serve the interests of society, and above all to safeguard the interests of individual patients and clients.

Equally underlined is that 'each registered nurse, midwife and health visitor is accountable for his or her practice'.

It becomes clear from these statements, and on reading the Code, that nurses are charged with providing a service at professional level: they must provide a quality service. However, in view of the present uncertainty about the reality, in terms of the existence and use, of the key elements of nurses' role, e.g. authority and autonomy to make nursing decisions coupled with the disproportionate levels of responsibility and accountability, what does the provision of a quality service of care mean in practice? Is it possible for nurses to act with confidence in an environment which to a greater or lesser extent has become unclear and insecure, particularly at front-line level where there is 'concern because of the lack of the necessary authority in the ward sister's role to control the environment for patient care'? (DHSS, 1981). Can the ward sister or staff nurse be accountable, be answerable for work or decisions about work, if they lack the necessary authority and autonomy in their role to permit them to make valid decisions about patient care?

Accountability is seen (RCN Working Group, 1983) as 'the basis of professionalism'. For this accountability to be acceptable, the clinical nurse should, 'assume responsibility for assessing patients' nursing needs, planning care, making decisions and judgements and taking independent action'. The authors of the report say, 'she is thus professionally responsible and answerable for her practice' (para.2.1, p.5).

Many observers have also commented on criteria which they see to be central to nurses operating at a professional level. In this respect, for me Professor Baroness McFarlane, summarises the situation:

> the calibre of entrants to nurse training, the reform of nursing education to provide a knowledge base to enable nurses to assess nursing needs and prescribe nursing care together with a knowledge base to enable nurses to act on a colleague basis with doctors as medical

technology becomes sophisticated; and the equipping of nurses with different kinds of thought mechanisms i.e. a move from expository learning towards insight learning, thus enabling nurses to use a decision-making process, to use knowledge as a basis for judgements about care. These are the competencies of the self-actualising individual. (McFarlane, 1983).

The self-actualised person becomes 'more of what he is capable of becoming, making full use of unique talents and potential and realising more fully the higher needs of esteem, cognition and self-actualisation' (Kramer, 1974).

Kramer when discussing 'professional socialisation' of the nurse refers to an 'index of professionalism'. The index is basically intended to obtain a 'differential assessment of how professional nurses are in terms of a comparison to some sort of professional criteria'. The index consists of the sum of weighted scores, from 0 to a maximum of 5 on nine indicators which include: professional courses undertaken since qualifying, the number of professional journals subscribed to, the number of professional books bought since qualifying, the number of hours per week spent on professional reading, activity and membership in professional organisations, publications in professional literature, professional speeches given, offices held or leadership roles within professional organisations and the extent of professional activity within the employing organisation. These criteria relate closely to those expressed by senior nurses at a recent seminar (DHSS, 1981).

In the light of the comments and observations by independent observers together with those of professional and statutory bodies, on the essential criteria of the nurse professional, it seems clear that in nursing many of these criteria are absent. Therefore, how can the situation be corrected to enable nurses to control nursing practice?

Rendering a service at a 'professional level' entails the provision of the necessary back-up in the form of clinical, managerial and educational support. In addition, in order to assume full accountability for patients' and clients' care, nurses must be prepared educationally and skillwise (in decision-making, communication, leadership and counselling). The full acceptance of accountability by nurses at ward/community level and the effective discharge of the major implications relating to the legal, administrative and clinical aspects, which are explicit in that accountability to patients, clients, relatives, peers, together with statutory and professional bodies, will depend substantially on the quality of nursing management, i.e. the guidance, support, sensitivity and understanding given by nurse managers at middle and top levels, in acknowledging the demands placed upon their colleagues together with a clear understanding of their vulnerability, during the period of transition, from a role which is virtually devoid of authority and autonomy to one in which the nurse is empowered with the requisite authority and autonomy to make essential decisions on patient and client care.

Essentially, the process of the professional development of the nurse must start at the point of entry to the profession, by ensuring an acceptable educational standard of entry to enable subsequent educational development and training of the nurse to occur more readily. To enable the improved education of nurses, the knowledge and the skills provided, and the methods of teaching used must be appropriate to the activities and judgements required of nurses, i.e. to solve nursing problems and to prescribe and make judgements of integrity in relation to the practice of nursing. Also, attention must be focused on the most appropriate setting to enable this educational preparation of the nurse to take place. Opinion now seems to favour institutes of higher education (WHO, 1966; Maillart, 1973; UKCC, 1984). Also, a greater measure of research-mindedness should be fostered at basic and post-basic levels within nursing by including as part of the curriculum teaching related to research findings and reports and by 'encouraging and enabling nurses who show an interest in research procedures to engage in direct research into clinical nursing' (Briggs, para.373, p.109).

Some Paradoxes of Professionalism in the Context of Mayeroff's Components of Caring

There continues a conflict between the paradoxes and the orthodoxies in nursing: to date the paradoxes are in excess in nurses' quest for true professionalism. In the words of a great leader of nursing:

> The great paradox of nurses being professionals and nursing being a profession is that the nursing profession is ambivalent. On the one hand nurses look at supply and demand, and say all they can afford is a workforce of techncial aides. But then they take on the vocabulary of caring and ennuciate the moral values associated with it. (McFarlane, 1983)

In the context of the *Code of Professional Conduct* (UKCC, 1984), it is interesting to note that the nurse must 'take account' of the values and beliefs of patients and clients; but, in practice, how much regard will be paid and credibility given to patients'/clients' values, beliefs and rights? Also, how much credence is placed on the acknowledgement and relevance of interprofessional and intraprofessional relationships among health care professionals? In the absence of a true understanding of each other's role and functions, there can only be negative effects on the delivery of care. Regrettably, the Code (paras.5,6) gives little, if any, reassurance on these vital issues.

In the context of Mayeroff's (1971) philosophy on caring, these 'ommissions', their non-acknowledgement in the Code, must be deemed to be short-comings in so far as professionals can only operate successfully on the basis of sound interprofessional and intraprofessional relationships.

In Mayeroff's *Components of Caring*, the Code is somewhat tame on 'autonomy', 'humility' and 'honesty', which involves an acceptance of dependence on others and an awareness of personal limitations (paras.3, 4). Likewise on 'knowing' — one's powers and limitations which includes general and specific knowledge, knowing what patients'/clients' needs are and responding to them — the code is equally restrained, e.g. 'take every reasonable opportunity to' (para.3). However, the code is emphatic about such central issues as acknowledging limitations of competence. On 'trust', 'hope' and 'courage', the code is quite realistic, appropriate and informative (paras.5, 7, 10, 12).

On components such as: 'alternating rhythms', discovering if what was expected (goal) matches what was achieved (result) and maintaining and/or modifying behaviour (care plan) accordingly; 'patience', tolerance of a certain amount of confusion and floundering and participation with the patient; 'hope', an expression of a sense of the possible; and 'self-actualisation', by helping the patient to grow, the nurse grows in meeting patients'/clients' needs, these are dealt with fairly clearly under paras. 1, 10 and 12 of the Code.

In this way, through sound selection and subsequent development, guidance and support, the talents of nurses can be developed and utilised, optimally; their level of responsibility and degree of autonomy could be more appropriately met, thus accentuating and enabling their professionalisation and self-actualisation together with providing the patient with a more acceptable professional level of service.

References

Batey, M.V. and Lewis, F.M. (1982) Clarifying autonomy and accountability in nursing service. (Parts 1 and 2). *Journal of Nursing Administration, XII*(9), 13–18; (10) 10–15

Bloch, D. (1977) Criteria, standards, norms — crucial terms in quality assurance. *Journal of Nursing Administration, VII*(7), 20–30

Butcher, R. and Stelling, J. (1969) Characteristics of professional organizations. *Journal of Health and Human Behaviour*, no.10, pp. 3–15

Cohen, H.A. (1981) *The Nurse's Quest for Professional Identity*. Addison-Wesley

DHSS (1977) The Extending Role of the Clinical Nurse — Legal Implications and Training Requirements (HC(77)22). DHSS, London

——— (1981) Seminar: Professional Development in Clinical Nursing — the 1980s

Engel, G.V. (1970) Professional autonomy and bureaucratic organisation. *Administrative Science Quarterly, 15* 12–21

Goode, E. (1969) The theoretical limits of professionalism: in Etzioni (ed.) *The Semiprofessions and Their Organisation*, Free Press, New York

Goodlad, S. (ed.) (1984) *Education for the Professions*. SRHE & NFER-Nelson, University of Guildford, Surrey

Hall, Dame Catherine (1983) Professional Regulation for a Newly Integrated Profession (Conference Paper). King's Fund Centre, London

Hall, R.A. (1968) Professionalization and bureaucratization *American Social Review, 33,* 92–104

Hingley, P. (1984) Stress: A report of King Edward Hospitals Fund. *Nursing Standard*, no.352, p.3

HMSO (1972) Report of the Committee on Nursing (Briggs). Cmnd. no.5115. HMSO, London

Kramer, M (1974) *Reality Shock*. C.V. Mosby, St Louis

McFarlane, Baroness (1984) Still a long way to go before image meets reality. 'Images and Reality', 5th Royal Marsden Hospital Nursing Lecture. *Nursing Mirror, 159,* (10), 6

Maillart, V. (1973) Higher education in nursing. *WHO Chronicle, 27,* 242

Mayeroff, M. (1971) *On Caring*. Harper and Row, New York

Nurses, Midwives and Health Visitors Act 1979, Eliz. II (Chapter 36). HMSO, London

Nurses, Midwives and Health Visitors Rules Approval Order, Eliz. II (1983) HMSO, London

O'Connor, J.G. and Meadows, A. (1976) Specialization and professionalization in British Geology. *Social Studies of Science, 6,* 77–89

RCN (1943) Nursing Reconstruction Committee (Horder). RCN

——— (1964) A Reform of Nursing Education (Platt). RCN

——— (1979) Implementing the Nursing Process. RCN

——— (1981) Towards Standards (Discussion Document). RCN

——— (1983) Towards a New Professional Structure for Nursing, RCN

Rogers, C.R. (1974) *On Becoming a Person*. Constable, London

Rowbottom, R. *et al.* (1973) *Hospital Organisation*. Heinemann, London

United Kingdom Central Council for Nursing, Midwifery and Health Visiting (1982) Education and Training (Working Group 3). UKCC, London

——— (1983) Code of Professional Conduct for Nurses, Midwives and Health Visitors. UKCC, London

——— (1984) Code of Professional Conduct for Nurses, Midwives and Health Visitors, 2nd edn. UKCC, London

WHO (1966) WHO Expert Committee on Nursing (Fifth Report). WHO

Wieland, G. (ed.) (1981) *Improving Health Care Management: Organization Development and Organization Change*. Health Administration Press, Ann Arbor, Michigan

Advised Further Reading

Alonso, R.C. (1971) A study of commitment orientations among professional personnel: nurses commitment to the profession, clinical speciality and employing organization. *Dissertation Abstracts International, 31,* March

Bosanquet, N. (1981) The price of professionalism. *Nursing Times, 77*(4), 1325

Bowman, M.P. (1980) The Education and Training Needs of First-Line Nurses. Unpublished MEd thesis. University of Newcastle upon Tyne

Cang, S. *et al.* (1981) An emerging model for ward sister roles in general hospitals. Health Services Organisation Research Unit, Brunel University

Chapman, C.M. (1977) *Sociology for Nurses*, Bailliere Tindall, London

Cohen, H.A. (1982) Higher education in nursing. *WHO Chronicle, 27,* 242

Craska, N.L. (ed.) (1978) *The Nursing Profession: Views Through the Mist.* McGraw-Hill, New York

Dent, H.E. (1983) Consequences of professionalism. *Nursing Times, 79*(41), 6

DeYoung, L. (1976) *The Foundations of Nursing,* 3rd edn. C.V. Mosby, St Louis

General Nursing Council for England and Wales (1979) Statement on Alleged Professional Misconduct and Industrial Action. GNC

Hancock, C. (1983) The need for support. *Nursing Times, 79*(38), 43–5

Hopping, B (1976) Professionalism and unionism: conflicting ideologies. *Nursing Forum, XV*(4), 372–83

Jones, E. (1983) What makes a professional. *Nursing Mirror, 156*(11), 24–5

McCloskey, J.C. (1981) The professionalization of nursing: United States and England. *International Nursing Review, 28*(2), 40–47

Martin, A. (1982) 'Easy does it'. *Nursing Mirror, 152*(18), 30

Peplau, H. (1977) The changing view of nursing. *International Nursing Review, 24*(2), 43–5

Pyne, H.R. (1982) Professional discipline in nursing. *Medical Education International Ltd,* no.36, pp.1540–1

Radical Nurses Group (1981) What is professionalism? *Nursing Times, 77*(17), 714

Revans, R.W. (1964) *Standards for Morale: Cause and Effects in Hospital.* Oxford University Press

Robinson, J. (1983) The game of professionalism. *Nursing Times, 156*(17), 9

Rowbottom, R. *et al.* (1973) *Hospital Organization.* Heinemann, London. Chapter 5

Stanley, I. (1983) Where do we stand with doctors? *Nursing Times, 79*(38), 46–8

7 STANDARDS AND QUALITY OF CARE IN NURSING

Aims:

The aims of this chapter are:

1. To examine the concepts of 'standards' and 'quality' in care.
2. To relate the concepts of 'standard' and 'quality' to the care of patients and clients.

Learning Objectives

The purpose of this chapter is to enable the reader to:

1. Understand the concepts of 'standard' and 'quality', in the context of patient care.
2. Appreciate ways in which standards and quality of care can be achieved.

A widening range of professionals, especially since the reorganisation of the National Health Service (1974), together with the many technicians and technologists, are concerned with the patient — directly or indirectly — in affecting his treatment and care. These professionals together with the services offered, if they are to be effective, need to be co-ordinated and focused on the patients to ensure their effect is optimised in securing their management and care. In this respect, the senior nurses play a vital role, because of their unique postition in being close to the patient round-the-clock, in co-ordinating these activities as well as effecting communication with and ensuring participation by patients and their immediate families, in assessing and establishing their problems and in effecting their care. Despite good intentions and sound practice, optimal care together with a quality service, may not always be possible — or achievable.

Background

The history of declining standards of care is dated. Concern about standards was mentioned as far back as the early 1940s (Horder Report, RCN, 1943). The Horder Committee considered how best to model nursing education so as to ensure the preservation of the highest standards of care. Yet, in 1985 there continues to be grave concern among nurses, together with nursing statutory and professional bodies, about declining standards.

Since the Second World War attempts have been made regularly by governments of differing political complexion together with statutory and professional bodies to identify the root causes of declining standards, and to find ways to establish as well as maintain standards and quality of care. For example, reports such as Platt (RCN, 1964), Salmon (1966), Mayston (DHSS, 1969), Halsbury (DHSS, 1974), Briggs (DHSS, 1972), the *Grey Book* (DHSS, 1972) and Merrison (HMSO, 1979), to mention but a few, have examined issues such as the education, training and development of staff together with the management and organisation of the NHS. Even though these reports give sound guidelines and include useful ideas on how to ensure the continuing viability and integrity of the Health Service — and nursing — too often their expressed structure and philosophy was either misunderstood, misinterpreted, ignored or was found to be wholly unsuitable, e.g. the structure and management arrangements proposed in the Salmon Report and the *Grey Book*, were, retrospectively found to be unsuitable; this particularly applies to the structure proposed by the latter.

Evidence

There is much evidence expressing concern about declining standards of nursing care; the areas of risk in hospitals and in the community are largely due to the increased workloads (Merrison Report, paras.13.5, 13.6, p.185). (This aspect will be discussed more fully in Chapter 8.) Among the impediments highlighted by the Merrison Commission were the Salmon and Mayston Committees' recommendations and their alleged tendency to withdraw good clinical nurses into administration. The particular reasons included 'untrained staff in charge of wards, neglect of basic nursing routines, inadequate supervision of learners, employment of agency staff, increased workloads and abandonment of patient care programmes' (para.13.5, p.185). Even though not defining 'standards' this report clearly identified 'causes' for declining standards. Also, the fact that student and pupil nurses form some 25 per cent of the total nursing staff employed in the hospital service, which not surprisingly produces conflict between patient and educational needs, and that the number of qualified teachers has been slow to expand: a high wastage rate has kept the ratio of qualified teachers to learners constant at about 1 to 25 since 1972 (paras. 13.5, 13.6, 13.47, 13.54). In this context, Maillart (1973) makes the point that nurses, like other professionals, need a secure base from which to operate successfully, for their personal satisfaction and security and the ultimate good of the patients/clients. According to Maillart: 'The dependence of hospitals on student nurses to provide 60–80 per cent of the nursing services shows how illusory the educational experience is.' This view continues to be upheld in so far as recently it was stated that, should the enrolled nurse training cease (a final decision on the future of the enrolled nurse has yet to be taken by the UKCC), an estimated increase of 60 per cent of untrained/unqualified staff would be required to ensure adequate clinical manpower (*Nursing Standard*, 1980).

Fundamental Problems

Currently, there is much debate about a shortage of nurses. Also there is a high level of stress associated with the practice of nursing; stress which in part may be associated with nurses' endeavour to maintain standards of care against mounting odds (Hingley, 1984).

For a variety of reasons, i.e. improved knowledge of patients and clients of their rights, press publicity of unacceptable practice by the health care professions, the sustained and on-going debate by statutory and professional bodies and the evidence highlighted in many reports, the subject of declining standards of care is a matter of concern — and priority of solution, in the 1980s.

Some fundamental problems in the context of inadequate standards of care highlighted by the Briggs Committee included: the ambivalent position of the nurse in training as both learner and worker; and the dual role of the hospital — provider of nursing care for patients and provider of education for nurses — also, rates of pay, basic conditions of service and a generally applicable career structure are determined nationally within the NHS, yet recruitment, contracts of service and detailed conditions of employment and deployment are determined locally. Therefore, the efficiency of the nursing workforce depends on the interrelationship between national, regional and local policies. Also, when establishing policies which will ensure that nursing resources meet the needs of a changing workload and workforces, the impediments are many, and sometimes can be great. In essence, there are no generally applicable scientific criteria which can be readily adopted by senior nurse managers in determining establishments and, as a result, 'they have to bargain, often crudely, for a reasonable share of the budget and to spend their allocation in accordance with subjective judgements related to the circumstances and availability of staff and other resouces'. (Briggs report, para.445, p.130).

Also, the advent of the *Trade Union and Labour Relations Act* (1974/76) provided an upsurge of industrial relations activity in the NHS and in nursing which has expanded the statutory rights of employees: coupled with this is the increased interest of nurses in trades union activity which has made demands on nurses' time and which correspondingly reduces the time spent in nursing patients (RCN, 1978).

The main areas of concern (which were originally expressed by the RCN to the Merrison Commission) in hospitals are untrained staff left in charge of wards and the inadequate supervision of learners, the neglect of basic nursing routines and employment of agency staff. And in the community: increased workloads which according to the evidence (Merrison report, 1979) cause severe pressure on nursing staff with the consequent curtailment of time allocated to patients and learners and, most important, the abandonment of patient care programmes because of the need to cope with emergency cases and high dependency patients (paras.75–80, pp.33–34).

The principal causes underlying this concern are extensively examined in an RCN document (1978) and in *Nurse Alert* (RCN, 1984). They include manpower, finance, technological change, and changes in conditions of service.

Manpower. The nursing service for its integrity and continuing viability requires properly trained and educated nurses whose job must always be the proper care of its patients. To secure this objective the correct recruitment, selection, induction, education, training, development and deployment of nurses is a priority. In addition, the role, authority, accountability, job-satisfaction and career progresion (for those who desire it) are vital prerequisites to ensuring staff morale, organisational integrity and sound patient care. It becomes obvious that if the bulk of care which patients receive is carried out by untrained, unqualified and relatively unsupervised nurses, as too frequently happens at present, the lot of patients is going to be unhappy and unproductive and will lead to a decline in the quality of care provided in their day-to-day care and rehabilitation.

Finance. Cash limits on public expenditure, of which the health service is no exception, have side-effects on manpower and the provision of resources and subsequently affect standards of care. In this respect, the continuing imposition by government of financial cuts has resulted in no growth in real terms as well as posing a serious threat to the maintenance of standards and quality of care.

Technological Change and Education. The need to up-date nurses in new skills and knowledge — and the way this is effected, usually off-the-job — clearly places further pressure on resources with the effect of depleting the wards of staff.

The basic education of the nurse continues to be fragmented (no continuous plan of training to meet basic and post-basic students' needs, because of inadequate numbers of nurse teachers). Various estimates of the shortage of teachers prevail, with a deficit of some 3000 teachers being common (GNC Department of Statistics, 1980). Also there is inadequate supervision of nursing students in the clinical situation, arising directly from the absence of a realistic number of nurse teachers; the advised and actual ratios of teachers to learners being: advised ratio 1:15; actual ratios 1:22 (GNC Annual Report, 1980/81). The inadequacy of nurses' supervision on the wards affects the reinforcement, through application of learners' skills and knowledge.

Changes in Conditions of Service. A variety of situations such as the shorter working week, additional statutory leave entitlement of nurses together with the effects of the *Employment Protection Act,* e.g. maternity leave provisions, and *Trade Union and Labour Relations Act* 1974, e.g. the hours that staff are away from their work when engaged in trade union activity or when undertaking the necessary training, affect and aggravate an already difficult manpower situation. The situation is compounded by nurses' concern relating to such central issues as inadequacy and/or inappropriateness of their education, training and development at basic and post-basic level, and their status, their 'subordination' by the medical and, indeed, paramedical professions. In addition, the lack of appropriate awards in the form of scholarship, career prospects and remuneration does little to maintain nurses' morale and improve their job-satisfaction.

Achieving optimum standards of nursing care together with ensuring quality of performance must be the central goal of every nurse practitioner and the priority of every nurse educationist and nurse manager.

Even though aspirations of quality care are not novel, securing effective and acceptable standards of care for the majority of patients and ensuring a quality service in this era of advanced medical technology is as yet an unachieved goal. The nursing approach, despite marked improvement — a more individual problem-solving approach — to these elusive ideals continues to remain subjective in assessing and evaluating patient care. There continue many impediments (RCN, 1978, 1984). Basically, nursing objectives are vague, unrealistic and unreliable: they are not based on assessment and evaluation of care in relation to defined criteria and standards. The results for the nurse practitioner, the nurse manager and, most importantly, the patient, remain disquieting and disabling.

A WHO Report (1966) stated that public pressure for the expansion of nursing care was creating a demand that could be met only by reorientation of nursing services. And that nurses were becoming increasingly aware that providing quality of service was a major problem. The report underlined that quality in nursing was exemplified by the nurse helping the patient to maintain or create a health regime that, if he were fit and well, he could carry out unaided.

When addressing a conference of Senior Nurse Managers, Dame Catherine Hall emphasised: 'It is in the interest of the professional practitioner to be "called to order" by her fellow professionals if she has somehow failed to maintain acceptable standards of professional competence or conduct'. (*Nursing Mirror*, May 1983). In the context of professional practice the General Nursing Council for England and Wales (Annual Report, 1981) highlighted prevalent nursing problems in the form of very serious allegations against nurses of abuse of drugs, unprofessional nursing practice and patient abuse which had caused the caseload of the Council's Investigating and Disciplinary Committees to increase.

The fact that cuts are reducing standards of care has frequently been highlighted, particularly in the areas of nursing the elderly, the physically handicapped, the mentally ill and the mentally handicapped. Also the now too often occurring closure of wards due to inadequate numbers of staff together with growing lists of patients awaiting 'non-emergency' care, are matters of deep professional and public concern. In this respect, a recent RCN report (1984) highlights the adverse regime that has been imposed on the service in the course of the past 18 months with the 'stop-go directives', e.g. July 1982, districts were asked to make efficiency savings of 0.5 per cent for the current financial year and for 1983/83: January 1983, regional allocations for 1983/84 showed a 1.2 per cent increase; June 1983, health authorities were asked to assume a growth rate of 0.5 per cent over the next 10 years; July 1983, revised cash units for 1983/84 were announced superseding those announced in Januray and reducing the figure of 1.2 per cent to 0.21 per cent.

In the wake of this stop-go policy, the RCN survey showed that 'uncertainty and anxiety was suffered by patients owing to shortage of beds and the resultant cancellation of admissions. Patients and relatives were often in an atmosphere of apprehension.'

Multiple Factors Interact in the Provision of Care

In this complex environment in which the care of patients takes place, many factors other than the provision of an appropriate organisational structure influence the circumstances under which nurses maintain standards and ensure better practice. For example, senior nurse managers must critically review the way nurses work, looking particularly at the nature of their deployment and supervision. Regular analysis of the tasks carried out by nurses must be undertaken so that the management structure which is employed relates to current needs and reflects new developments.

At a Nursing Process Workshop (October 1983) considerable emphasis was placed on important and crucial issues to improve the care of patients, e.g. the continuing use of research to monitor and improve care; the need to improve clinical practice with co-ordinated educational change; the use of nurse managers at middle-line to initiate and facilitate change; and, most important, the need to produce and to provide evidence to demonstrate improvement in patient care, through the agency of current practice, instruments and procedures.

In view of the well-documented shortcomings in assessing, evaluating and in delivering care to patients, is there any answer to this dilemma? What, if anything, can be done to improve the lot of the patient/client, in providing effective and efficient care? In essence providing a quality service.

The report *Nurse Alert* emphasises the rising standard of expectation for care in the context of 'patients being more literate, informed and expecting explanations and proper communication and, in this respect they expect to be able to understand their treatment'. 'Significantly', the report states, 'nurses complained about not having enough time to talk to patients'. Yet, the relevance of nurses' communication with patients has been highlighted by notable nurses and many researchers, over the years.

The Merrison report stated that the role of health workers is subject to 'many kinds of change', notably those brought about by developments in techniques in health care. Evidence (from Regional Medical Officers) supplied to the Royal Commission also stated that the character of health care is constantly changing, sometimes rapidly and extensively: 'This gives rise to a continuous process in which tasks and functions are redistributed between professionals' (para.12.26).

These issues make realising standards and quality of care all the more important and the more difficult.

So what is involved in establishing standards, to ensure quality of care?

Criteria, Standards and Quality

Defining and measuring the quality of nursing care, to date, has remained an elusive ideal, despite much effort and research, particularly carried out in Great Britain, Canada, Germany and the USA.

Nurses' concern about ensuring standards and quality of care has always been a priority. In my experience, nurses, in the main, strive unrelenting to ensure the comfort and well-being of the patients. However, the ever-present desire to maintain standards of care has acquired noticeable momentum during the past two decades: an aspiration that has been underlined by nurses, in the nursing press, and by professional and statutory bodies. This additional drive to set, achieve and maintain standards has been precipitated by such events and factors as increased and more complex medical technology which further taxes nursing resources and nursing expertise and inevitably tends to promote a more mechanised approach to patients and their care with the tendency to reduce the all-important human contact (dehumanising care) so necessary in ensuring patient/client care. Also, the emphasis on quality of care is rooted in the explosion of nursing knowledge, as distinct from medical knowledge, producing the accelerated professionalisation of nurses by improved education, training and development of nurses stimulated and progressed through a deliberate approach to solve the profession's problems, giving improved enlightenment to patient care, through research and evaluation.

A Framework for Nursing: Traditional and Current Perspectives

Nursing as practised over the years has undergone changes in its emphasis and practice. The approaches that have been prominent during the past sixty years include that of the 'medical' approach which essentially was based on 'cure' rather than care with the total approach to the patient being fragmented and isolated, through the intervention and existence of many independent professionals. As always, nurses provided a round-the-clock service and attempted to draw the professional strands together in an attempt to ensure satisfactory and continuous care.

Regrettably, at this time the emphasis was more on the 'task' and 'cure' rather than on the 'patient' and 'care'.

Improved education of nurses together with greater emphasis in the syllabus on the behavioural and social sciences (even though still inadequate this has been accentuated in the recent ENB syllabus, 1985) produced further searching among nurses and other health care professionals, in their quest for improved practice. Also, relevant to this change was the reorganisation — integration — of the NHS in an attempt to obviate barriers between different groups and professionals responsible for care, i.e. the hospital, local authorities and general practitioners. The emphasis was on a 'team' approach to care — clinically and managerially. Underlying this approach was the philosophy of making care more accessible, manageable — and, most important, more human — in meeting patient/client needs. The team approach to care both within the hospital and in the NHS as a whole continued to prove unsuccessful as evidenced by further adjustment of the organisation and professions responsible for care. Also the dilution of nursing by the increased dependency on untrained and unqualified personnel to maintain a service for patients/clients proved a major handicap to team nursing.

The most recent thinking and practice in the care of patients and clients is based on a 'holistic', individual approach to care: in essence, a systematic, problem-solving approach. The intention is to effect nursing care through meeting individual patients'/clients' needs. Its essence is to humanise care by dehospitalising patients — enabling their independence and securing their self-actualisation by utilising their abilities. This approach in addition to involving the patient must also involve the family — certainly the patient's close relatives, if practicable.

Inevitably, to be effective, this approach, places great emphasis on the number (individualised based) and quality of nurses, and the competencies, in terms of clear accountability, for ensuring a 24-hour service together with their authority and autonomy to make nursing decisions. In this context, Hegyvary (1982), when discussing primary nursing, patient-centred practice, states four characteristics which include accountability, 24-hour responsibility for delivered care; autonomy, the authority to make decisions relating to nursing care; co-ordination, providing a link between health care professionals; and comprehensiveness, ensuring care throughout 'a specific time period'.

Any attempt at measuring the quality of care must, as a prerequisite, establish criteria and standards. One point is obvious: the end product of health care must be judged on whether the patient is better as a result of the treatment/care which is given.

In the context of the nursing process, criteria are specific, i.e. they relate to the individual patient and the particular problem/s presented: in essence, the criteria are fashioned to meet individual patients needs.

The setting and achieving of standards must combine the efforts of clinical nurses, nurse managers and nurse educators. Nurses cannot work in isolation, but must operate within a framework of mutidisciplinary understanding and support. A WHO report (1966) gives similar emphasis to multidisciplinary support when discussing 'quality in nursing': 'The services of the wide range of professionals are helpful only to the extent that they are co-ordinated'. And, 'all health workers, but particularly physicians and nurses should observe and listen to the patient and communicate with each other in assessing his health problems'. Even though standards for nursing practice are usually linked to the professionalism of the nurse, 'they can also be used to monitor professional performance for quality, in order to be licensed and maintain accreditation, as in the USA as well as being used in those countries without an accreditation system to serve as guidelines in policy, planning and education.' (van Maanem, 1984).

Nursing standards in the UK are generally linked with the accreditation of nursing as a profession, in the context of the education, training development and practice of nurses. For example, the *Code of Professional Conduct for Nurses* (1984) underlines; 'each registered nurse, midwife and health visitor shall safeguard the interests of individual patients and clients'. In this respect ways to enhance 'the professional work and life of recently registered nurses, with regard to the individual responsibility for the effective practice of nursing' was the subject of a DHSS seminar (1981) which concluded that such factors as professional development, accreditation, participation in research, publications, peer group reviews and teaching expertise, are prerequisites to sound practice.

Prerequisites to evaluating quality of care include establishing criteria and standards. These are 'points of reference' (van Maanen, 1984).

Block (1977) emphasises the importance of ensuring that basic terminology is clear and accurate, before attempting to evaluate health care. She suggests that quality assurance methods must stem from 'precise, universally acceptable definitions'. In her paper she discusses 'criteria' and 'standards'. The concept of 'criterion' is expressed as, 'the value-free name of a variable believed or known to be a relevant indicator of the quality of patient care'.

A 'standard' is defined as, 'the desired and achievable level of performance corresponding with a criterion, against which actual performance is compared. It carries the connotation that there is one score or one value on a variable that must be obtained if the quality of care is to be judged to be satisfactory.'

The relationship of criteria and standards is illustrated with examples which relate to the clinical setting. For example, using the criterion of 'pain', the 'standard' would be 'patient has little or no pain'; using the criterion 'condition of wound', the standard would be 'absence of infection'. And using the criterion of 'temperature', the standard would be 37°C.

In a comprehensive analysis of medical care (McLachlan, 1976) it is stated: 'The term quality of care is being increasingly used often by doctors and their potential patients. The meaning given to it is not always the same and when it is accompanied with proposals for assessment, sometimes evokes emotional responses.'

The quality of care is an important component of nursing output. However, as yet, there is no consensus among nurses for measuring output. But pressure from peers, clients, together with statutory and professional bodies, to know how well patient care is being delivered, ensures that the issue of quality of care is constantly highlighted.

The subject of standards of care together with the difficulty of measuring standards and quality was highlighted in the Merrison report (1979) where the impreciseness of health together with the lack of a clear and commonly accepted definition of health, creates problems for attempts to assess efficiency of a health service by measuring the health of a population or by making historical or international comparisons (paras 3.14, 3.15 and 3.18, pp.20 and 22).

Nursing standards are how well an individual nurse meets an individual patient's nursing needs. Also, to set and achieve standards, clinical nurses rely on others, particularly nurse managers for resources such as manpower and money, and nurse educators for professional knowledge and expertise (RCN, 1981).

The report also uses such phrases as: 'nurses develop their own standards of care'; 'the profession must agree on acceptable levels of excellence'; 'agreed standards of care provide a baseline for measurement'; and 'standards of care influence nursing practice and nursing education'.

More recently an RCN report (1983) links 'high levels of clinical expertise' and 'the authority of the ward sister to manage the clinical environment' with the improvement and maintenance of standards of nursing care (paras. 2.3 and 2.5, pp.5 and 6).

The *Code of Professional Conduct for Nurses* (UKCC, 1984) refers to 'safe standards of practice' underlining the registered nurses' professional accountability (paras. 10 and 11).

What, in practice, does 'a reasonable standard of care' mean to a nurse and to a patient? How do nurse practitioners and nurse managers know when the care of their patients is satisfactory? Is optimum? Is the assessment of the standard and quality of care largely subjective — based upon little more than personal intuition and experience? More important, can the standard and the quality of care which a patient receives be assessed? Is there a measure, an index, to inform nurses of the fabric — standard and quality — of care given?

One of the main difficulties in establishing an index for standards and quality of nursing care, is the absence of a definition of nursing with sufficient specificity. This point is highlighted in a WHO report (1966):

> There is no accepted definition of good nursing practice. In a broad sense, 'quality of nursing care' is concerned with helping the patient with his daily pattern of living or with those activities that he normally performs without assistance. The most important condition conducive to achievements of quality is contact with nurses whose work exemplifies good patient care.

A Working Committee of the Royal College of Nursing (1979) identified 'good nursing care' in terms of 'nursing behaviour'. They concluded that purposeful nursing behaviour includes: 'The selection and prescription of nursing actions to meet the patient's needs; the carrying out of specific nursing work; a systematic review to see if the nursing actions have met the patient's needs. "Good" nursing care was agreed by the committee as planned, systematic and focused care which implies a continuous and dynamic pattern of assessment, planning, action and review.' What do nurses do, how do they perform it and what effect does this have on the patient?

Quality of Care

Quality is a degree of excellence. Ensuring quality service and quality care embodies many elements. In the context of nursing care 'quality' relates to the integrity, sensitivity and humanity of nursing activities and interventions, which include nurses' approach to patients: is it done with interest, enthusiasm and enlightenment? Or is it apathetic? Is there true interaction with the patient? Are relevant aspects of care and hospital procedure explained in a clear precise way in relation to their plan of care and treatment, with due regard to the patient's fears, worries and anxieties? Or is communication only at minimum level — vague and incomplete? Is there time to talk to and discuss matters with patients and their relatives — unhurriedly? Are patients' needs being acknowledged?

Met? In fact are nurses fully aware of how best to meet the patient's needs — especially their social/emotional needs? Is the patient cared for physically? Are patients and their relatives given emotional support? Are they comforted? What is done by nurses and other health care professionals to demistify, simplify and clarify, the hospital routine and ritual for the patient? Is the patient's self-actualisation — independence — enabled? In essence, what is done to dehospitalise the patient? Are nurses encouraged to be creative in relation to patient care plans? Are new approaches to care fostered? Are nurses sufficiently involved in the preparation and evaluation of care? And how up-to-date are nurses in their knowledge and skills? What means are available to them to get up-to-date with technology and practice that affect patient care? Lectures? Seminars? Conferences? On-the-job development? Action-learning? Reading?

The resulting quality and/or improvement of care is dependent on how well or badly nurses expedite these processes. This quality, is formalised in the 'nursing competencies' and by the *Code of Professional Conduct*.

How can Standards be Achieved? Maintained? Approaches

To maintain and improve standards and quality of care, many factors need to be taken into account. For example, basic education and training needs, to take cognisance of the demands and sophistication of the service within which nurses will practice on completing their training. In addition, fewer demands for ensuring a service must be placed on nursing students: the philosophy of the new education structure, which hopefully can be realistically implemented, has in the main got it right, i.e. phased responsibility for the nursing student with no clinical accountability. The latter, even though highly desirable, is difficult to envisage in the context of the present situation in hospitals where there continues to be substantial reliance on either untrained and/or unqualified staff to provide essential care for patients. To implement the new structure would obviously require more experienced, qualified nurses to ensure the supervision, training and support of nursing students. Also there must be rationalisation of post-basic education to ensure it is aligned with the needs of patients (nursing competencies require constant updating), staff, and the particular demands of the job. In this context a DHSS Seminar (1981) linked the complex issues of enhanced career prospects, status, and financial reward with potential improvement in standards of nursing. The *Code of Professional Conduct for Nurses, Midwives and Health Visitors* which links workload with professional competence and standards, underlines the need for nurses to have regard to the workload as well as the pressures which their colleagues are experiencing and to take appropriate action if these are seen to endanger them and/or their practice (para.9). In addition, it emphasises that nurses must be accountable for their practice and, in this way, take every reasonable opportunity to update and improve their professional knowledge to ensure competence of practice as well as to accept responsibility for assisting their peers and subordinates to develop professional competence. Also, they must have regard to the environment in which care is delivered together with the available resources for ensuring care, and make known to senior nurse management if these endanger safe standards of practice (paras.2, 7 and 8).

The issues which are involved in measuring and controlling quality were much debated by the Merrison Commission (Chapters 12 and 13). The report underlined, 'that when attempting to measure quality of care, the first thing is to establish standards' (para.12.45, p.173). However, this is by no means easy, for many reasons — primarily 'health' is not a precise concept (Merrison report, 1979). One approach to measuring the quality of care is to assess the outcome of a particular treatment or care on the patient or client. Are the patients/clients better as a result of their treatment and/or care? However, this also has problems, central to which is the impreciseness of health. In addition, uncertainties about whether and how the patients/clients have improved together with the reason for that improvement, as well as whether they have been well cared for, is difficult to establish.

Currently, when attempting to establish quality and standards of care three approaches, all of which are linked, can be used.

First, data about 'input': i.e. the resources used which include staff — trained or untrained, qualified or unqualified — together with their qualifications and the institutions in which care is delivered, particularly their equipment and its ready accessibility, can be assessed.

Secondly, it is necessary to establish data about 'process': what is done to the patient/client which includes such vital factors as diagnosis, care and after-care.

Thirdly, the 'outcome': the effects of treatment and care, or the lack of these and their effects can be scrutinised.

These three processes are linked in so far as a successful outcome depends substantially on sufficient and correct input of resources together with their transformation and effects on patients/clients through the use of the appropriate medical and nursing processes.

A technique which has been used to assist the evaluation of quality of care, is that of ensuring the outcome of treatment, i.e. the randomised controlled trial (RCT) which is a method of obtaining a bias-free result in comparing the treatments or a treatment with no treatment. There are obvious practical problems associated with this approach, e.g. if a doctor taking part in an RCT believes that his patient would benefit from the treatment under examination, he must either withdraw the patient from the RCT or suppress his own views. However, despite certain shortcomings about RCTs, the Merrison Commission says: 'There is little doubt that their more widespread use could eliminate procedures whose benefits are accepted because they have never been systematically challenged.' And, 'it would be a major advance if health departments would as a matter of routine promote the testing of new and expensive services before their introduction' (paras.12.48 and 12.49, p.174).

As well as these approaches and techniques for evaluating outcome, a most important though basic consideration is the use of reliable, legible and complete patient/client records to facilitate the study of treatment and quality of care.

To ensure quality of care, as well as concentrating on techniques for evaluating output, methods must also be adopted with the aim of improving the performance of individual health care professionals. As most NHS professions are hierarchically organised, the junior staff will normally look to their superiors for guidance, support, praise and correction. However, medical consultants and general practitioners have autonomy. There is no one to tell them not to prescribe a particular drug or to undertake a particular procedure. Also, in practice there are limits to which senior nurses can supervise their subordinates. In addition, currently nurses are seeking autonomy for nursing decisions. In practice this independence is prized by the health care professions. However treasured or well founded, independence may pose problems in ensuring a quality service. For example, professionals exercising their own judgement may not be aware of how their performance compares with that of their colleagues. Most important, health care professionals must be aware of their interdependence when attempting to provide a quality service. To obviate some of these problems some form of checking is required. This can be done by the use of 'professional audit', medical and/or nursing together with research into clinical, medical and nursing methods and staff appraisal schemes. The audit can be particularly useful in ensuring quality, particularly the more informal 'peer review' which has the advantage that it is not imposed by an external body and 'obviates any difficulty about applying national standards which may be ill-defined' (Merrison Report, para.12.52, p.175), by enabling clinical decisions to be checked, errors to be identified and, through discussion and change (if indicated) effect improvements in performance and quality. In this way, the assessment of quality of care must take cognisance of 'specific measures, accountability or control mechanisms based on the measures and performance ratings of the nurse' (Jelinek and Dennis, 1976).

In attempting to establish quality of care, there is 'significant social and geographical inequity in the services offered to patients and clients' (Merrison Report, para.3.12, p.19). In addition, because health is an imprecise concept, in practice the state of health of individuals varies from the 'ideal' through different degrees of nurses; also, currently there is difficulty in defining how many and what type of workers are needed in the NHS. To compound the problem roles of staff remain unclearly and inadequately defined, therefore the level of training and education remains unclear, and there is also a high degree of professionalism which, in itself provides manpower problems — difficulty in using staff flexibly. The cumulative effect of these factors makes it extremely difficult to establish standards for, together with the quality of, care offered (Merrison Report, paras.2.2, 3.12 and 12.57). In this situation even though it is vital, in the interest of an effective service, to establish standards of care in an attempt to measure/assess quality, this becomes extremely difficult.

So how can this important goal of ensuring quality be achieved? The three stock approaches to assessing quality of care include;

1. Examining data about 'input' (structure), e.g. the availability and accessibility of resources and a profile of staff which includes their expertise and experience;
2. Process (throughput), e.g. what is done to the patient, which includes an examination of the nursing, medical and paramedical processes; and
3. Outcome (output), e.g. the effects of these processes — diagnosis, treatement and care — on the patient/client.

Clearly, these processes must be examined in concert, as they are intimately linked, e.g. a satisfactory, anticipated outcome of treatment and care will depend on the relevance, availability and integrity of resources used and their effective processing, to establish the quality of the service.

A Royal College of Nursing discussion document (1981) identifies eight key factors as prerequisites for the professional control of standards of nursing care. They include a philosophy of nursing; the relevant knowledge and skills; the nurse's authority to act; accountability; the control of resources; the organisational structure and management style; the doctor/nurse relationship; and, the management of change. It also recommends an approach to standards of care. In this respect it underlines the importance of identifying and meeting patients' nursing needs by identifying goals. In this context, as well as providing good nursing care, the report suggests, on the basis of individual needs, that of necessity care should be individually planned; that care should be systematically recorded, reviewed and evaluated; and that nurses should accept accountability for their nursing action.

In planning care on an individual basis, even though nurses must rely on other professionals for information about medical diagnoses and the plan of medical care, in the final analysis they must be responsible for their assessment of the patient's problem and making decisions about nursing care. To do this, nurses must have clear, decisive and unambiguous authority, accountability, responsibility, and autonomy. These important elements of role, as well as being highlighted by the RCN as being important to the provision of effective and efficient care to patients, are also highlighted in a DHSS seminar (1981) which made clear their relevance in relation to the satisfactory work of nurses, at each level of the nursing organisation, stating that at each level accountability should be matched by the necessary authority. The seminar also underlined that, in addition to having the necessary authority, the full responsibility of the sister's role (which had been eroded) should be restored and that they should have adequate assistance, so that they are enabled to function effectively in the environment in which patient care is delivered. Linked to this was the concern that proper financial reward together with educational and professional development opportunities should be ensured to enable nurses to develop their careers in clinical posts with direct responsibility for patient care, to enable them to maintain high standards of care.

Certain views expressed at the DHSS seminar on how to ensure quality care resemble closely the findings of a study carried out into 'direct patient care' in the USA (Colavecchio, 1982) which links manpower issues together with interpersonal relationships and the level of recognition for the uniqueness of the practice of nursing, with ensuring a quality nursing service. In addition, lack of essential staff was seen as the major problem in retaining nurses at the bedside; but factors such as not enough time, limited recognition of nurses' status, inadequate salary, repetitive routines, lack of input by nurses into policy making, together with their limited authority and power to change patient care were also underlined as being relevant.

In view of the many impediments to the provision of a quality service, i.e. maintaining realistic-demanded standards, can care be effectively evaluated?

Evaluation

The evaluation of nursing practice (in-patient) is succinctly described in a WHO report (1979).

The concept of evaluation of health care is stated as embracing a systematic process to determine the extent to which an action or sets of actions were successful in the achievement of predetermined objectives. The process involves measurements of adequacy — the allocation of activities and resources in manner and quantity sufficient to permit the achievement of desired objectives; efficacy — the benefit to the patient of the services, or treatment advocated or applied; effectiveness — the ratio between the achievement of the programmed activity and the desired level — that which had been proposed would result; and efficiency — the ratio between the result that might be achieved, through the expenditure of specified resources, and the result that might be achieved through a minimum expenditure.

Why Evaluation?

Essentially, evaluation is a deliberate attempt to collect and communicate information about (in this instance) the service/care being evaluated. To do so in an effective, reliable manner must include the employment of deliberate methods which enable representative sampling which will permit unbiased assessment of the activity being measured. It is an empirical investigation which is sometimes called 'reality testing' (Campbell, 1969).

The purpose of this investigation is to provide nurse managers, the decision makers, with information to enable them to select an appropriate course of action to the 'measurement' of care.

Evaluation in nursing, e.g. evaluation of the nursing process, is based on (ought to be based on) a systematic examination of predetermined objectives which are based on patients' needs and operationalised through the plan of nursing care. The evaluation of care is a process which to be effective must be conducted in a systematic manner. Evaluation is wholly dependent on the examination and assessment of determined objectives which, ostensibly, are based on patients'/clients' needs. Central to the process of evaluation is the notion of measurement, i.e. measurement of the adequacy, efficacy, efficiency and the effectiveness of the care process, which implies an acknowledgment of criteria and standards (measures of performance which are both desired and achievable).

These objectives must be realistic in their definition and must be testable. In this way objectives must be based on criteria — acceptable standards of performance, which are defined for each objective and which will subsequently act as indicators of whether or not these objectives, standards, are met. In this respect, criteria are both special and measurable (referenced), quantitatively and qualitatively. Standards denote long-term goals of nursing care, aspired for by nurses, managers (planners), practitioners and educationists. In effect, they represent desired and achievable levels of performance, corresponding with criteria against which actual performance is compared.

Evaluation includes pre-formative measures of initial goals which is effected during the planning stage and which can be changed if desired; formative measures taken during the implementation of the plan to determine the progress and integrity of the objectives set and which entails continual interchange of information: at this stage, modification of the care plan/programme may be indicated; and summative, which relates to final plan/programme outcomes.

Using a systems approach to care, nursing can be viewed as having an input/structure — resources, time, knowledge, skills, expertise; an output/process of transformation achieved through the nursing process, medical process and paramedical process; and an output which can be demonstrated through patient/client behaviour and staff satisfaction. In this context, standards can be set to measure the adequacy, efficacy, effectiveness and efficiency of any or all of these processes. Structuring and process can be tested by establishing care plans which are realistic, valid and reliable and which are based on sound information. Patient outcomes are more difficult to establish but may be evaluated in terms of the physical, social and psychological changes desired and achieved. However, to do this effectively, these changes must be related directly to patient needs for nursing care and to well-defined objectives which are quantifiable. However, in addition, such important intangibles as the patient's will to make progress, the effects of family relationships, and the family's psychological state, should not be excluded from assessing outcome. Approaches such as Maslow's theory of adaptability, of coping, 'may prove useful as a means by which nurses conceptualise nursing and develop better ways of providing care' (WHO, 1979).

Research

In view of the importance of ensuring quality of care to patients, by virtue of their right, can this be readily achieved in the light of the many uncertainties which relate to 'health', 'care', 'manpower', together with the complexity of the environment in which the care and management of patients takes place?

Establishing criteria which enable nurse managers, at all levels, to establish the standard of quality of care provided to patients and clients, continues to occupy considerable nursing time.

Recently (Ball and Goldstone, 1984) devised a package, 'Criteria for Care', which is a set of operational tools to help the nurse manager to improve the level of nursing service and manage the resources available to best effect. In essence, the package provides a framework to enable nurse managers make decisions and identify desired objectives to establish, maintain and improve patient care.

The authors state that the system provides an information framework for the solution of questions such as:

What percentage of their time should nurses spend on direct care? How much direct care should be delivered to patients in a particular dependency group? What ratios should exist between the amounts of direct care to be given to patients in each group? And, what level (or 'quality') of care should be achieved?

The system is intended to assess current nursing workload on medical and surgical wards together with analysing the demands made upon nurses by that workload. To meet these objectives the system provides the means of obtaining data on nursing workload and nursing activity together with the level of patient care being achieved. In addition, it provides an information matrix which enables nurse managers make decisions about the most effective deployment of staff, and, most important, about optimum levels of staff required, to ensure and maintain a high (desired) standard of care.

To effect these objectives, information is obtained on ward profile, i.e. ward policies, staff/patient allocation etc.; measures of workload and nursing activity which includes classifying patients into four dependency categories. In addition, nurse activity sampling is carried out, nursing activities being categorised as direct care, indirect care, associated work and personal/miscellaneous activities. Also, direct patient care sampling, i.e. the amount of direct care which is given to patients in each dependency category (I, II, III and IV).

The measures of output/performance are based on the level of care being given which is elicited through the use of a quality of care instrument 'monitor' and a nursing staff satisfaction questionnaire. The nursing staff satisfaction questionnaire is based on a series of questions which are related to their level of satisfaction with patient care currently being provided on their ward as well as their satisfaction with current staffing patterns.

The information thus obtained forms the basis of an information framework, based on the present functioning of the ward, which enables nurse managers make decisions on such vital issues as nursing policy, nurse staffing and the most effective deployment of nursing staff.

The main function of this system is to enable nurse managers to effect with confidence, 'decisions relating to the quality and standards of nursing care'. To ensure this central objective, the system provides a means of monitoring the effect of changes in patient dependency, nursing policy, the increase and/or decrease of nursing staff numbers on the delivery of care, the spread of workload over different shifts, i.e. day, evening and night and the excellency and/or deficiency in the delivery of care.

The system relates to other nurse manpower systems in so far as it uses similar measures of workload.

Research into standards and quality of care and the means of establishing these continues in the USA and the UK. The 'quality' of the care delivered to patients is difficult to establish, largely because of the many factors already discussed as well as the fact that standards and quality of care continue to be based on the experience of the nurse. In reality, their roots lie in intuition and subjectivity. Therefore, what is needed is an instrument/index that is easy to use and understand and, most important, provides nurses with useful and relevant information on the care they give their patients.

The Rush Medicus Methodology

The Rush Medicus Methodology is an instrument developed jointly by the Medicus Systems Corporation and Rush College of Nursing. The instrument meets the requirements of comprehensiveness, speed and ease of scoring and application, according to its authors. In essence the Methodology, which is used for monitoring quality of nursing care, is an observational instrument for acute care, compiled and refined from the best process criteria extracted from nursing literature. The criteria are organised according to the nursing model of the nursing process and are based on assessment, planning, implementation and evaluation.

'Monitor'

Goldstone and his colleagues have carried out extensive research into the Rush Medicus Methodology: The modified anglecised version is published as 'Monitor' (Goldstone, 1983). 'Monitor', provides an index of nursing actions and provides evidence of nursing judgement and decision making. It also enables an index of the day-to-day process of care, and in this respect it can become a useful tool for management and control of patient care. It is patient orientated, simple to use, and it is organisationally feasible.

Essentially, 'Monitor' consists of quality-related items which lend themselves easily to a scoring system based on 'yes' 'no' responses. It is based on a master list of over 200 criteria, split into four sub-lists each appropriate to patients of different dependency levels, i.e. Category I patients (self-care), Category II (average care), Category III (above average care) and Category IV (maximum or intensive care) (*Nursing Times*, August 1984).

Because the responses demanded are yes/no there is minimal score for subjectivity in the final score, which is the percentage of 'yes' responses. It is a useful method for evaluating quality of nursing care as practised in medical, surgical and paediatric units.

The methodology relies on observation of patients and the environment in which they are being nursed, patient interview, nursing staff interview, and an examination of the appropriate patient nursing records. The criteria for 'measuring' quality hinge on the extent to which the nurse focuses on the patient's needs. The care plan is based on the assessment of the patient's needs or problems. The criteria for assessing the implementation of the care plan depend on checking that care is provided in accordance with that plan.

The main sections of 'Monitor' are akin to those of the nursing process, i.e. planning nursing care (based on an assessment of the needs of the patient), implementing and monitoring the plan (establishing whether the plan agreed, in terms of its objectives, is met); adjusting the plan according to the patient's response to the care provided; and evaluation of the plan.

The instrument is regarded by the authors, following extensive research and 'feedback' from nurse managers and nurse practitioners, as being 'both valid and reliable'. The authors have considerable experience with this index of care and argue that it is a most useful tool for the nurse managers, enabling them to make proper decisions on the quality of care offered, and, most important, readily detecting and remedying any faults in the service to patients. The index is part of a wider information framework published by the same authors which is aimed at manpower requirements analysis.

In the following chapter the concept and the issues relating to manpower will be discussed.

References

Ball, J. and Goldstone, L. (1984) Criteria for care. *Nursing Times, 80*(36), 55–8
—— and Collier, M.M. (1984) *Monitor: An Index of the Quality of Nursing Care for Acute Medical and Surgical Wards.* Newcastle upon Tyne Polytechnic Products Ltd
——, ——, —— (1984) Criteria for Care (The Manual of the North West Nurse Staffing Levels Project). Newcastle upon Tyne Polytechnic Products Ltd
Block, D. (1977) Criteria, standards, norms. *Journal of Nursing Administration*, Sept. pp.20–30
Campbell, D.T. (1969) Reforms as experiments. *American Psychologist, 24*(4), 409–29
Colavecchio, R. (1982) Direct patient care: A viable career choice? *Journal of Nursing Administration, 11*(8), 17–22
DHSS (1969) Report of Working Party on Management Structure in the Local Authority (Mayston). HMSO. London
—— (1974) Report of the Committee of Inquiry into Pay and Related Conditions of Service of Nurses and Midwives (Halsbury). HMSO, London
—— (1972) Management Arrangements for the Reorganised National Health Service (Grey Book). HMSO, London
General Nursing Council for England and Wales (1979/80) Annual Report, GNC
—— (1980/1) Annual Report. GNC
Goldstone, L.A. (1983) 'Monitor', Newcastle upon Tyne Polytechnic Products Ltd.
Goldstone, L.A. and Ball, J. (1984) The quality of nursing services. *Nursing Times, 80*(35), 56–8
—— and Collier, M. (1982) Nursing manpower requirements: a framework for rational discussion. *Health Services Manpower Review, 8*(3) 6–9
Hall, Dame Catherine (1983) Nurse Managers Warned of the Risks to Maintain Standards. *Nursing Mirror, 156; 19*, 11
Hegyvary, S.T. (1982) *The Change to Primary Nursing: A Cross-Cultural View of Professional Nursing Practice.* C.V. Mosby, St Louis
Hingley, P. (1984) Stress: A Report of King Edward Hospitals Fund. *Nursing Standard*, no. 352, p.3
HMSO (1972) Report of the Committee on Nursing (Briggs). Cmnd. no. 5115. HMSO
—— (1979) Royal commission on the National Health Service (Merrison). Cmnd. no. 7615. HMSO
Jelinek, R.C. and Dennis, L.C. (1976) *A Review of Evaluation of Nursing Productivity.* US Dept of Health, Education and Welfare
—— Houssman, R.K.D., Hegyvary, S.T. and Newman, J.F. (1976) *A Methodology for Monitoring Quality of Nursing Care.* USDHEW Publications. Health Resources Administration, Bethesda, MD (HRA) 76–25
McLachlan, G. (ed.) (1976) *A Question of Quality: Roads to Assurance in Medical Care.* Oxford University Press, Oxford
Maillart, V. (1973) Higher education in nursing. *WHO Chronicle, 27*, 242–4
Ministry of Health, Scottish Home and Health Dept (1966) Report of the Committee on Senior Nursing Staff Structure (Salmon). HMSO, London
Nurses, Midwives and Health Visitors Rules Approval Order (1983) no.873. HMSO, London
RCN (1943) Nursing Reconstruction Committee (Horder). RCN
—— (1964) A Reform of Nursing Education (Platt). RCN
—— (1978) An Assessment of the State of Nursing in the National Health Service 1978. RCN
—— (1979) Working Committee on Standards of Nursing Care and Related Matters. (Interim Report). RCN
—— (1981) Towards Standards (A Discussion Document). RCN
—— (1983) Towards a New Professional Structure for Nursing. RCN

—————— (1984) Nurse Alert: A Report of the Effects of the Financial and Manpower Cuts in the NHS. HMSO, London

Trade Union and Labour Relations Act 1974, Eliz II. HMSO, London

Trade Union and Labour Relations Act (Amendment) 1976, Eliz II. HMSO, London

United Kingdom Central Council for Nursing, Midwifery and Health Visiting (1983) Code of Professional Conduct for Nurses, Midwives and Health Visitors. UKCC, London

—————— (1984) Code of Professional Conduct for Nurses, Midwives and Health Visitors, 2nd edn. UKCC, London

Van Maanem, H.M.Th. (1984) Evaluation of nursing care: Quality of nursing evaluated within the context of health care and examined from a multinational perspective. in
· Willis, L.D. (ed.) *Measuring the Quality of Care.* Churchill Livingstone, Edinburgh

WHO (1966) WHO Expert Committee on Nursing (Fifth Report). WHO

—————— (1976) The Nursing Process (Report on the first meeting of the Technical Advisory Group. ICP/HMD 049(1). WHO

—————— (1979) Evaluation of Inpatient Nursing Practice. (Report on a Working Party, 4). WHO

Advised Further Reading

Alkin, M.C. and Fitz-Gibbon, C.T. (1975) Methods and theories of evaluating programs. *Journal of Research and Development in Education,* 8(3), 1–15

Ball, J.A., Goldstone, L.A. and Collier, M.M. (1984) *Criteria for Care.* Newcastle upon Tyne Polytechnic Products Ltd

Bennett, M. (1984) *Quality of Nursing — Strained or Thrice Blessed?* Royal Melbourne Hospital Oration, Oct.

Commission of the European Communities (1981) Advisory Committee on Training in Nursing. Report on the Training of Nurses Responsible for General Care. (R82/5/A). EEC

De Geyndt, W. (1970) Five approaches for assessing quality of care. *Journal of Hospital Administration,* Autumn, pp.183–4

Goodlad, S. (ed.) (1984) *Education for the Professions.* SRHE and NFER Nelson, University of Guildford, Surrey

Lapsley, I. (1979) The use of accounting information in consensus management teams, *Business Finance and Accounting (UK),* 6(4), 539–58

McLachlan, G. (ed.) (1964) *Problems and Progress in Medical Care.* Oxford University Press, Oxford

Revans, R.W. (1964) *Standards for Morale: Cause and Effect in Hospitals.* Oxford University Press, Oxford

Rezler, A.G. and Stevens, B.J. (1978) *The Nurse Evaluator in Education and Service.* McGraw-Hill. New York

RCN (1981) Towards Standards (A Discussion Document). RCN

Taylor, D. (1984) *Understanding the NHS in the 1980s.* Office of Health Education, London

Willis, L.D. and Linwood, M.E. (eds.) (1984) *Measuring the Quality of Care.* Churchill Livingstone, Edinburgh

Yura, H. and Walsh, M.B. (eds.) (1978) *Human Needs and the Nursing Process.* Appleton-Century-Crofts, New York

8 INFORMATION, MANPOWER AND PRODUCTIVITY

Aims

The aims of this chapter are:

1. To discuss information systems.
2. To examine some approaches to the study of manpower.
3. To examine the nature of productivity and its relationship to standards and quality of care.

Learning Objectives

The purpose of this chapter is to enable the reader to:

1. Appreciate the relevance of information to manpower planning.
2. Understand some approaches to manpower problems and their effects on the delivery of patient care.
3. Understand the concept of productivity in the context of the delivery of care.

Background

The day-to-day management of the NHS is devolved to Health Authorities which employ staff, provide buildings, equipment and, most important, ensure that patients receive the optimum standard and quality of care.

The NHS does not delegate detailed control over the management of its service to a public corporation, which would have to operate like businesses, being obliged to find a large part of their own capital and resources. In this respect, the NHS is not subject to having to meet a target rate of return on capital.

In practice, the size of the NHS, the power of the Health Authorities and the influence of the health professions mean that central Government cannot administer the Service in a detailed way. In fact, 'The size and complexity of the NHS budget renders it impracticable for the DHSS to control expenditure in great detail.' (DHSS 1977).

The NHS has a staff of 1.2 million and a budget of £17,000m. In this respect, the NHS is the largest employer in the country and as such it is affected by such central developments as the control of salaries and wages and an expansion of trade union membership among professional and auxiliary workers.

Currently, it is impossible (because of lack of knowledge) to say how many workers the NHS needs and of what type. In addition, roles are not always clearly defined, consequently the educational, training and management needs of staff are difficult to predict and prescribe with accuracy, therefore the function of management, i.e. matching resources to needs, is frustrated or made impossible.

However, in this unclear situation one point is paramount: manpower accounts for over 70 per cent of total NHS costs. (Griffiths, DHSS, 1983, para.35, p.23).

The emphasis of treating patients whenever possible without admitting them to hospital as well as discharging them as soon as reasonably possible has very definite implications for nursing and midwifery. In effect it means that within hospitals the pace and intensity of work have stepped up because a greater proportion of the patients are in need of active treatment. The fact that greater emphasis is being placed on more highly dependent patients in the work of the community health services, has resulted in a growing need for more nurses.

There are no adequate data relating to the overall balance between nursing and midwifery demand at national level. In addition, the variations, some of them sizeable, in local staffing problems, suggest that inadequate attention is paid locally to determining criteria for staffing needs. Also, there are not only regional variations, but very often there are variations in the same kind of hospital; and chief nursing officers tend to think in terms of budgetary rather than of manpower ceilings (Briggs, HMSO, para.405, pp.117–118).

Many factors combine to establish higher levels of need for health care professionals in clinical nursing, nurse management, education and research. The central factors include, longevity, higher living standards as well as the higher consumer (patient) aspirations and expectations in relation to information, rights, and the standard and quality of care and service provided. Also, new and improved technology together with the rapid out-dating of scientific knowledge — with its direct effects on patient management and care together with the increased dependence on specialists, nurses, doctors, para-medicals — and increased patient turnover, have had major effects on nurse manpower particularly in relation to nurses' work, deployment, education and training.

The evidence, giving areas of risk in hospital and in the community due to increased workload and/or staff shortages, is defined in a number of official documents and reports which include statements such as:

Standards of patient care have been put at risk in hospital and in the community as a result of financial restraint, increased workloads and manpower shortages. In the community increased workloads cause curtailment of time allocated to patients and learners as well as abandonment of patient care programmes. (RCN, 1978)

Supply and Demand

The factors which affect the supply/availability of nurses are many, varied and include the image of the nursing profession and the status of nurses; these can directly affect the recruitment of nurses. Where nurses have been successfully recruited, what happens to them subsequently together with the nature of the environment in which nursing is practised will have a major influence on them completing training and/or their retention as part of nursing manpower subsequently.

Therefore, the factors which nursing management, together with professional and statutory bodies, the NHS as a whole, neglect at their peril, include initially ensuring, by every available means, that the image of nursing which is presented to the public and peer professions is that which accentuates the worthwhileness of the profession, its updatedness and its integrity. In this respect those aspects which require investigation, analysis and activation include ensuring the right people, by education, commitment (ethic) and personality, are selected to train as nurses. Following selection nurses must be given a suitable period of induction — a settling-in period — followed by counselling and appraisal, to establish their commitment. Those who continue in nursing must be trained and educated using up-to-date methods of education and ensuring their optimum participation in the subject of nursing intellectually (by the use of a problem-solving, Gestalt-type approach as opposed to a wholly expository approach) as well as practically. During the period of studentship, there must be far less reliance on nurses to meet service needs: there must be increasing responsibility with minimum accountability (clearly, in the present situation, it seems to me unrealistic for nursing students to be totally devoid of accountability). Also, a proper nurse counselling service (long overdue and much needed) must be established, at the very least within each DHA so that nurses can receive proper support as well as be able to externalise their fears and anxieties in confidence and with trust.

On completion of training nurses must continue to be afforded scope to up-date, develop and actualise (fulfil through the full use of their talents and abilities) themselves. Above all, they must be afforded proper career prospects as well as conditions of service appropriate to their training and demands.

The re-entry of qualified nurses to the profession must be properly explored and developed, particular attention being paid to their up-dating and conditions of employment to effect their integration into the full-time nursing workforce.

Organisational, technological, social and personal changes have mark-ed and wide-ranging effects on the NHS and nursing and, as a result, nursing and other health care professions must progress, otherwise their professional viability and integrity will be threatened.

Burns and Stalker (1966) underline the problems and the difficulties of organisation which are faced with change, often finding it difficult to adapt to the change. Therefore, 'one of the principal responsibilities of management is to develop organisations to meet the challenge of the future' (Kenny, *et al.*, 1979). This responsibility, they say is exercised by assessing the resources and opportunities available, defining objectives and, most important, efficiently managing the resources allocated to meet these goals.

The most important resource to any organisation is its staff. Therefore, their correct education, training, development and deployment is a prerequisite to their commitment to the organisation and to ensuring the success of its objectives.

The Real Issues

The history relating to nurse manpower dates back to the publication of the Athlone Report (RCN, 1937) which was set up particularly to enquire into the recruitment, training, and conditions of persons engaged in nursing and to advise on measures for the purpose of maintaining an adequate service. Six years later, in 1943, the Nursing Reconstruction Committee (Horder, RCN, 1943) had the task of surveying the present and future demand for and supply of nurses as well as to advise on methods of recruitment.

A recent report (Taylor, 1984) states that certain occurrences raise questions as to the Government's intention and efforts to control NHS resource use whilst simultaneously raising its productivity. In this context, the report cites events such as adjustment to budget (1983) with consequent loss to the Health Services equivalent to £140m, together with attempts by the Secretary of State to reduce manpower levels, despite the fact that industrial action involving nurses, ancillary workers and other groups (1982) had resulted in increased waiting lists to unprecedented and unacceptable levels.

The standard of service provided to patients and clients is dependent on a variety of elements, events and people, all of which affect the care and the ultimate rehabilitation and recovery of the patient. Elements which affect the standard and quality of care and management of patients relate to the organisational/authority structure within which nurses operate, the framework of industrial relations, the nature and quality of nursing education and training, at basic and post-basic levels, together with the adequacy or stringency of resources and the actualisation of nurses.

Among the elements of a quality service, the most important and expensive element (often the largest proportion of the operational budget is concerned with staff) is that of 'manpower'.

As well as being the most costly resource employed by the NHS, manpower is also the most valuable. Resource constraints, the need to contain expenditure, and the emphasis on local accountability for performance have served to focus interest on size, utilisation and cost-effectiveness of the workforce, and in this context an understanding of the composition, distribution, performance and cost of the labour force is a prerequisite for the formulation, implementation and evaluation of local and national plans and strategies for the provision of health care.

The translation of plans into manpower budgets, strengthens the discipline of negotiations for resources. In this respect, sound information, knowledge and skills relating to all aspects of nursing manpower are indispensable for the nurse planner and nurse manager.

Information: A Prerequisite to Manpower Planning

A recent report on the collection and use of information about manpower in the NHS (Körner, NHS, 1984) has, as its main aims, the control and efficient use of manpower together with the strategic planning and policy development and the determination of conditions of service and accountability. The report underlines that rigorous assessment of prospective manpower requirements and equally rigorous retrospective accounting for the use of manpower resources lie at the heart of effective manpower control (para.2.15, p.10).

In view of the emphasis which, currently, is placed on the acquisition and use of concise and relevant information by managers in the NHS, which is highlighted by the many Körner reports, it may prove helpful to the reader to provide a brief examination of their philosophy and recommendations in enabling nurse managers to secure and use information to make realistic decisions about the use of resources: the paramount intention being to secure an efficient and effective health service.

The DHSS and other central bodies need information about employees for three main reasons, i.e. policy development and planning, for considering future staffing levels and the distribution of training resources: to support negotiations on terms and conditions of service: and for accountability reasons to enable an assessment by the Secretary of State (who is accountable to Parliament) of the policies set together with the priorities identified for the use of NHS resources and, most important, to ensure the efficient and effective use of those resources, by Health Authorities.

The *Grey Book* (DHSS, 1972) made it clear that members of authorities should devote their limited time to major issues of policy planning and resource allocation and to enable them effect the monitoring and control of performance, they should require their officers to present them with argued and supported alternatives for the major issues requiring their consideration, (para.1.29, p.17).

The report (Körner, 1984d) also emphasises that the information which is available is sometimes 'unreliable, of doubtful relevance, out of date, and with gaps especially about the community's needs for health services and the effectiveness of services in meeting these needs', and suggests that 'improvement of the information made available could be done by 'a systematic assessment of what information is needed at each management level and by the establishment of an expert information function at Area and Regional levels' (para.3.34, p.55). The report underlines the fact that good information will not lead to effective monitoring unless positive use is made of it by each management level.

The Merrison report continues the theme of 'good information' by underlining its importance for planning, (para.6.23, p.57).

The whole question of resource allocation and control, based on an information system, dates to the Resource Allocation Working Party (RAWP, DHSS, 1976). The RAWP used population, adjusted for age, sex, marital status, standardised fertility ratios and standardised mortality rates as the basic measures of need. (They recommended that revenue funds should be allocated according to relative need for health care.) This approach was subject to much criticism, particularly the use of mortality rates as a measure of morbidity, the failure to include, or allow for, family practitioners' services and the fact that it failed to take account of factors which may be important locally in determining the need for resources, e.g. occupational status of the population and social deprivation.

The Perrin Report (DHSS, 1978) advised that NHS authorities should 'give urgent attention to improving stores management and control systems and to additional staffing and training, and improved systems should be provided for central purchasing functions' (para. D).

Study of Information Requirements: The Körner Reports

The DHSS undertook a study of information requirements of the health services and subsequently issued a Consultative Document (1979). The document proposed a joint NHS/DHSS Steering Group 'to provide a permanent forum for considering information matters'.

In 1980 an NHS/DHSS Steering Group was set up with the broad terms of reference to examine the field of NHS statistics. Three years later saw the publication of the First Report (Körner, NHS/DHSS, 1982) on the collection and use of information about manpower in the National Health Service.

Common to the Körner reports is the use of 'minimum data sets', i.e. the minimum amount of data common to all posts and employees in relation to skill, location and position where work is carried out, volume of work and costs of the post. This minimum data is deemed to be necessary to provide the necessary information for management to enable it to make decisions and to effect its responsibilities about employees and posts. In essence, manpower control and planning. In addition in the absence of nationally recognised arrangements for recording data about NHS posts minimum data sets will allow more realistic comparisons to be made between different district health authorities on a national basis. Even though the use of computer systems and information technology are implicit in the Committee's recommendations to effect an integrated manpower information system, the collection of minimum data would initially (according to the authors) be well within the practicability of a non-computerised, manual system.

To date, the published reports relate to information about:

1. Hospital clinical activity (1982);
2. Community health services (1983);
3. Patient transport services (1984a);
4. Paramedical services (1984b);
5. Maternity services (1984b);

6. Finance (1984c);
7. Manpower (1984d);
8. Services for and in the community (1984e,f);

Current debate on the central information-gathering systems in the NHS indicates a degree of dissatisfaction by professionals on some of the inherent inconsistencies in the statistical information gathered. In addition, at local level, hospital or ward, the relevance of such statistical information in relation to the work of hospitals together with its significance to the management care and treatment of patients, is constantly argued. Some of the problems are epitomised in the areas of 'bed states' and 'bed occupancy' which limits useful analysis. Also, some doubt exists as to the accuracy of the methods of collecting this information thereby questioning its ultimate reliability and statistical significance. In this context, the SH3 annual hospital returns are questioned in relation to usefulness, e.g. the information obtained is essentially related to events rather than patients: there is no way of determining the number of re-admissions or of identifying the patient. Also, information is incomplete and there is a lack of integration with other sources. Most important, the outcome of patient care is unknown (Yates, 1982).

The volumes of statistics arising from the information gathered are great and may be limiting to the manager in their interpretation, and usefulness, as they are out of date (two or three years) before being published.

Paradoxically, it could be said that NHS managers and professionals, at all levels, are suffering from a dearth of confusing and outmoded information which, if anything, may limit their progress in day-to-day management and/or strategic planning. This paradox poses many questions. For example; Do the many reports of Körner correct these anomalies? Will the volumes of information collected merit the employment of more researchers and analysts? Will the average professional continue to remain uninitiated as to the usefulness of the information provided? Or will the information be presented in a straightforward manner, readily interpreted by all? Will there be information 'overload' rather than information 'deprivation'? Clearly, not only the professionals, but, most important, patients, their relatives and the general public at large require further demystifying of information. It is their right.

The Reports

The Körner reports (NHS/DHSS 1982–84) relate to information about 'Hospital Clinical Activity'. The Committee's concept of 'clinical activity' is not explicitly patient-orientated and the Steering Group's main concern is with information for health services management. It does not really tackle specifically the information needed by professionals to evaluate the results of their care, i.e. about the occurrence of disease or about the health needs of populations, except in so far as these can be inferred from data about hospitals episodes. Most important, according to some observers, it does not make recommendations about describing health status or the clinical and social outcomes of the use of health services. These 'omissions' are regarded as limitations to a report inquiring into health service information and offering prescriptions for its development (Beveridge, 1983).

Not all views on the philosophy and recommendations of the Körner reports have misgivings and are negative. For example, comments on the Community Health Services report (1983) make clear that 'activity statistics are of equal interest to nurses, adminstrators and treasurers and should be standard management material in unit and district management terms'. Also it is stated that the report 'contains innovative concepts which lift the community health services out of their inherited legislative straight-jacket and illuminate them afresh'. Most important, the report tidies 'the woolly thinking behind the use of the team "community health services", with a clear distinction being made between "services to the community" and 'patient care in the community'. (Bussey, 1983).

In addition, it is acknowledged that the report provokes much forward thinking about managers, particularly in the context of using information to inform local groups regularly about their work. Also, where fieldworkers and managers have easy access to the same information, the potential for role change is great, thus enabling fieldworkers to become more involved with managing productively the problems of the service they provide (rather than responding to centralised decisions), if they have regular flows of information about their service (Harries, 1984).

The effects on innovation in the community, together with the credibility of the report to fieldworkers, is echoed by another observer (Webster, 1984) who states that the report 'offers innovative approaches to the whole area of community health services statistics', as well as stating: 'the report (part 1), is of particular interest to health visitors and midwives, particularly its programmes which are related to prevention and intervention'. Webster also suggests that part II of the report, which is substantially about people who receive care outside of hospital, 'should provide district managers with information which enables them to think of patient care services as a whole'.

The reports are seen as having special value to midwifery managers, namely those of 1982, 1983, and that on manpower (1984d) (Gee, 1984). In the context of their usefulness, the 1982 report is seen to provide positive effects in that it underlines that maternity information differs from other types of information on care in that recordings start with one individual and end up with two or more. And, that information about the birth is required to plan other services, e.g. child health. In addition, the report on community health services, acknowledges:

> that information about maternity patients should be collected on the antenatal services including those provided on hospital premises; that information should be collected on the support services for domiciliary confinements; there should be a District summary for the DHSS antenatal care; and a minimum data set i.e. midwives counting the numbers of antenatal consultations and data about the emergency support provided for domiciliary confinements.

Paramedical staff, especially physiotherapists, are concerned about the unit of measurement, 'patient contact', in so far that:

> it has no fixed value and is not related either to staff hours or to workload generated. It is a count of the number of occasions on which a patient comes face to face with one or more paramedical staff. (Williams, 1983)

There is disagreement, 'that patient contacts will measure activity and workload'. In this respect, it is argued that, 'an occasion of undefined length, involving one or more staff, cannot be a unit of workload measurement.

From an analysis of some comments on the Körner reports, it is clear that there remain doubts among some professionals as to the usefulness of the philosophy and recommendations, practically, of some reports. Also, some disquiet is indicated with certain aspects of the reports which are regarded as being inadequate and/or creating too much information. In addition, one professional body, the RCN, has shown its concern stating that the plans to collect information in the NHS 'could concentrate on administrative quantative material to the detriment of care quality, where the emphasis is on number crunching' (Keighley, 1984). Most important, the RCN fears, in conjunction with certain Körner reports, that the Griffiths report (DHSS, 1983) (which advocates the appointment of general managers) 'will produce in many nurses the belief that such information gathering will permit judgements based purely on management/administrative needs to outweigh the health care needs'.

However, despite the misgivings of some observers, there would seem to be a general acknowledgement of the merits of these reports in so far that they contain clear and unambiguous concepts as well as being innovative. Also, they are seen to clarify the present unclear labelling, particularly in the 'community services' as well as to stimulate more positive thinking in relation to the collection and use of information by managers in so far as many professionals can be involved more realistically and imaginatively in the decisions they take — and their effects. Most important, it is envisaged that a clarification of the concept of productivity, which even though much desired is greatly disputed by health care professionals, will result. In this way the use of minimum data sets will permit managers to make decisions commensurate with their responsibilities, thereby ensuring that targets can be aimed for more realistically and more accurately by permitting comparisons to be made between units, districts and regions.

The recommendations made, if they provide a demystification of present procedures for information collection, interpretation and use, and thereby enable an improved understanding of the work situation by managers and workers, allowing more informed decisions to be taken in relation to patients and clients, will have been worthwhile. However, these effects can only be hopefully anticipated: the real effects will become known only retrospectively.

In the final analysis, the Körner reports must be seen by all nurses, other health care professionals and administrative staff at least as a major positive move towards encouraging and enabling the viability of the Service. Also, they must be viewed within the context of a parcel of guidelines which include the Merrison and Griffiths reports in general and the EEC Nursing Directives and the *Nurses, Midwives and Health Visitors Act* 1979, all of which have the central purpose of ensuring a quality service to patients and clients.

Already, health authorities have been asked to implement their main recommendations of Körner by April 1987.

The Körner Report: Implications for Manpower

The 'Third Report on the Collection and Use of Information about Manpower', (1984d) emphasises that to achieve effective manpower control, necessitates rigorous assessment of prospective manpower requirements together with rigorous retrospective accounting for the use of manpower resources. This is most important, since often the largest proportion of operational budgets is concerned with staff:

> The translation of plans into manpower budgets (as well as financial ones) strengthens the discipline of negotiations for resources and similarly the requirement to monitor manpower out-turn against agreed budgets focuses the attention of managers on the economical and efficient deployment of staff. (NHS/DHSS, 1984d, para.2.15, p.10)

The rationale of this report is embodied in such statements as: control involves deploying staff in a manner to 'maximise productivity while simultaneously minimising costs and monitoring staff use and output along the chain of accountability'. And, 'that managers assess their performance against agreed objectives as well as against the performance of comparable centres of activity regionally and nationally'. In this way the report believes that variances can be pinpointed and then be subjected to detailed investigation. The control of manpower, it is suggested, can be more explicit and formalised in the evolving concept of national performance indicators and in the reviews of regions by ministers and of districts by regions (paras.1.7, 1.8, 1.9, p.6).

The report underlines the complexity and the cost of manpower to the NHS and, in this respect states that staff costs amounted to over £6,000m and the organisation spanned about 5,000 'different combinations of grade and area of work' in the financial year 1982/83. It further emphasises, 'pressures to increase staff numbers' and, in this context, identifies contributing factors such as 'improvements in diagnostic and treatment techniques with attendant higher specialisation, the quest for quality care, the growing number of elderly and reductions in working hours'. The report also contrasts the 'pressures' which are associated with present resource constraints, i.e. the need to contain costs and expenditure and the emphasis on local accountability, all of which 'focus interest on the size, utilisation and cost-effectiveness of the workforce' and which demand knowledge of 'relative and absolute sizes of different groups, their deployment, their output and their remuneration' to ensure the 'prudent use and effective control of manpower'.

A prerequisite for the formulation, implementation and evaluation of local and national plans and strategies for the provision of health care is an understanding of the composition, distribution, performance and cost of the labour force. To effect this understanding through improved and reliable information, the Körner Committee propose the 'routine collection of a series of minimum data sets to provide, at reasonable cost, the basic information which authorities and their officers need to discharge their responsibilities' (para.1.1, p.5). In this way, it is hoped that the information on which officers base their decisions is relevant, reliable and, most important, is readily available.

The scope of the report, in reviewing the information about health services manpower has been to identify the data necessary for the 'control and efficient use of manpower; annual and strategic planning and policy development; determination of terms and conditions of service; and accountability' (para.1.3, p.5). The types of data about health service manpower which is central to the report include 'data about the distribution and costs of posts' together with 'data about the characteristics, input and cost of employees' (para.1.10, p.6).

The report states that data about individual posts as well as about planned staffing levels are basic components of manpower control, and in this way are central to forming the basis of health service planning. It also recommends, in terms of information content about posts, data about skill, location/position where work is carried out and about the costs of the post. It recommends that the skill content of hospital-based posts be identified by specialty (specialties) and the grade of the post and that the skill content of community-based posts be identified by the grade of the post and its location. In addition, the volume of work involved in the post should be identified in terms of worked hours, budgeted hours and paid hours. And the costing of posts should be done using the local budgetary control and costing system (paras. 2.3, 2.5, 2.6, 2.13 and 2.14, pp.9 and 10).

Establishing a Framework for Nurse Manpower

Nurses form the major part of the NHS workforce. Therefore, as a direct consequence it makes good management sense to ensure their proper regulation and deployment thus enabling a more effective nursing service which provides security and satisfaction for patients and clients as well as providing nurses with a reasonable degree of job satisfaction.

To establish a framework for manpower planning leads inevitably to a consideration of the information needed in this process. Nurse manpower planning can take place at various levels in the health service structure, i.e. at national level, at regional, district, hospital or ward level.

At national level, the DHSS monitors manpower groups, including nurses, examines manpower requirement in particular sectors and develops national manpower models.

In addition to finding the information to establish a framework for planning, there still appear to be problems with integrating and standardising systems operating at different levels, and in giving local managers access to the information they need. Also, the most serious problem which is central to measuring nursing activity, 'is that different results will be obtained according to the quality of care which is being delivered'. (ORS, DHSS, 1983a). This report discusses various approaches to establishing patient dependency.

Patient Dependency

Patient-nurse dependency studies are undertaken for many reasons which include those that relate solely to patient classification systems; those that relate to the application of classification systems for the assessment of workload; those relating to patient dependency leading to deployment and establishments; and those that relate to deployment and/or establishments (Wilson-Barnett, 1978).

Top-down Approach

The 'top-down' approach examines relationships between measures of manpower, e.g. numbers of staff and measures of activity and/or cost. Frequently, this approach is used for strategic planning when manpower and activity are related to cost constraints and strategic priorities.

An example of a study using this approach is that of the 'Trent Nursing Formula' which relates nursing manpower to measures of activity, such as medical and surgical beds and extra throughput.

'Bottom-Up' Approach

This approach is based on how much nursing care patients need, i.e. patient-dependency; its central approach is to find ways of classifying patients which relate to the amount of care they need. In essence, nursing manpower is directly related to tasks performed. In addition to the use of patient-dependency in the 'bottom-up' approach, another approach to quantifying the nursing care required by patients includes doing so directly from a patient care plan with frequencies and times against each item of care.

The main studies using this approach include the 'Aberdeen Formula'; the classification used by Barr (1965) for general medical and surgical patients and which encompasses both basic and technical care; and the research of Rhys Hearn (1974).

Multi-Factorial

When determining staffing needs many complex factors must be seriously considered. Factors which are central to this exercise include the extended training requirements of nurse learners, arising from the provisions of relevant EEC nursing directives; the reduction in the number of hours which nurses work and the provisions of the *Trade Union, Labour Relations Act, Employment Protection Act* and the *Health and Safety at Work Act*, all or some of which may reduce the time spent by nurses in actual care. These factors need to be acknowledged and compensated for by nurse managers, to ensure even distribution of the workload.

Estimating Nurse Manpower

Probably the most widely used method of estimating demand has been via norms or simple ratios, e.g. nurses per bed or community nurses per head of population as they have the advantage of being simple to use; but their disadvantages are many and they are not flexible enough to take account of particular local circumstances; they are misleading if applied in the wrong context; and they are based on subjective assumptions. However, in practice, 'most people concerned with manpower planning in the NHS are unlikely to use documents as their primary source of information'. Instead training initiatives, meeting of people with similar interests and informal communication are the main methods by which 'good practice' is disseminated (*Nurse Manpower*, DHSS, 1983a, paras. 1.23/5.9).

But, are these informal ways of acquiring information about such an important and key subject as nurse manpower, acceptable, valid, reliable and useful for nurse managers, to enable them to make important decisions about the staffing of their hospitals?

And how, in the absence of vital information, can decisions by managers be made on such vital questions as how many nurses are needed? In essence, how can nurse manpower be assessed?

There have been many studies which provide perspectives on ways to assess and plan nurse manpower, some of which have recently been evaluated (DHSS, 1983a).

The Operational Research Service of the DHSS (1983) has developed a 'demand' formula for use in examining national demand for nursing staff. The formula consists of the construction of a numerical relationship between the total stock of hospital nursing manpower (whole time equivalents including a proportion for learners) and activity rates. These rates are in general cases and lengths of stay for the acute sector, and occupied beds for the non-acute sectors. The activity rates used include surgical cases, surgical length of stay, medical cases, medical length of stay, births, etc. The authors see the value of the model as its use to examine differences in staffing levels between areas, or after adaptation, districts.

The more well-known studies on nurse manpower which have been assessed for their appropriateness and usefulness in nursing include the Rhys Hearn method (1977). The Rhys Hearn method is based on a prescription of 'ideal care' as seen by nurses in charge of wards. In the original studies nurses in charge of wards were asked to prescribe 'direct care' for their patients. In this context, direct care was defined as those items of nursing care which can be related directly to the needs of individual patients. Indirect care was determined from observations over a number of geriatric wards and was expressed in hours per patient per day.

The staffing requirements (for the wards studied) were calculated from prescriptions of direct care weighted according to 'dependency factors' or patients' individual characteristics.

The main advantage of this approach is seen as it being patient-centred and therefore more acceptable to nurses as it is related to process rather than being task-orientated. The main disadvantages relate to the amount of data gathering and the general complexity of the approach.

Aberdeen Formula (SHHD, 1969, 1974, 1976, Cameron, 1979)

The Aberdeen Formula is a formula for calculating nursing workload as a basis for staffing. It was primarily developed as a result of research into nursing work which was undertaken in the North Eastern Region of Scotland.

The formula is based on five categories of activity, i.e. basic nursing, technical nursing, administration, domestic work and miscellaneous activity. The average number of patients in the various categories is recorded in a four-week period, and the equivalent number of fully bedfast, totally helpless patients is computed by using the appropriate factors for each category. The upper and lower limit figures for basic technical nursing are entered, and a mean figure for basic technical nursing is calculated. The mean of the figures used for administration and domestic work is utilised to calculate the workload for these groups of activities. These three figures are totalled and a percentage added to cover miscellaneous duties, depending on whether tea and coffee breaks are taken in off-duty time (4 per cent) or not (6½ per cent). This figure is then quoted as the weekly workload for the ward plus or minus approximately 5 per cent. This method proved to be complex and laborious. As a result the formula was simplified by taking the average dependency of the patients for a given specialty and applying this to the average number of actual patients in the ward. This is then combined with the use of an average figure for basic and technical nursing resulting in a formula for calculating nursing workload.

Essentially, the philosophy underlying the approach of Rhys Hearn is that of a detailed system of dependency assessment in which emphasis is placed on the needs of individual patients. Also, basic and technical care are treated separately; times, for each item of care measured by 'dependency factors' which influence these times, e.g. obesity, confusion, etc.

The formula is thus expressed: $W = N [F (B + T) + A + D + M]$ represents weekly average workload in hours; N, relates to the average number of patients in the ward; F, the average dependency factor for ward specialty; B, basic care in hours for totally bedfast patients; T, represents technical care as a percentage addition to basic nursing; A, administrative time per patient; D, domestic duties per patient; and M, miscellaneous duties per patient.

Barr Groupings (1964, 1965)

The Barr Dependency Groupings was developed for use in general and medical and surgical wards. Initially, three dependency groups were devised, self, intermediate and intensive care, aimed at examining the efficiency of hospital care and the measurements of workload.

The dependency groups are identified in terms of basic and technical care as well as making allowances for elderly patients.

An alternative approach to manpower planning is by use of GRASP (Meyer, 1984) (Grace Reynolds Application and Study of Peto).

GRASP has been adopted by hospitals in the USA and Canada, providing acute, long-term and specialty care.

The system does not classify patients into dependency groups, but instead, assesses the number of hours of nursing care each patient will need each day. In this way, the instrument permits individualised data which provide the basis for patient distribution, staffing, quality assurance, budget and cost accounting.

The GRASP system incorporates Pareto's Law, i.e. where a relatively small number represents the majority. When applied to nursing activities the initial research showed that of 'the many hundreds of possible direct care nursing activities, on average 40 to 50 will account for 85 per cent of the nursing time provided to any patient'. Therefore, it was possible to develop a tool for these nursing activities, 'to predict accurately the nursing time required by any given patient' (Meyer, 1984).

The workload measurement tool which combines specific nursing activities and their values, requires that each day the nurse notes the item/s that will apply to the patient that day. Usually 8 to 10 items are totalled for each patient, their time values being expressed in tenths of hours, i.e. the care hours required for each patient are calculated and similarly the total care hours for individual patients.

The significant nursing activities are determined either by study, i.e. all possible nursing activities are listed and data are collected usually over two weeks, to establish how often each activity is repeated over 24 hours: or by consensus, i.e. the use of knowledge or experience from which reasonably accurate estimates can be made.

The GRASP system is described as 'a proven method of measuring and managing nursing workloads'.

In summary, the authors of Manpower Planning (DHSS, 1983a) state that much of the work on patient-nurse dependency has been conducted by nurses themselves and that in spite of the large volume of work, much of it is repetitious. Also, the design of studies undertaken is often confused and statistically dubious. In addition, the lack of application of many studies may derive from the fact that the nursing role is complex, only some of it is measurable, and that all studies carry assumptions about nursing standards based on subjective judgements. Most important, the authors state that some studies have confused objectives, leading to an inappropriate choice of methodology (paras.5.14 and 5.15, p.4).

The authors also emphasise that in attempting to quantify the complexity of manpower issues a variety of factors need to be considered, many of which are very difficult to quantify. Therefore, any attempt to produce a single figure of nursing staff required will never be acceptable on bases of scientific method and professional judgement. They say 'it may be more realistic, therefore, to determine the ranges within which staffing levels are ideal, adequate or affordable, the simpler the models the easier it is to identify, check and where necessary update the assumptions they contain'. The authors suggest areas of activity where much could be gained by investigating further, such areas as the cost of employing different types of nurse manpower, i.e. young and mature learners, full and part-time nurses, bank or agency staff and the impact of the geographical location of training courses, the flow of information between the NHS and the independent sector, the potential supply of qualified nurses who are not currently working for the NHS and the impact of career structures within the NHS on supply in different specialties.

The words of Merrison (HMSO, 1979) are significant: 'Uncertainties about whether and how far a patient has improved and what his improvement has been due to, or whether he has been well cared for, will be reflected in difficulties of establishing standards or norms for staffing and procedures.' (para.12.45, p.173).

Clearly, in the light of the overwhelming evidence, it is difficult to devise sensible manpower strategies without first defining and eventually measuring nursing work to be done. At present, discussion and decisions about budgets and establishments start and finish in terms of numbers and nurses and numbers of hours, and there is usually no separate consideration of nursing work that has to be done, or alternative ways of doing it to prescribed standards of performance, and of relative costs. Also, an outstanding deficiency of nursing manpower policy at present is that there is little or no incentive for the 'manager' to utilise manpower more efficiently (Griffiths, DHSS, 1983b, para.9, p.13).

Nurse managers are entrusted with securing and maintaining the best deal for their patients: ensuring and enabling quality of the nursing service. To do this effectively, they must ensure the proper interviewing, selection, induction, training, support and deployment of staff. (These issues are fully discussed in Chapters 10 and 11.) In addition, clinical nurses must be fully involved in the determination of their own workloads if they are to be responsible for the standards of care for patients in their charge. Most important, nurse managers must have sufficient information of the correct type at their disposal to bid and argue for greater resources to ensure an effective and efficient nursing service.

Nursing Productivity: Concept

In view of the foregoing analysis of nursing manpower, can it be realistically assumed that productivity can be enhanced by the more enlightened and effective use of resources? If this is so, how can managers optimise the physical, creative and intellectual abilities of their staff to secure this objective as well as to enhance staff job satisfaction through their self-actualisation?

Management is about people and is related principally to changing or regulating their behaviour. In any organisation a priority is getting staff to work in the most effective and efficient manner: in essence, ensuring, maintaining and optimising productivity. In industry this is done to effect a profit which will sustain the continuing viability of the industry. In health care professions, productivity is related to ensuring the effective and efficient deployment of staff in their efforts to secure a high standard and quality of nursing care. There is no profit motive.

Currently, the delivery of nursing care to patients, through the transformation of nursing resources, is enshrined in a framework known as the 'nursing process' (discussed in Chapter 4). This process includes assessing and determining nursing productivity, on a patient-to-nurse (one-to-one) basis which is relatively straightforward in so far as the nurse responsible for nursing care and the patient receiving it are readily identified (if quantification is thought to be necessary and useful) in terms of time spent by the nurse, the resources used and the ultimate change in the patient's behaviour. Assuming satisfactory measures/indices of nursing input and output exist, nursing productivity would be a function of these for any nurse aggregated by the number of patients.

In reality, determining nursing productivity in hospitals, or in the community, is complex and problematical because of the many variables which impinge on the nursing environment, at ward or community level. For example, productivity is determined by, and is subject to, such variables as the team approach to nursing, the use of unqualified and/or untrained staff. Also the unclear role of the nurse and their diffuse accountability for patient/client care poses problems for nurse managers which are difficult to untangle. The complex environment in which nursing takes place together with the blurring of nurses' clinical boundaries particularly in relation to their responsibility and the extent of their authority to act, make even a crude assessment of nursing productivity difficult.

'The study of productivity is, the study of how to deliver the best nursing care in the most appropriate manner at the lowest cost. It is the relationship between the amount of acceptable output produced and the input required to produce that output' (Jelinek and Dennis, 1976).

The concept of nursing productivity embraces key factors, all of which are associated with the provision of quality care: they include, quality of role together with the status of the role occupant, the degree of authority and autonomy of nurses for nursing decisions and their working relationship with other health care professionals. Role clarity has been found which is central to productivity, is 'directly related to work satisfaction and, conversely, unclear role contributes to staff turnover and staff tension' (Lyons, 1970; Hurka 1972).

The primary concern of nurses and nurse managers is the delivery of quality care to patients and clients in the most effective, efficient and humane manner.

The efficiency of using nurses to do this is increased by either reducing the number of nurses achieving the same result, or achieving a larger result by using the same number of nurses — or a combination of the two.

When an increase in output is required the objective is not more expenditure of energy or working harder: it simply means achieving better results for the same effort. As this is/ought to be the prime objective of all organisations, how can it be done?

Work done by Jelinek and Dennis (1976) suggests that what is needed in the hospital/community context to determine nursing productivity is, 'a framework that is defined in terms of the nursing organisation'. The authors continue: 'Because performance and utilisation measures are becoming increasingly important to a wide variety of health care related groups, it is important that an easily understood concept such as productivity be established for nursing services.'

The inputs to patient and client management are many and include both human and non-human resources, e.g. staff, nurses, doctors, paramedicals and ancillary staff; staff expertise, knowledge and skills, education, training, technology, finance, buildings and time.

The outputs include changes in the behaviour of patients and clients together with staff satisfaction and enrichment through job enrichment and career progression prospects.

Despite clearly defined inputs, modes of conversion/transformation and output, the paramount problem that is presented in the care and management of patients is a noticeable lack of accepted objectives together with measures/indices in evaluating the standard and quality of care. Therefore, credible feedback to effect any desirable change in output is absent. In addition, the multi-professional team approach to the delivery of care makes it difficult, if not impossible, to attribute in a precise manner, outcomes specific to interventions by any particular group of professionals.

The organisation of health care is inevitably influenced — positively or negatively — in its work and productivity by the nature and characteristics of the community (the environment) in which it exists and operates, as well as by the national and local political and social policies which clearly, whether positively or negatively orientated, can affect such central issues to productivity as finance, manpower, and working conditions and morale.

Increased productivity is dependent on a variety of factors including the setting of clear realistic and achievable management objectives, developing, implementing and monitoring management plans. Also, it includes the control of expenditure, ensuring a clear general management role (identifiable individual/s). In addition, productivity involves the proper leadership and motivation of staff by providing a rich working environment with incentives. Most important, it necessitates a workforce that is properly trained, educated and developed in current trends and developments.

Jelinek and Dennis regard as central to productivity, input, technology and output. They also see the environment as defining and/or affecting the primary factors, e.g. the guidelines and constraints imposed by the hospital, the health care system as a whole, and external influences such as government.

Despite the massive expenditure on the NHS generally, there is little emphasis on the 'productive' aspect. However, as major resources are utilised by the NHS and nursing it is imperative that managers are aware of and control how these resources are utilised to optimise their effect on the patient care.

The Griffiths Inquiry (discussed in Chapter 2) was about the use and management of manpower and related resources in the National Health Service. The Inquiry see, as part of the role of the NHS Management Board, a two-fold function, i.e. the achievement of consistency and drive of the Health Service, first by giving leadership to the management of the NHS and secondly by controlling staff performance. To effect these functions, Regional Health Authorities and District Health Authorities, through their respective Chairmen, are recommended to extend the accountability review process through to Unit managers and to identify a General Manager who would have overall responsibility for management's performance together with reviewing and reducing the need for functional management structures and initiating major cost improvement programmes. The Personnel Director would have the particular responsibility to overcome any lack of incentive of staff by rewarding merit, reviewing the remuneration system and conditions of service for management and taking action, as appropriate, on ineffective performance. The Personnel Director would also have to ensure that a policy for performance and career development operates, assess the alignment of management training of different staff groups with the needs of the Service, review procedures for appointments, grievance and appeal, and dismissal, and identify any conditions of service which are not cost effective. In essence, the Griffiths report is concerned with sound management practice which is directly related to the effective and efficient use of resources, both human and non-human, which has as its focus, 'the concern to secure the best deal for patients; the best value for the taxpayer;

and the best motivation of staff' (para.3, p.11).

Clearly, these initiatives and proposed policy are targeted at ensuring productivity, and, in this context the report recommends the use of management process to provide the necessary leadership to capitalise on the existing levels of dedication and expertise and to stimulate, initiate, and effect a constant search for cost improvement. The intention is to sharpen the process of decision taking and implementation, as well as to review the effectiveness and efficiency of such action. It proposes that hospitals and units take all their own day-to-day management decisions and that, 'real output measurement, against clearly stated management objectives and budgets, should become a major concern of management at all levels'. (para.7, p.12).

On incentives, the report underlines as paramount to sound performance, securing proper motivation of staff by reviewing incentives, rewards and sanctions and suggests the use of merit awards, redeployment of the non-efficient performer and using dismissal, as a last resort.

This view of motivation has some significance for management. For example, if management has provided for the physiological and safety needs of its employees and in doing so has caused the motivational emphasis to move up to the social and ego needs, unless it provides opportunities for satisfying these needs, its employees feel deprivation which is reflected in their behaviour.

Herzberg's (1966) 'Motivation — Hygiene' theory sheds light on the productive process and, in this context he states: 'A hygiene environment prevents discontent with a job, but, cannot lead the individual beyond a minimal adjustment consisting of the absence of dissatisfaction. A positive 'happiness' seems to require some attainment of psychological growth.'

In most cases, the hygiene factors fail to provide for positive satisfaction because they cannot lead to this psychological growth. To feel that one has grown depends upon achievement in tasks that have meaning to the individual and since the hygiene factors do not relate to the task they are powerless to give such meaning to the individual.

The motivation-hygiene theory of job attitudes began with an in-depth interview study of over 200 engineers and accountants working in industry in Pittsburgh (1959). These interviews probed sequences of events in the working lives of the respondents to try and determine the factors that were involved in their feeling exceptionally happy and exceptionally unhappy with their jobs.

The findings of the study indicate that the factors involved in job satisfaction — motivators (satisfiers) — are separate and distinct from those that are involved in job dissatisfaction.

The Griffiths report sums up its philosophy on manpower and productivity in the NHS by indicating the views held that, 'the NHS is different from business in management terms, not least because the NHS is not concerned with the profit motive and must be judged by wider social standards which cannot be measured. These differences, the report states, can be greatly overstated. It continues, 'the clear similarities betweeen NHS and business management are much more important. The NHS does not have a profit motive, but it is enormously concerned with the control of standards' (paras.1 and 2, p.10).

What is the reality of productivity when discussed in the context of the delivery of health care?

The Griffiths inquiry makes it clear, both implicitly and explicitly, that productivity is central to ensuring a viable health service and, in this context, managers should concern themselves with such central issues as quality of service, meeting budgets, cost improvement, motivating and rewarding, and productivity. The point is also made that the presence of a general management process would be enormously important in ensuring that the same level of care could be delivered more efficiently at lower cost, or a superior service given at the same cost. Productivity is seen to be related to central issues such as setting precise management objectives with the clinical and economic evaluation of practices together with the devolution of responsiblity to units and, above all, implementing a general management process, i.e. 'providing the necessary leadership to capitalise on the existing level of expertise and dedication, as well as to stimulate initiative, urgency and vitality' (para.9, p.13). Griffiths sees performance review, based on management budgets, which involve all health care professionals, including clinicians, playing a vital part in improving performance and productivity, and, in this respect, strongly advises, 'real output measurement, against clearly stated management objectives and budgets, becoming a major concern of management at all levels (paras.6 and 7, p.12).

Regrettably, because of the lack of a clearly defined general management function (para.4, p.11), 'whether the NHS is meeting the needs of the patient, and the community, and can prove that it is doing so, is open to question' (para.2, p.10).

Even though health care professionals 'produce', i.e. the inputs to the health care system — staff experience, knowledge, skills, motivation and effort together with time, money, equipment and technology — is processed and hopefully ultimately 'produces' improved/rehabilitated patients and clients, the problems of indicating in a tangible and quantitative way productivity in the NHS is difficult, certainly when attempting to draw parallels with that of industry. The reasons for this include: the broad goals of the health care system 'are abstract, there is diffuse authority, a low interdependence of professionals' and an absence of, or few, indices or measures. This situation is clearly different from industry where there are 'concrete goals, formal authority, task interdependence and performance measures.

Finally, it has taken twelve years (since the publication of the *Grey Book*, DHSS, 1972) to again highlight the problems, inadequacies, non-use and/or non-availability of credible information to enable managers to make sound decisions; therefore, can it now be realistically assumed that health care professionals, at all levels of management, will acquire and use in a positive way the recommendations of Körner? More to the point, where relevant information is available, will it be used with skill and wisdom, to ensure that decisions on matters relating to patient care, manpower and planning, are soundly based and expedited with confidence; The answers to these questions can only be revealed retrospectively.

References

Barr, A. (1965) Measurement of Nursing Care. Doctorial Dissertation, Reading University
Beveridge, C. (1983) Limitation of Körner: Who is counting the human factor? *Health and Social Services Journal*, XCIII, no.4869, 1256–9
Bussey, A.L. (1983) Körner and the community health services in context. *Community Medicine*, 5(4), 327–9
Burns, T and Stalker, G.N. (1966) *The Management of Innovation*. Tavistock
Cameron, J. (1979) The Aberdeen Formula: Revision of nursing workload per patient as a basis for staffing. *Nursing Times, Occasional Paper*, 75(49). (Updating of the Aberdeen Findings 1974 and 1976)
DHSS (1972) Management Arrangements for the Reorganised National Health Service (Grey Book). HMSO, London
——— (1974) Organisation of Work in Hospitals (Third Report) (Cogwheel), HMSO, London
——— (1976) Sharing Resources for Health in England: Report of the Resource Allocation Working party (RAWP). HMSO, London
——— (1977) The Way Forward, HMSO, London
——— (1978) Management of Financial Resources in the National Health Service (Perrin). Royal Commission of the NHS Research paper no.2. HMSO, London
——— (1979) Information requirements on the National Health Service. DHSS, London
——— (1982) Health and Personal Social Services Statistics for England. HMSO, London
——— (1982) Nurse Manpower: Maintaining the Balance. DHSS, London
——— (1983a) Nurse Manpower: Planning: Approaches and Techniques. HMSO, London
——— Inquiry into the State of the National Health Service (Griffiths). DHSS, London
Gee, A. (1984) The Körner Report: New Directions for Midwives. *Nursing Times*, 80 (23), 48–50

Harries, C. (1984) How data can make a manager of you. *Health and Social Services Journal, XCIV*(4887), 291–2

Herzberg, F. (1966) *Motivation to Work.* Wiley, New York

Hurka, S.J. (1970) Career Orientation of Registered Nurses Working in Hospitals. *Hospital Administration*

HMSO (1972) Report of the Committee on Nursing (Briggs). Cmnd. no.5115, HMSO, London

——— (1979) Royal Commission on the National Health Service (Merrison). Cmnd.no.7615, HMSO, London

Jelinek, R.C. and Dennis, L.C. (1976) *A Review of Evaluaion of Nursing Productivity.* US Dept of Health, Education and Welfare

Keighley, T. (1984) College concern over Körner Group's Report on information. *Nursing Standard, 376,* 1

Kenny, J. *et al.* (1979) *Manpower Training and Development,* IPM, London

Lyons, T.F. (1970) Reducing nursing turnover, Hospitals, *JAHA*

Meyer, D. (1984) Manpower planning: an American Approach (GRASP). *Nursing Times,* 80(34), 52–4

NHS/DHSS (1982) Collection and Use of Information about Hospital Clinical Activity (First Report), HMSO, London

——— (1983) Community Health Services Information (Interim Report). HMSO, London

——— (1984a) Collection and Use of Information about Patient Transport Services (Second Report). HMSO, London

——— (1984b) Information on Paramedical Services and Maternity Services (Fourth Report). HMSO, London

——— (1984c) Collection and Use of Financial Information in the National Health Service (Sixth Report). HMSO, London

——— (1984d) Collection and Use of Information about Manpower in the Community (Third Report). HMSO, London

——— (1984e) Collection and Use of Information about Activity in Hospitals and in the Community (Fourth Report). HMSO, London

——— (1984f) Collection and Use of Information about Services for and in the Community in the National Health Service (Fifth Report). HMSO, London

RCN (1937) Interim Report of the Inter-Departmental Committee on Nursing (Athlone). RCN

——— (1943) Nursing Reconstruction committee (Horder). RCN

——— (1978) An Assessment of the State of Nursing in the National Health Service. RCN

Rhys-Hearn, C. (1974) Evaluation of patients' nursing needs: predictions of staffing. *Nursing Times Occasional Paper* published in four parts, 19 and 26 Sept. and 3 and 10 Oct

——— (1977) Nursing workload determination: Development and trials of a package. *Medical Information, 2,* 2

Scottish Home and Health Dept (1969) Nursing Workload per Patient as a Basis for Staffing. Report by the Work Study Dept of the North Eastern Regional Hospital Board, Scotland Scottish Health Service Studies, no.9 (Aberdeen Formula). SHHD, Edinburgh

Taylor, D. (1984) *Understanding the NHS in the 1980s.* OHE, London

Webster, X. (1984) Körner and the community. *Nursing Times, 80*(72), 51–2

Weiland, G.F. (Editor) (1981) Improving Health Care Management: Organization Development and Organization Change. Health Administration Press, Ann Arbor, Michigan

Wilson-Barnett, J. (1978) *Review of Patient-Nurse Dependency Studies.* Nursing Research Liaison Group. DHSS

Williams, J. (1983) Körner: Massaging the figures. *Health and Social Services Journal, XCIII* (4869), 1258–9

Yates, J. (1982) *Hospital Beds: A Problem for Diagnosis and Management.* Heineman Medical, London

Advised Further Reading

Abel, P.M. *et al.* (1976) Nursing manpower 1: A sound statistical base for policy making. *Nursing Times Occasional Paper, 72*(1), 1–4

Althaus, J.N. *et al.* (1982) Nursing staffing in a decentralised organisation. *Journal of Nursing Administration,* (part 1) *XII*(3), 34–9; (part 2) *XII*(4), 18–22

Ball, G. and Goldstone, L. (1984) Criteria for care. *Nursing Times, 80*(36), 55–8

Batten, J. (1982) *Expectations and Possibilities.* Addison-Wesley, New York

Bloor, J. (1984) Manpower planning: an American approach. *Nursing Times, 80*(45), 52–4

Bramham, J. (1982) *Practical Manpower Planning,* 3rd edn. Institute of Personnel Management (UK)

Brown, R. (1983) Unfair dismissal cases as pointers to management performance: the NHS experience. *Personnel Management (UK), 15*(7), 25–7

Christman, L. (1982) Can we measure quality? *Nursing Times, 78*(21), 867

Cobin, J. (1983) Combining computers with caring. *Nursing Times, 79*(41), 24–6

Cox, A. (1984) The Körner Report: What's in it for us? *Nursing Times, 80*(21), 47–9

DHSS (1972) Organisation of Medical Work in Hospitals (Second Report) (Cogwheel). HMSO, London

———— (1982) Nurse Manpower: Maintaining the Balance. HMSO, London

Fulmer, R.M. (1983) *The New Management.* Macmillan, New York

Godfrey, M. (1978) Job satisfaction — or should that be dissatisfaction? How nurses feel about nursing. *Nursing, 78, 8(4),* 90–102 April 1978 (Part 1)

Goldstone L.A. and Collier, M. (1982) Nursing Manpower Requirements: A framework for rational discussion. *Health Services Manpower Review, 8*(3), 6–9

Hersey, P. and Blanchard, K.H. (1982) *Management of Organizational Behaviour: Utilizing Human Resources.* Prentice-Hall, New Jersey

Hunt, J.W. (1981) *Managing People at Work: A Managers Guide to Behaviour in Organizations.* Pan Books, London

Hurka, J.S. (1972) Career Orientation of Registered Nurses working in Hospitals. Hospital Administration (Fall)

Jelinek, R.C., Haussman, R.K.D., Hegyvary, S.T, and Newman, J.F. (1976) A methodology for monitoring quality of nursing care. USHDEW Publication. Health Resources Administration, Bathesda, MD, 20014 (HRA), 76–25

Johnson, M. (1981) Managing the load. *Vocational Education, 56,* 42–4

Joiner, C. and Hafer, J.C. (1983) Reward preferences of nurses: A marketing concept viewpoint. *Journal of Health Care Marketing,3*(2), 19–26

Latham, G.P. (1981) *Increasing Productivity through Performance Appraisal.* Addison-Wesley, New York

Meltzer, H. and Nord, W.R. (eds) (1981) *Making Organizations Humane and Productive: A Handbook for Practitioners.* Wiley-Interscience. New York

Milligan, B. (1974) Patient-Nurse Dependency and Workload Index. King's Fund Project Paper no.2 (2nd edn)

Oates, J. (1984) Nursing implications of the first Korner report. *Nursing Times, 80*(21), 45–6

Pavett, C.M. (1983) Evaluation of the impact of feedback on performance and motivation. *Human Relations, 36*(7), 641–54

Rose, M.A. (1982) Factors affecting nurse supply and demand: An exploration. *Journal of Nursing Administration, XII*(2), 31–4

Rosenbaum, B.L. (1982) *How to Motivate Today's Workers: Motivational Models for Managers and Supervisors.* McGraw-Hill, New York

Wilson-Barnett, J. (1978) *Review of Patient-Nurse Dependency Studies.* Nursing Research

Liaison Group, DHSS

Wieland, G.F. (Editor) (1981) Improving Health Care Management: Organization Development and Organization Change. Health Administration Press, Ann Arbor, Michigan

Yura, H., Ozimek, D. and Walsh, M.B. (1981) *Nursing Leadership: Theory and Process*, 2nd edn. Appleton-Century-Crofts, New York

9 STRESS

Aims

The aims of this chapter are:

1. To examine the concept of stress.
2. To discuss the concept of 'burnout'.

Learning Objectives

The purpose of this chapter is to enable the reader to:

1. Appreciate the concept of stress.
2. To relate the phenomenon of burnout to health care professionals.

Stress and Burnout

Having examined the environment in which nursing takes place it is evident that many problems of an educational, social, emotional and manpower nature are highlighted which cause stress, to a greater or lesser extent. Recent work by O'Hanlon (1981) suggests that subjects showing high levels of performance under suboptimal conditions are most under stress.

Concept

Stress is the 'rate of wear-and-tear on the body caused by life' (Selye, 1956). Selye found that certain physiological changes occur in stress which he refers to as 'general adaptation syndrome' which is exemplified by 'the alarm reaction, stage of resistance and the stage of exhaustion'. The latter stage follows the continual exposure of the person to stress, possibly resulting in 'burnout'.

The physiological manifestations of stress are well chronicled and are due essentially to the release of adrenaline and nonadrenaline. They include a rapid pulse rate, usually raised blood pressure, increased respiration rate, increased muscular tension, increased urinary output, glycosuria, lack of concentration, agitation, restlessness and sweating.

Cause

The Briggs report underlines many causes of stress and anxiety among nurses. The main causes relate to the changing nature of medical care which has added to the strain imposed on nursing staff by causing anxiety about errors in medicine dosage, fears of machinery, the constant tension in intensive care units, the ethical problems of abortion, transplantation and resuscitation, uncertainty over rapid decisions to be made in times of crisis and the care of an increasing number of patients with mental disorders (para.581, p.176).

The sources of stress are many, and include major and/or frequent organisational changes, which affect staff and their jobs, i.e. working conditions, status, role, policies and procedures. This situation is exemplified in nursing and the NHS by changes precipitated through the Salmon, Mayston, Merrison and Griffiths (DHSS, 1983) reports, which by their frequency, and recommendations, made major demands on staff — physically, socially and emotionally. Also where there is a lack of relevant information about one's job, i.e. how to do it, its demands, and how well or otherwise it is being done, this can be a major source of stress, especially to junior and inexperienced nurses. (In this context job appraisal, performance evaluation together with subsequent regular feedback to staff is an important recipe for success.) Other sources of stress (many of which are associated with repeated change) include loss and/or diminished status of the person together with an absence of leadership, or new leadership, which may be more demanding on performance and productivity.

Professionals in the NHS have been subjected to repeated organisational change, over the past two decades, which was initiated through the agency of reports such as Salmon (1966), Mayston (1969), Cogwheel (1967, 1972, 1974), *Grey Book* (1972), Merrison (1979), Griffiths (1983). In addition to the effects of these changes, nurses have also had to cope with the changes which were precipitated through the EEC Nursing Directives (1977) and the *Nurses, Midwives and Health Visitors Act,* 1979.

Stress in nursing is accentuated by factors which include excessive reliance on untrained and unqualified staff, and this together with the increasing complexity and demands of medicine, greater patient expectations, a more rapid patient turnover and increased numbers of consultants has meant greater pressure on ward staff. The feeling of pressure is accentuated by the nature of nursing with its many and continuing physical, emotional and social demands. In addition, many nurses are young, nursing students may be away from home for the first time and additionally may have personal and domestic problems. The environment in which nurses work, by its very nature, contains varying levels of emotional stress and anxiety (Revans, 1964). In addition, patients, relatives, and indeed colleagues, make heavy emotional demands on nurses which may compound their own stress and anxiety. Also, new technology, and its effects on the management and care of the patient can cause stress and anxiety about the possibility of errors in drug administration and apprehension about the use and management of new machinery, as evidenced in the Briggs report. There are special tensions associated with working in intensive care units together with the many ethical/moral dilemmas which are associated with nurse decision making on issues as contraception, abortion, euthanasia, transplantation, dialysis and the resuscitation of patients. There may also be uncertainty over clinical decision-making, particularly those decisions that have to be taken urgently; the increased turnover of patients, the restriction on resources and 'the effort required by nurses to maintain standards of care, often against heavily weighted odds' (Hingley, 1984). The compound effect of these can produce an intolerable level of stress for the nurse, possibly leading to burnout.

Burnout

The subject of burnout is currently much discussed in nursing because of its disabling effects on nurses together with reducing their efficiency and effectiveness in delivering care.

The phenomenon of burnout has been highlighted recently, but the syndrome has been known for many years. Many writers in the USA have written on different aspects of burnout. Among the prominent are Shubin (1978), Harrison (1980), Johnson (1981), Paine (1981) and Wimbush (1983).

Burnout in the 1980s has become a major problem as well as posing a hazard to the nurse. Because of the stressful nature of their work, and frequently being devoid of a counselling service (there are only three accredited counsellors for nurses in the UK) nurses at all managerial levels, but particularly those at the front-line level, as well as those who are working in the more intensive wards or units, e.g. acute surgical, ITUs, CCUs, theatre and accident and emergency departments, are prime targets.

Concept

Essentially, burnout results from constant emotional pressure due to intense and prolonged involvement with people which results in draining one physically, emotionally, mentally and socially.

Burnout can be defined as:

> a state of mind that frequently afflicts individuals who work with other people (essentially but not exclusively in the helping professions) and who pour in much more than they get back from their clients, supervisors, and colleagues. It is accompanied by an array of symptoms that include, general malaise; emotional, physical and psychological fatigue; feelings of helplessness and hopelessness, and a lack of enthusiasm about work and even about life in general' (Pines, 1981).

Burnout in nursing is substantially due to factors such as the effects of unsocial hours, the demands of the job and high level of anxiety (Revans, 1964), which is present at operational level (ward or community), financial constraints and the inevitable lack of resources, high attrition rates together with absenteeism caused by 'sickness' which make additional demands on the remaining nurses, in their attempt to maintain standards and quality of care. Also, lack of support by colleagues and/or senior nurse managers and nurse educationists by not providing the necessary physical resources, lack of proper education and training in the knowledge and skills required by nurses to enable them to cope with new technology and other demands of their job, together with a noticeable lack of counselling to cope with nurses' problems, fears and anxieties and an insensitivity by colleagues and senior nurse managers to the real issues which confront the less experienced, less mature nurses particularly (though not exclusively) at operational level. These latter deficiencies were highlighted in an official report some five years ago (GNC Annual Report, 1979/80, p.18). Nowadays, nurses are charged with the responsibility of preventing these serious occurrences (UKCC *Code of Professional Conduct*, 1983, paras. 11 and 12).

Aggravating Factors

The causes of burnout in nurses, in addition to those already mentioned, include an intolerable workload resulting from too many patients/clients and too few trained nurses and a lack of supportive services. In addition, the complex and demanding nature of nursing and the unclear role of the nurse make it difficult, if not impossible, for nurses to meet the demands of their role. Also there is inadequate preparation for role and insufficient support and counselling to help nurses cope with their many clinical, educational, managerial and personal problems. There is a lack of real authority to permit nurses to make nursing-related decisions. Also there is an imbalance between the demands of the accountability and responsibility of nurses in relation to their authority to make those important nursing decisions. Therefore, these constant pressures to which nurses are subjected can lead to physical, mental and emotional exhaustion; ultimately producing the disabling condition of burnout.

The professions which are prone to burnout are the health care and teaching professions whose members are constantly 'giving' rather than 'getting'. These professionals are required to show empathy, be sensitive — tolerant and supporting of the needs and problems of others — and, as a result of their professional education and training, maintain a constant high standard of service.

Burnout is prominent in jobs which are 'emotionally taxing and with a client-centred orientation'. The syndrome of burnout is exemplified by physical exhaustion which includes weakness, loss of energy and unnatural, unusual and excessive fatigue. In this situation, even though the person is tired — exhausted — they may be unable to sleep. The physical presentation also may include generalised muscle tension as shown through the occurrence of headache and backache. As a direct consequence of this extreme exhaustion inevitably the person is prone to accidents and illness.

The emotional manifestations, especially those of depression, hopelessness, frustration and isolation, are precipitated by loss of the coping behaviours and in the extreme may lead to suicidal tendencies.

The mental and social signs of burnout include constant complaining about colleagues' work, and toward life in general: the person constantly demonstrates negative rather than positive attitudes. This is often coupled with feelings of inadequacy and inferiority. In essence, the person's finite energy has been expended producing psychological and physiological exhaustion which results in the inability of the person to fulfil their role.

Wimbush (1983) summarises the condition: 'The nurse avoids any emotional investment in her patients and professional objectivity vanishes'.

Effects

The effects of burnout are personal, organisational and economic. The effects on the nurse have already been discussed. However, the organisational and economic effects also are important.

In organisational terms, there may be attrition and absenteeism which in turn can produce both short-term and long-term manpower problems resulting in further stress. Additionally, because of staff shortage more nurses may need to be recruited, inducted and trained. Most important, because of the physical, social and emotional effects of burnout on the nurse the resulting effects on patient care can be far-reaching.

Conversely, in addition to its negative and destructive aspects, burnout may also have positive consequences for the person which include becoming aware of problems, examining demands imposed by the environment, learning about one's strengths and weaknesses and, as a result, reorganising one's priorities, identifying one's strengths as well as one's weaknesses. The positive effects may also present in identifying and developing coping behaviours. To optimise the positive effects, one must face reality by acknowledging that a problem/s exists and take the appropriate action to diffuse the situation.

Management

What can be done to prevent or correct the situation? What, in effect, is central to the management of stress?

The management of stress is the dual responsiblity of the individual and the organisation (Figure 9.1). Oskins (1979) found that ICI nurses choose, 'poor staffing patterns and working with high percentages of inexperienced 'floating' or pool nurses', the most stressful of situations.

The many causes of stress should be identified, prevented if possible and/or corrected. This includes addressing issues of manpower and, in this context, approaching in a positive manner the interviewing, selection, induction, education and training of staff which are as vital prerequisites to sound nurse performaance, close examination must be given to the definition of the nurse's role. Also factors which negate against job satisfaction, e.g. poor working conditions, lack of status, inadequate salary, inappropriate or inadequate education and training, lack of support, and diminished career prospects must be examined and corrected.

The organisation of nursing should be more realistic in terms of the needs and demands of nurses, more personalised and more humanised. The authority of nurses should relate to their level of responsibility and accountability. The demands of the nursing role should be balanced with the education and training of the nurse and the needs of patients and clients. Stress and anxiety prevention and/or alleviation methods should be developed. A counselling service, much discussed, should be readily available for all nurses together with ensuring regular discussion groups/workshops where nurses can discuss and externalise their stress.

Figure 9.1: Framework for Stress Management Planning

STRESS MANAGEMENT RESPONSIBILITY

	Individual	Organisation
Removal or avoidance	— Self awareness — Personal planning Time management Life/career planning — Supportive relationships	— Full two-way information flow — Identify and change stressor norms — Decision making, policy formulation, etc. — Reassignments
Immediate response	— Conflict skills — Influencing skills — Assertiveness skills — Problem-solving skills — Alter expectations — Supportive relationships	— Problem identification ↓ Diagnosis ↓ Problem solving — Employee education — Employee assistance programmes
Long-term protective	— Effective self management Nutrition Exercise Relaxation — Supportive relationships	— Actively support/ encourage good self management practices by organisation members — Integrative support groups, task forces, etc.

(left vertical axis label: Type of Response)

Source: Marshall and Cooper (1981). Reproduced by permission of Gower Publishing Co. Ltd.

A more comprehensive and positive approach to the education of nurses to inform them of the problems relating to stress should be undertaken as well as adopting a more positive psychological vetting of nurses on selection in an effort to screen those potentially prone to stress and anxiety.

In view of the damage to the nurse, patient, and to the organisation, resulting from intolerable levels of stress, both management and professionals have a major preventive role.

Management primarily must ensure the proper resourcing of jobs. It must also monitor staff to detect any unacceptable level of stress. In addition, it must support staff by all means available, i.e. by ensuring their proper induction, training and development, avoiding undue work demands, and ensuring adequate resources, and by counselling them when necessary. Most important, management must use the potential of their staff — their skills, knowledge and expertise, thus increasing their job satisfaction, security, performance and enabling their self-actualisation. Also, management must monitor the environment in which staff work. (*Code of Professional Conduct*, UKCC, 1983, paras, 4, 10 and 11).

Professional and statutory bodies together with management, must ensure that nurses' role, in terms of its responsibility, authority, accountability and autonomy is realistic, appropriate to the demands of the job and receives appropriate recognition by ensuring the education of nurses to meet its demands; together with affording role occupants appropriate status and conditions of service.

Even though the role of management is central to enabling nurses to cope with stress, of equal importance is the part played by individuals. In this respect, professionals must discuss and share problems and support their colleagues (*Code of Professional Conduct*, paras. 5, 11). Above all, they must develop coping behaviours — skills to enable them cope with high levels of stress.

In the following chapter the subject of interpersonal skills will be discussed, skills when developed, and used, e.g. communication and counselling, can help immeasurably in the reduction of stress.

References

DHSS (1969) Report of Working Party on Management Structure in the Local Authority Nursing Service (Mayston). HMSO, London
——— (1972) Management Arrangements for the Reorganised National Health Service (Grey Book). HMSO, London
——— (1972) Organisation of Medical Work in Hospitals (Second Report) (Cogwheel). HMSO, London
——— (1974) Organisation of Medical Work in Hospitasl (Third Report) (Cogwheel). HMSO, London
——— (1983) Inquiry into the State of the National Health Service (Griffiths). DHSS, London
EEC (1977) Legislation. *Official Journal of the European Communities, 20,* no.176
GNC (1979/80) Annual Report. GNC
Harrison, W.D. (1980) Role strain and burnout in child-protective social workers. *Social Service Review, 54,* 31–44
Hingley, P. (1984) Stress: Report of King Edward Hospitals Fund. *Nursing Standard, 352,* 3
HMSO (1972) Report of the Committee on Nursing (Briggs). Cmnd. no5115. HMSO, London

———— (1979) Royal Commission on the National Health Service (Merrison). Cmnd. no. 7615. HMSO, London

Johnson, M. (1981) Managing the load. *Vocational Education, 56*, 42–4

Marshall, J. and Cooper, C.L. (eds.) (1981) *Coping with Stress*. Gower, London

Ministry of Health and Scottish Home and Health Dept (1966) Report of the Committee on Senior Nursing Staff Structure (Salmon). HMSO, London

———— (1967) Reports of the Joint Working Party on the Organisation of Medical Work in Hospitals (Cogwheel). HMSO, London

Eliz II, *Nurses, Midwives and Health Visitors Act* 1979 (Chapter 36). HMSO, London

Oskins, S.L. (1979) Identification of situational stressors and coping methods by intensive care unit nurses. *Heart and Lung, 8*, 953–60

O'Hanlon, J.F. (1981) Boredom: Practical consequences and a theory. *Acta Psychologica, 49*, 53–82

Paine, W.S. (1981) The burnout phenomenon. *Vocational Education, 56*, 30–3

Pines, A.M. *et al.* (1981) *Burnout: From Tedium to Personal Growth*. Free Press. New York

Revans, R.W. (1964) *Standards for Morale: Cause and Effect in Hospitals*. Oxford University Press, Oxford

Selye, H. (1975) *Stress Without Distress*. Hodder and Stoughton, London

Shubin, S. (1978) Burnout: The professional hazard you face in nursing. *Nursing, 8*, 7

United Kingdom Central Council (1982) Professional Conduct (Consultative Paper). UKCC

———— (1982) Education and Training. UKCC

———— (1983) Code of Professional Conduct for Nurses, Midwives and Health Visitors. UKCC

Wimbush, F.B. (1983) Nurse burnout: Its effect on patient care. *Nursing Management*, Jan. pp.55–7

Advised Further Reading

Batten, J. (1981) *Expectations and Possibilities*. Addison-Wesley, New York

Brown, R. (1983) Unfair dismissal cases as pointers to management performance: The NHS experience. *Personnel Management (UK), 15*(7), 25–7

Cooper, C.L. (1981) *Psychology and Management*. Macmillan, New York

Duffy, E. (1962) Activation in N.S. Greenfield and R.A. Sternbach (eds.) *Handbook of Psychophysiology*. Holt, New York

Ellenburgh, F.C. (1981) More than a bandaid for burnout. *Clearing, 55*, 153–4

Joiner, C. and Hafer, J.C. (1983) Reward preferences of nurses: a marketing concept viewpoint. *Journal of Health Care Marketing, 3*(2), 19–26

Lader, M (1970) in O.W. Hill (ed.) *Modern Trends in Psychiatric Medicine*, no.2. Butterworths, London

Latham, G.P. (1981) *Increasing Productivity Through Performance Appraisal*. Addison-Wesley, New York

Meltzer, H. and Nord, W.R. (eds.) (1981) *Making Organizations Humane and Productive: A Handbook for Practitioners*. Wiley-Interscience, New York

Pavett, C.M. (1983) Evaluation of the impact of feedback on performance and motivation. *Human Relations, 36*(7), 641–54

Rose, M.A. (1982) Factors affecting nurses supply and demand: an exploration. *Journal of Nursing Administration, XII*(2), 31–4

Rosenbaum, B.L. (1982) *How to Motivate Today's Workers: Motivational Models for Managers and Supervisors*. McGraw-Hill, New York

Sanders, A.F. (1983) Towards a model of stress and human performance. *Acta Psychologia, 54*, 61–97

Yura, H. and Ozimek, D, and Walsh, M.B. (1981) *Nursing Leadership: Theory and Process*, 2nd edn. Appleton-Century-Crofts, New York

10 INTERPERSONAL SKILLS: RELEVANCE TO NURSE MANAGEMENT AND PATIENT CARE

Aims

The aims of this chapter are:

1. To discuss the particular inter-personal skills of communication, decision-making, leadership and counselling.
2. To examine the role of inter-personal skills in the management of:
   a. Patient care and
   b. Staff efficiency and effectiveness.

Learning Objectives

The purpose of this chapter is to enable the reader to:

1. Understand the nature of inter-personal skills.
2. Apply these skills to the care of the patient and the management of staff.

Inter-personal Competencies

Clues to the actual and/or potential demands made on nurses are identified in a report published five years ago (NSC, 1980). The report identifies spheres of training and education which could feature in management development programmes and, in this respect underlines the subjects of communication, committee work, interviewing, performance review, counselling, labour relations and ethics. It also underlines areas of legislation which relate to health and safety, drugs, abortion, transplants, mental health, confidentiality and the extended role of the nurse (paras.13, 14 and 15).

This chronicle of activities which trained nurses may encounter in the course of their job, inevitably will produce problems and will require decisions to be made. The successful handling of these problems require of nurses specific and substantial knowledge and skills.

For the hospital or community nursing service to function optimally and sensitively, i.e. to meet patient/client needs as well as to ensure the job-satisfaction of nurses, the performance of its activities requires certain inter-personal and inter-professional skills to be acquired, delivered and used. In this respect inter-personal competence can be deemed, 'the ability to control the responses of others, and which depends upon a variety of factors, both positive and negative, e.g. the learning of role prescriptions, role behaviours, intelligence and cue sensitivity; also, role rigidity (role-based) and general motivation' (Weinstein, 1969, Hurley, 1978).

Establishing a relationship between the quality of nurse performance and patient/client outcomes must always be the central goal of the nursing profession. For example, the more closely selection procedures can be related to ultimate criteria of care and of the job, 'the more useful they are to the nursing profession because they will reflect quality of professional performance' (Rezler and Stevens, 1978). Thorndike (1963) underlines, 'it is impossible to choose valid predictors of criteria when the criteria of success are ambiguous or imprecise'.

Inter-personal skills need to be developed and sustained to ensure the quality of inter-personal, i.e. nurse-patient/client, nurse-nurse, and nurse-professional, experiences.

Skills tend to differ from one management level in the NHS to another, e.g. nurses at all levels need to be able to work effectively with others as well as to communicate, lead, appraise and counsel staff. Also, at front-line level, the mastery of skills such as those requiring the ability to use essential knowledge and information, to use appropriate methods and techniques in the performance of one's job, are important to ensure the success of the care programme. Whereas at top-line management level skills including the ability to formulate policy, to plan and monitor activity and performance, are prerequisites to satisfactory and successful job performance. In addition, Mott (1972) includes a reference to 'a fourth requisite skill which emerges at top-management — institutional skill i.e. the ability to handle relationships with outside organisations and to create and formulate policy'.

Patients, clients, relatives and nurses 'need information when it is important, rather than at a time convenient to their superiors' (Revans, 1964).

In the work situation, nurses need to be motivated, be given leadership, be supported and counselled and have their work and progress assessed and appraised. However, as a prerequisite to establishing a suitable nursing workforce, proper interviewing, selection and induction procedures must be engaged.

Therefore, to enable nurses at all levels of nursing to perform optimally, many skills need to be acquired, developed and used.

Nurses at ward/community level are principally concerned with the care of the patient. The management of patients, in effecting this care, of necessity demands establishing a close rapport with the patients, and their families. The essence of this rapport — the nurse-patient nurse-relative relationship — is good communication.

The patient has needs which have to be understood and met: this understanding and meeting of needs relies substantially on the interaction of the patient with the nurse. Patients may have fears and anxieties which need to be clarified and allayed. Nurses, in the care of patients have to institute a care regime: to do so effectively requires the interaction of patients and guidance of their relatives. Central to the success of this interaction is the establishment of effective links with the patient and their relatives which can only be done substantially and effectively through conversation and observation.

In general terms, inter-personal skills include the important and indispensable qualities of respect for oneself and others, the ability to see things from another's point of view, confidence in oneself and in one's relationships with others, sensitivity towards the feelings, values, attitudes and ideas of others, the capacity to establish a firm set of values and, most important, acceptance of responsibility for one's actions and decisions.

In addition to personal and social skills, nurses need to acquire numeracy skills to help understand and cope with technical studies and projects; manipulative skills which are related to a range of practical tasks which they perform in the context of their job; and process skills, e.g. the ability to identify, formulate and tackle systematically and imaginatively new problems.

The nurse is responsible for much more than carrying out specific nursing procedures; nursing also helps 'to provide for those activities that make life more than a vegetative process, e.g. social intercourse, recreational and productive occupations' (WHO, 1966, para.3.1). To fulfil this vital and demanding role clearly nurses must master as a basic prerequisite to all others, the skills of communication.

Communication

Patients have many needs which must be met and satisfied. Among their needs is the need to be spoken and responded to in a way which shows them that they are important as well as being part of the group. Nurses and patients need other people in which to reflect, to share, their views, values and goals, understand their needs and to listen to their worries, fears and anxieties.

The ward or community climate, whether it is rigid or more relaxed, can enhance or block communication among staff and between staff, patients, clients and their relatives. Therefore, the attitudes shown by all staff who work at this operational level can affect the social-emotional climate, which if favourable may increase the anxiety of staff, ultimately hindering patient recovery (Revans, 1964). In this respect, communication is a prerequisite to the successful care of patients and clients in enabling their reassurance and lessening their anxiety.

Concept of Communication

In real life communication goes on in all directions all the time. However, in most organisations of which the National Health Service is an important example, communication tends to occur in three directions — downwards, upwards and horizontally. Some observers agree that communication occurs (in hierarchical organisations) downwards more often, and with more ease, than upwards: this is partly due to the resources, authority and influence of staff and their aptitude, ability and persistence to initiate and direct communication.

Communication skills enable people to communicate with each other through a variety of means, as in language (verbal), gesture (non-verbal), reading, writing, drawing, and more broadly through the creative arts.

The essence of good communication is getting the message to the right place/person at the right time, being understood as initially intended, and receiving a response. The reasons for communication are for personal, social and emotional reasons as well as to ensure information to enable people to do their job effectively.

'Anxiety is enhanced by uncertainty. Uncertainty is magnified by communication failure. The difficulties of communicating and of being communicated with are highlighted by unrealistic ideas of one's own role, knowledge, status and other features of the self' (Revans, 1964). Revans also states: 'Low morale particularly among nursing staff, tended to be associated with communication problems.'

As the job of the nurses increases in complexity, there is a corresponding need for more information. Miller (1960) emphasises: 'Only so much information can be processed by a system in a given time.' In this context, Wieland (1965) says: 'Higher information loads cause the system to break down, to show strain, or to engage in various coping mechanisms, which can produce relative inefficiency.' He also states that, 'as job complexity increases, supervisors will become overloaded and eventually management will feel pressures to create additional levels of supervision, thus reducing the span of control'.

Getting the message to the right person at the right time and receiving a response seems simple enough and yet this process in hospitals and in the community is commonly reported as a problem. Certainly it is now commonplace in the NHS and nursing to attribute organisational problems to 'failure of communication'. Basically, there are two main and very important reasons for communication in a hospital which have their roots in the social-emotional aspects of patients, clients and staff and the tasks, the job, being performed.

First, patients have a need to be noticed, spoken to, and generally responded to in a way which shows them that they are still part of a group and that their status and sensitivity primarily as human beings and secondarily as patients, is acknowledged. Essentially, patients need nurses in which to reflect, in order to live a full life, have their needs met, during their stay in hospital. The essence of this has its roots in the nurse-patient relationship which has as its centrepiece, communication.

Secondly, to carry out tasks efficiently, to perform one's job effectively, nurses must receive, and react to, information to enable them to perform their job with sensitivity, accuracy, effectiveness and efficiency.

In addition, the Griffiths Inquiry (DHSS, 1983) underlines the relevance of 'better communication as a prerequisite to ensuring a happier working environment and more satisfied staff' (para.27, p.20).

In the context of this environment, nurse managers have to get work done through other staff — nurses, other professionals and non-professionals. To effect this, they must pass on instructions and information: in effect they must communicate. In this situation, close rapport between staff at ward, hospital and the community operational level as well as at different levels of management, i.e. district, region and national levels, is clearly central to ensuring understanding, confidence and efficiency of staff in the day-to-day working and viability of the total organisation.

Communication in nursing can be viewed as being nurse-patient/client and nurse-relative orientated together with being of an intra-professional and inter-professional nature. It may be of an informal nature. The need for ensuring effective lines of communication is important in all hospital situations; but it is of special importance in large organisations, e.g. the NHS, where breakdown is likely because of the complexity of the organisational structure, i.e. a hierarchy of authority which, despite many attempts at its simplification, continues to have a complex committee structure and the extended line between front-line and top management.

Theory and Process of Communication

The basic rules of communication relate to such factors as what is said — this should be precise and clearly expressed; when it is said — an opportune moment should be chosen, when information can be clearly given and understood; how it is said — avoid voice inflections or mannerisms which indicate personal feelings.

Verbal communication is, 'a transactional process involving a cognitive sorting, selecting, and sending of symbols in such a way as to help a listener elicit from his own mind a meaning or response similar to that intended by the communicator'. Central to this process is the ability to perceive, receive and interpret verbal and non-verbal stimuli. Therefore, for communication to be effective, its reception and interpretation is dependent on many factors which include physiological (integrity of the senses and the CNS), psychological (absence of fear and bias), and environmental (absence of noise, interruptions), which to a greater or lesser degree, affect the integrity and viability of the stimulus. In addition, such factors as the complexity of the communication (its length and the nature of terminology used), its timing, lack of understanding of the communicator in relation to the target person/group, and/or the ability of the person to respond, if required, can enhance the integrity and the interpretation of the message.

The communication process is standard and embraces a cycle of events which include encoding, structuring the information at source, in a manner that enhances its transmission; decoding, relating and translating the information by the recipient, which is dependent on such factors as the integrity of the specialist part of the CNS and the extent or limitation of the knowledge and experience of the person.

Listening is a most essential part of the communication process not least because where the nurse fails to listen and pay attention to what the patient/client is saying, information might be lost, particularly emphasis that is placed on words or phrases which provide vital clues which otherwise may be missed and/or misinterpreted.

As well as the use of words as the common form of communication, additional factors in non-verbal form are constantly conveying information as to one's attitudes and feelings. These include such things as body contact, posture, physical closeness to others, and facial expression together with gestures, pauses, emphasis on omissions from speech and hesitations. Argyle (1972) sums up the situation of non-verbal communication: 'When a person is emotionally aroused he produces diffuse, apparently pointless, bodily movements. While a person speaks he moves his hands, body and head continuously, and these movements are closely associated with speech, and form part of the total communication.'

Impediments

Difficulties in transmitting information arise all the time. Even though this is more true of large, complex organisations, they can also affect small and less complex units. Essentially what happens is that impediments in the chain of communication can act as barriers to the acceptance, understanding or response (appropriate action) to the information. These impediments may be present in the source, origins of the communication, the method which is chosen to transmit the communication and in the person/group receiving communication. For example, the person sending the information may be seen to be biased, may be unpopular or even disliked by the target/group. Also there may be personality problems between the persons/groups involved. Similarly, the department from which the communication originates may be seen to be biased, may be distrusted or, as in the case of certain bureaucratic departments, a sea of information — often in the form of circulars, may (no doubt for sound reasons) be seen to be relevant at source; but, for many reasons, may not be met with similar enthusiasm by the potential target group. Additional impediments may reside in the communication itself in so far as its length, terminology — choice of words — mixing of many items of information and a general lack of clarity, precision and focus. Also, additional emotional factors may superimpose such as fear (consequences of the information), disinterest (not relevant to us) and dislike (dissatisfaction/disagreement with the source). Most important, the environment, and its staff for which the communication is intended, may in addition to being hostile to source have further difficulties in the form of overworked and anxious staff (no time, interest and/or energy to appreciate what is being said or written).

Because of these impediments, serious side-effects may result which can lead to a dislocation or a disruption of inter-professional and intra-professional integrity coupled with frustration, hostility and low morale of staff, predisposing to patient/client errors which may prove costly in terms of the well-being of patients and clients and the job satisfaction of staff.

Communication, as a prerequisite to quality care is indisputable, and, in this way, plays a vital role in helping patients/clients cope with their problems as well as enabling nurses make decisions about these problems.

Problems: Decisions: Concept

In organisational terms decision making embraces processes such as defining and setting goals, selecting options and defining a plan. The effective delivery of nursing care requires conscious planning of desired outcomes or goals; selecting a suitable option, the most satisfactory nursing approach; and most important, ensuring the effective use of resources to achieve the goals set.

Essentially, a decision is a commitment to take a course of action. A decision situation exists where there is an alternative choice. It embraces processes such as defining goals, selecting options and defining a plan (important in the nursing process).

Decisions have been divided by Lyden and his colleagues (1969) into four basic categories which include:

Strategic: key decisions which set the basic pattern of a plan.
Tactical: decisions relating to the detailed application of effort in the execution of a care idea, e.g. the planning of a care programme for a patient.
Programme: decisions which follow directly from the choice of strategy e.g. decisions relating to an aspect of the care plan. And
Policy: decisions which specify a decision, rule, or guide, indicating how certain situations are to be handled, e.g. decisions made by top management, region or district.

Fulmer (1978) says that there are meaningful differences between problem solving and decision making. He makes the distinction: 'problem solving is the process that allows the manager eventually to make a decision'. And, 'the best decision maker in the world is bound to fail if the wrong problem has been isolated to decide about'. Drucker (1975) expands this latter observation: 'The most common source of mistakes in management decisions is the emphasis on finding the right answer rather than the right question.'

A problem can be said to be present if a state of affairs is sufficiently unsatisfactory to stimulate somebody into taking action. Many writers on organisation have underlined the centrality of problem-solving to the manager. Revans (1972) states: 'To managers everywhere, not only in hospitals, the first object of attention is the immediate problem, the pressing problem. The manager's principal perception is not of objectives nor of resources, nor of good, nor of means, but of problems. In this context, Wieland (1980) refers to 'innovative roles - roles demanding problem-solving activities in which one attempts to bring about change; and which may place one in conflict with those who stand to profit from maintaining the status quo'.

Problems in the NHS and nursing are many and tend to be due to industrial growth, advances in technology and organisational change; therefore, what action can nurse managers take to help resolve problems, in an orderly, economic and scientific way?

Problem-solving in the NHS

A characteristic of the health service is that the provision of health care is often a team activity. Different skills have to be combined in various ways to meet the needs of individual patients; different professionals must come together to plan and co-ordinate their activities to meet complex objectives.

The teams are consensus bodies, i.e. their decisions need the agreement of the team managers. They share joint responsibility to the authority for preparing plans and making delegated planning and operational decisions.

However, 'teams may become ineffective through failure to initiate ideas and lack of drive to carry them through' (*Grey Book* (DHSS, 1972), para.1.27, p.17).

The Griffiths Report (DHSS, 1983) underlined the 'lack of clearly defined general management function throughout the NHS i.e. the responsibility drawn together in one person, at different levels of the organisation, for planning, implementation and control of performance' (para.4, p.11). The report also says: 'Consensus management can lead to lowest common denominator decisions and to long delays in the management process' to 'sharpen up the process of decision taking on matters where there is disagreement and on implementation, by identifying personal responsibility to ensure that speedy action is taken' (para.15, p.17).

Most important, the report emphasises, 'the present lack of a stringent approach and the current emphasis on functional management mean that staffing is too heavy and there is unnecessary delay in decisions being taken and activity carried out' (para.29, p.21).

Nurse managers, at all levels, constantly need to be sensitive to their immediate environment and be aware of potential problems. For example, all senior nurses need to be constantly aware of the principal aims and objectives of the organisation; ensure that practices and procedures

are up-to-date, valid and reliable and, most important, that effective
monitoring and controls are established and maintained so that variations, digressions and irregularities of practice can be readily appreciated.
Also, they need to be constantly vigilant and observant and when potential problem areas are discovered they should regard them in a positive
way, and analyse and resolve them.

Peter Drucker states: 'Whatever a manager does he does through making decisions. These decisions may be made as a matter of routine. Indeed, he may not even realise he is making them.'

Regrettably, the information relating to most problems and decisions
is not usually realistically 'labelled' and classified; all that may be
available is a collection of indistinct and sometimes confused information and ideas.

Because of the complexity of ward organisation and patient care,
together with new developments and advances in science in general, and
medical technology in particular, problems of a complex and varied
nature constantly confront the nurse. They include situations which relate
to the ethical issues, i.e. problems associated with abortion, euthanasia
and the use of life-support apparatus. In addition, they may arise from
organisational issues, e.g. problems of communication, inter-professional
and intra-professional relations, together with those problems which are
associated with the provision (or lack of) and the use of resources. Also,
bearing in mind the nature of the work that is undertaken at ward or
community level, that is caring for patients or clients, many problems,
which have their roots in patients'/clients' and staff emotions, may arise.
These are just some of the situations which confront the nurse in charge
of the ward, and which usually require prompt decisions.

The ability to make the right decision is important for many reasons.
For example, the wrong decision can be wasteful of resources and may
prove costly to the person and to the organisation. This is certainly true
of decisions taken within the ward. For that reason major decisions require careful planning, discussion and subsequent monitoring to ensure
the desired, intended, effect is achieved. This is the essence of the nursing
process which is a problem-solving (patients' problems) approach to
care.

Problem-solving Framework

A basic and somewhat general approach to decision-making is included
in the following outline. This approach includes many steps, the first
of which is deciding if a problem does exist. If a problem does exist

it is important, within reasonable limits to define it; this is done by collecting all information concerning the problem. Having collected the information critically appraise it: discard irrelevant facts and scrutinise further what, at this stage, appear to be relevant facts. Define and examine and evaluate alternatives — different but acceptable courses of action. Compare and contrast the advantages and the disadvantages of the preferred alternatives considering carefully all aspects of any proposed plan before a final approach is decided. Focus on the agreed final approach. Implement the plan. Observe and evaluate the consequences of the plan/decision so that further corrective action can be taken, if desired. Finally, ensure feedback to the person/group/organisation to obviate repetition of the problem.

A detailed framework for problem-solving, prepared by Gay and Cameron (1967) follows. The framework is based on a 5-point approach.

Identification of the Problem

In this stage the following issues need to be clarified by asking certain questions: Is there a problem? What information about the problem is available? Is this information indicative of a situation needing corrective action? In effect, does a problem present? If so, define the problem and identify its source — roots, i.e. whether technical, organisational or human. Endeavour to discover whether the problem is a symptom of a deeper cause. If so, a more extensive search will be required before proceeding further, to identify the true problem.

Preparation for Solution: Reality: Constraints

Rarely is a solution to a problem forthcoming and straightforward. Therefore, many questions must be asked in the important preamble, if the process is to succeed uneventfully; and if the final 'solution' is to be successful. For example, what are the limitations in the situation? e.g. time, money, equipment, manpower; is enough expertise available to be able to deal with the problem? Is there enough expertise about the system itself? Enough about the background? If not, can this information/advice be obtained from other sources? Is there sufficient authority to deal with the problem? If not, how can the necessary authority be obtained? Alternatively, should the problem be passed up to the appropriate authority level? Should the problem be delegated to a subordinate? Most important, is there bias in regard to the situation? the person?

The Solution

Thoroughness, in the first two phases, in terms of attention to detail, has an important bearing on the final result. The validity and reliability of the information obtained is central to the ultimate decision. Therefore, searching questions must be asked. For example, how can reports on the situation be evaluated? Are the sources of information reliable? Is there confirmation or conflict between different statements and/or reports? What inferences and judgements can be made from the factual statements? And, on the basis of the evidence now available, is there really a problem?

The general requirements of a successful problem-solving approach involve a combination of many factors which include:

1. The use of lateral thinking, expansion away from the problem. In essence, the ability to stand back and observe the whole problem. For example:

    A . . . . . . B, Problems as seen
    A . . . . B, Enlarge, move back in time
    A . . . . B, Enlarge, move forward
    A . . . . B, Optimum problem

2. Vertical thinking, which is both systematic and logical. In effect, this enables the manager to dig deeper into the problem.
3. An understanding of human needs. And,
4. An understanding of the technology.
5. Adopting a creative approach to help the generation of 'alternatives' which may help accelerate the finding of a solution.

Creativity To assist creativeness the problem-solver should maximise the space from which he may sample by pushing back any limiting boundaries as far as possible, e.g. eliminate the fictitious and real restrictions in so far as it is economically and organisationally justified and broaden one's own knowledge, particularly in the policy, practice or the technology in which the problem exists. Examine the alternatives in the context of acceptable solutions, to obtain as large and as diverse a group of ideas as time will allow. Search the space available by sampling as many areas as possible rather than allow ideas to cluster around one possible solution.

Creative, original, thinking is very important in problem solving. To enhance creative thinking use can be made of model building, a chart, mathematical formula or a formal verbal description. Brainstorming can also be used to produce a large number of ideas. Also, the process of synthesis which entails bridging things of a different nature and breaking problems into their component parts should be encouraged to assist the creation of possible alternatives.

The Search for Alternative Solutions to Problems. In producing alterntive solutions such factors as knowledge, the information available to draw on in generating ideas together with the effort exerted, how actively one seeks ideas and applies oneself to the task and the aptitude, the inherited qualities which contribute to creativeness are central. Also, for the method used for generating ideas, e.g. aids used and assistance sought, as well as change of the large number of alternative solutions to a problem, the particular ones a person will conceive depend on the extent upon change, i.e. the particular chain of ideas the person happens to pursue, or things one happens to see and hear during the period.

In the search for alternatives, starting from the present solution, the problem-solver generally proceeds from one point to another, which is known as the path of least resistance; the jump from one point to another tends to be relatively small, and the ideas tend to cluster around the present solution: real restrictions being least limiting and fictitious restrictions being most limiting. Many questions need to be posed. For example, what obstacles have to be overcome by the solution? What alternative solutions are there? How do the alternatives compare in respect of dealing with the major aspects of the problem, i.e. probable secondary problems created by introduction of the solution? Which is the best alternative? Does this best alternative leave some aspect of the problem unresolved? Will the best alternative create secondary problems? And, has the solution been checked against my definition of the problem?

Implementation of the Solution — Policy or Procedure: Decision-taking

The way the solution, policy, procedure or practice is implemented is central to remedying the problem. Questions that need to be asked by the manager, include: Have I selected the best person/s to implement the solution? Have I effectively communicated the necessary information in relation to the proposed solution? Is the necessary authority available to the person/s for the successful, smooth and uninhibited implementation of the new policy, procedure or practice?

Follow-up

Implementing the solution in the form of a policy, procedure or practice is, in itself, not enough to ensure success: the solution must be seen to be effective. If the initial problem was a symptom of a root cause, a decision must also be taken on how and when the root cause is tackled.

Finally, the manager must assess the value of the incident and its process of solution, to his own understanding, development and enlightenment as well as its meaningfulness in terms of organisational success.

Strategies for Decision-making

Strategies for decision-making are dependent on the nature of the manager, style of management and the problem presented. Managers may adopt different strategies to help in decision-making. These include:

1. *Autocratic:* In this style of management the manager makes the decision. Communication is one way. The manager attempts to enforce his decisions. This style has the obvious advantage of being economic in terms of time and other resources. However, staff may be aggrieved due to frustration of their ideas, skills and knowledge. It may lead to staff discontent and lack of job satisfaction.
2. *Democratic:* The manager allows his subordinates to make decisions. This has the disadvantage of being uneconomic in terms of time and other resources. Any decisions are based on consensus, a view frowned upon by Griffiths (para.15).

In McGregor's (1960) view a manager accepts certain assumptions about his subordinates. Theory X assumes the average person has an inherent dislike of work and will avoid it if he can; most people must therefore be coerced to make them work towards organisational objectives, and the average person prefers this. Managers, however, think of themselves as exceptions. Theory Y assumes people will use self-direction and self-control in the interest of objectives, and the average person prefers this.

The implications of these theories for decision-making are that in theory X, the manager is assumed to be the person best fitted to make decisions, whereas theory Y assumes that subordinates are capable of making at least some decisions.

Many decisions made by individuals or groups will affect others' daily lives. The extent and intensity of these effects may be insignificant; but if the decisions are wide-ranging, their influence may be substantial and long lasting for good or ill, on the person. Therefore, the responsibility for ensuring correct and just decisions in relation to persons, policies or procedures, is one about which all managers must strive. Organisational success together with individual success, job-satisfaction and happiness are substantially dependent on managers' success in achieving this goal.

The role of senior nurse as a decision-maker is linked to another important element in their role — that of leader.

Leadership

Leadership entails two sets of decisions: first, what should be done, i.e. the task and how it should be accomplished, and second, how subordinates are to be involved in task-related activities (Ullrich and Wieland, 1980). The concept of leadership is complex and much discussed. Leadership behaviour is essential to the manager and to the organisation in that 'it influences the ways which other organisational members behave' (Ullrich and Wieland, 1980).

Many prominent researchers throughout the years have attempted to analyse the elements of leadership, with varying degrees of success. Prominent among these researchers are Cooper (1966), Halpin (1966), Fiedler (1967), Likert (1967), Sergiovanni (1969), Mintzberg (1973), Argyris (1974) and Blake and Mouton (1964).

Leadership Behaviour: Concept: Perspectives

Early investigation into leadership behaviour concluded that individual qualities were predominant in the leader. Studies undertaken compared and contrasted leaders with non-leaders. These studies focused particularly on personality traits. In this context, Cartwright and Zander (1960) disagree with the trait theory and emphasise that leadership embraces actions by group members as 'setting group goals, building the cohesiveness of the group and improving the interactions among the members'. They conclude, 'leadership may be performed by one or many of the group'. However, some researchers suggest that the attributes of leadership are any or all of these personality characteristics that in any particular situation make it possible for a person either to contribute to a group goal or to be seen as doing so by other group members. Even though the ward/community sister or her deputy is the acknowledged, appointed, leader of the ward or in the community, a staff nurse, senior or enrolled nurse, or a senior student (given the appropriate situation and freedom to act), could demonstrate leadership behaviour, given the requisite professional expertise, skills, and most important, the encouragement and opportunity.

Despite isolating certain hallmarks, the concept of leadership still remains unclear. It is something of a paradox; where leadership exists, it may often remain 'unnoticed'. Yet, the absence of leadership from a group (ward, hospital, district or region) tends to create difficulties for the staff and for the organisation. In a major way lack of, or inappropriate, leadership can produce a state of uncertainty, due to lack of direction, motivation and personal security of staff. 'The organization looks to its head for guidance and motivation' (Mintzberg, 1973).

Leadership is a word that is used frequently but despite the fact that much research has been done on it and many views have been expressed, yet, there is little in the way of consensus about it. However, despite this uncertainty, there is agreement that leadership has something to do with influencing people, their behaviour, their willingness to follow. In essence, it entails manipulating the person or the group, causing them to follow. In this context, leadership implies a following. So why do people follow? Why do some people want to be led rather than want to lead? The answers to these questions even though not easy to find, invite certain assumptions about leadership behaviour. For example, leaders, apparently, do appear to have certain personality traits which make them attractive to others, particularly in respect of enabling them to lead, influence, persuade, or inspire others to follow — and, most important, to sustain group integrity in its cohesion, morale, and direction. Gibb (1954) states that the attributes of leadership are 'any or all of those personality characteristics that, in any particular situation, make it possible for a person either to contribute to achievement of a group goal or to be seen doing so by other group members'. Argyle (1958) in a study of groups of manual workers also found that groups under certain supervisors may produce 50 per cent more work than under other supervisors. Blake and Mouton (1964) formulated a 'Managerial Grid' (Figure 10.1) which gives some clues to leadership elements in that it depicts two dimensions of leadership, i.e. the concern of the leader for task (production) and/or concern for people (staff satisfaction).

According to Blake and Mouton, a manager's job is to perfect a culture, central to which aim is to promote and sustain efficient performance of highest quality and quantity which fosters and utilises creativity and stimulates enthusiasm for effort, experimentation and change. The character of leadership is a significant factor in the organisation's success or failure. Strong and effective leadership creates high involvement and shared commitment which stimulates people to overcome obstacles to achieving maximum results. The Managerial Grid provides a framework for learning some of this knowledge. It offers some guidelines for fitting this learning to concrete use in managing production through people.

Figure 10.1: The Managerial Grid

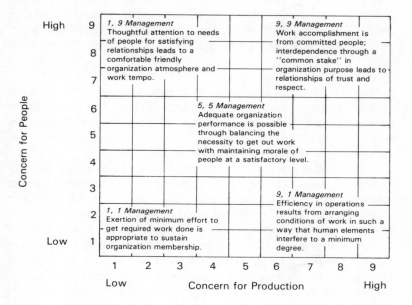

Source: Robert R. Blake and Jane Strygley Mouton (1984) The Managerial Grid. Gulf Publishing, Houston, p. 12. Reproduced by permission.

The grid provides a framework that embodies two concepts (concerns): concern for production and concern for people. At the top left corner of the grid the 1,9 style indicates a minimum of concern for production but maximum concern for people. Conversely, in the lower right corner is 9,1 style which indicates a maximum concern for production and a minimum for human aspects. In the upper right corner is the 9,9 style where concern for both people and production integrate. In the centre is the 5,5 style which indicates an intermediate (middle of the road) amount of both kinds of concern. In a 9-point system such as employed in the grid, 81 mixtures of these two concerns could be conceived. The character of 'concern' at different grid positions differs even though the degree may be the same; e.g. when high concern for people is coupled with a low concern for production, the type of concern for people expressed (that people be 'happy') is different from the type of high concern for people shown when a high concern for production is also evident, i.e. that people be involved in the work and strive to contribute organisation purpose. Finally, each of the five theories depicted in the grid defines a different set of assumptions regarding how individuals orientate themselves for managing situations of production that involve people. Each constitutes an alternative way of thinking and can be applied for analysing how a given situation is being or might be managed.

Leadership Style

Fielder (1967) suggests in order for a leader of a formal group to be effective he must 'maintain a certain amount of psychological distance between himself and the group'. He also suggests that 'the style of leadership for any given situation depends on leader-member relations, task structure and the position and power of the leader.

The central debate on leadership has tended to centre on leadership 'style'. Basically styles of leadership are of two main types, those that relate to people and those that relate to the task (Bowers and Seashore, 1966). Sergiovanni *et al.* (1969) say that 'it-depends' variables affect leadership style, i.e. one style of leadership may be effective in one situation and with one group but not in another situation or group. In essence, the style of leadership depends on the situation that exists in any given time. Secord and Backman (1974) suggest the current approach to leadership emphasises leadership behaviour, i.e. those actions that are functionally related either to goal achievement or to the maintenance and strengthening of the group. In this way, leadership frequently becomes specialised taking different forms or roles. One of these, the task role, requires the person to organise and direct the activities of members so that they are focused on achieving group goals with maximum efficiency. Strongman (1979) identifies factors characteristic of the leader which include, 'personal, the person talks more and participates more in the group and recovers from interruption faster, and interaction, the person initiates and maintains interaction, expansiveness'.

Over the years there has been considerable investment in research into leadership, yet, suprisingly, this has yielded little in the way of positive outcomes. For example, the debate on whether leaders are born, i.e. whether there are innate qualities — attitudes and abilities which are particular to the leader — continues unceasing. Or, are leaders made? The view that leaders are born still has some merit. Experience and practice in human relations, knowing how people act, respond, are motivated and are encouraged to be productive, are obvious elements of importance to the leader and, to some extent, can be acquired and developed through training and experience.

Experience in management is clearly, important to leaders in order to enable them to relate, interrelate and/or reshape conventions and events. In this way, education in management theory, particularly in the applied social sciences, is vital to enable managers to understand their role and functions fully — central to which is to help people to learn — change their behaviour and to understand why people behave in a particular way. However, due to the limited information available on leadership knowledge and leadership skills, together with being unable to identify the ideal characteristics of the leader and the nature of leadership, it becomes difficult to train and develop people, to provide them with a suitable knowledge base and develop appropriate leadership skills.

The contingency theory of leadership which is proven over the centuries, especially where national events of a serious nature occur, e.g. war, and demand a person of special ability to lead, is based on the idea that the 'situation' produces the leader.

There are different 'shades', styles of leadership; some work in one situation, others do not. Different work situations, because of the nature of staff and their work, require different leadership approaches. For example, some work situations require autocratic approach (telling) and some require a democratic approach (bringing out). Styles vary with the situation and may include accepting views or changing views (behaviour). In some situations, the totality of views may be greater than one's own. Each situation may be different and, in this respect, the skill of the leader is vital to judge the situation in so far as adopting the appropriate leadership style.

Leadership style can be identified by using a questionnaire, which takes account of leadership characteristics, the Leader Behaviour Description Questionnaire (Halpin, 1966). The questionnaire is in two parts; the first part relates to 'Initating Structure' and includes 15 items. In this section, which is based on a five-point scale, the respondent ticks one of five categories — A (always); O (often); Occ (occasionally); S (seldom); N (never), an example of which is: 'He makes his attitudes clear to staff: A, O, Occ, S, N'. The second part 'Consideration', also includes 15 items, which include the following example: 'He acts without consulting staff'. The original questionnaire by Halpin was adapted by Sergiovanni and his colleagues, and can be used to find one's leadership 'style'. There are 35 items which describe different aspects of leadership behaviour. The respondent circles each item according to the way he would be most likely to act as leader of a group — A (always); F (frequently); O (occasionally); S (seldom); N (never); e.g. 'A, F, O, S, N, — would allow members complete freedom in their work'. The respondent checks his score on two dimensions to find the style of leadership, Concern for Task (T) and Concern for People (P).

On analysis, a score on the 'T' dimension, concern for task, indicates an autocratic style of leadership; a score on the 'P' dimension, comcern for people, indicates a *laissez-faire* style of leadership. A balancing of 'T' and 'P' indicates shared leadership.

Value of Different Styles

Clearly, adopting an autocratic style may be both harmful and inefficient for the staff and for the organisation in so far as it may inhibit and constrain staff in the effective performance of their job, and reduce their job satisfaction and stunt their self-actualisation. Conversely, adopting a democratic style, when the work situation is better suited to an autocratic style, may have the undesired effect of accentuating stress where staff may be either unwilling or incapable of coping with added responsibility.

Role of Leader

The role of the leader is essentially threefold which includes acknowledgement of the individual, the group and group and/or organisational goals. All three overlap. The goals relate to the tasks of the organisation, what the group or the team are doing. This includes the selection and definition of goals and tasks as well as ensuring that they are agreed and/or known by the group. The leader must ensure that there is consent, i.e. the need to say 'agree', and that there is true consensus. Consensus may be indicated for many reasons which include the inability of members to articulate; or members may be 'fed-up'.

The leader must also ensure that group morale as well as individual morale is maintained. This is done by respecting individual sensitivity, acknowledging and, when possible, utilising the views and suggestions of the group. In addition the leader must communicate with staff, counsel them as required, support them and, most important, provide a working environment which is secure and which utilises their skill and expertise, optimally.

In the team situation the leader must acknowledge the need to provide support for the team, to ensure the goals of the organisation are met and the tasks of the organisation are accomplished. For success there needs to occur ossification between the task/s to be accomplished and the support made available. Finally, even though education plays an important role in helping the leader to understand the real issues involved in 'managing' people, ensuring that they develop and perform effectively, efficiently and with confidence, in the final analysis leadership is something you have to do, to find out for yourself. In this context, knowing yourself, understanding what others are trying to do, and most important, being able to assess with accuracy what others think of you, are important prerequisites to leadership.

Implications of Leadership for Nurses

What are the implications of leadership for the nursing profession? Clearly, to ensure its viability and integrity in the realisation of its goals the profession must foster effective leadership, that is initiate new ideas, motivate staff, establish effective communication systems, persuade, understand and involve nurses to the level required to enable them to function effectively in their job. The profession, through proper selection, education, training and development of staff, must secure a system which will ensure the nurturing of its members so that they are able to lead the profession at all levels, more especially nowadays with the exacting demands of complex organisational and discontinous change which is highlighted by new technology, together with greater social and educational demands.

It is the view of the Griffiths Inquiry, that the general manager, in addition to other functions, is to be responsible for the leadership of the authority's management team and in this respect will have to ensure (among other things) the provision of proper advice. (HC(84)13, para.4.3). The leadership role is seen as a driving force to ensure direct and personal responsibility for developing management plans, securing their implementation and monitoring achievement as well as being central to capitalising on existing high levels of expertise and dedication of staff in stimulating their initiative, urgency and vitality.

In this demanding situation the role of the teacher/manager is great and must include motivating, encouraging and guiding their students and staff to enable them to readily appreciate and realise agreed objectives — organisationally, clinically and educationally. In doing so, they must effect staff and student motivation by encouraging and fostering a general willingness to enter a work and/or learning situation and decide appropriate strategies to achieve the objectives set (Griffiths, para. 9 (a) (c)). In addition, they must assess balance and take cognisance of the needs of the staff and students and the demands of the work and/or learning environment (*Code of Professional Conduct*, UKCC, 1984, para.11). The nurse teacher/manager must distinguish between intrinsic motivation which is imposed by external agencies or conditions on the task or the student. The work must be arranged to enable staff and nursing students to achieve and have their status and worthwhileness recognised, and in this way help them to professional maturity.

In nursing the teacher and the manager intentionally or incidentally must lead, motivate, encourage, support, counsel and guide students so that they work and learn in a socially, psychologically and educationally secure environment and thus realise agreed goals. The teacher/manager according to Davies (1967) 'must balance two factors, that is, the need of the student in a learning situation, together with the demands of the learning situation, and the identified learning task. In this way they must strive to ensure more effective task involvement together with encouraging and enabling a productive learning outcome.' This approach is imperative to enable trained nurses and nursing students not only to achieve their goals, but, most important, to realise their aspirations in their quest for self-actualisation.

Interviewing: Concept

Interaction between people is taking place most of the time. However, it becomes necessary from time to time to formalise this interaction. This situation is exemplified in the 'interview'.

There are many forms of interview and they include those of selection, appraisal, termination and counselling. All of these forms relate to staff. However, in addition, there is the 'patient interview' now much discussed in the context of the nursing process and which is the chief method available to nurses by which information can be obtained from patients and their relatives, to enable them establish a framework for the nursing care plan.

Staff are the most important as well as being the most expensive (costwise) resource. The manager is concerned with the effective and the efficient use of the resources. The total cost of employing nurses is high, in terms of salary as well as the employment of other people and materials to provide them with many services. Therefore, the proper selection of staff must be viewed by managers as a vital prerequisite to organisational efficiency.

The way the health service in general and hospitals in particular select, develop, support and monitor individual performance really matters in terms of ensuring the happiness and self-actualisation of the person (job-satisfaction and career progression) as well as ensuring the continuing integrity and viability of the organisation by employing competent staff. With this in mind, nurse managers and nurse educationists have an important part to play in selecting the right staff, ensuring their proper development, and realising and using their professional and mangerial and other talents (Griffiths (DHSS, 1983), paras. 1, 3 and 9).

The interview can be of an informal nature, as in the exchange of information through discussion, or it may be formal as a prelude to selection (selection interview); counselling (counselling interview) when dealing with a problem; when reviewing performance (performance review or appraisal interview); and on termination of employment (termination interview) to isolate the reason for leaving.

Selection

What should interviewers know? To optimise the effect of the interview, which can be limited because of time constraint, a numerically large interview panel, lack of preparation by interviewers, and lack of briefing by panel co-ordinators, key areas need to be considered in advance.

The first task involved in filling a position is to define the job. This is known as job analysis and can be done on an eight-point scale which includes job title and grade together with the duties, responsibilities, working conditions, social aspects, salary and prospects of the potential employee. In addition to this, consideration must be given to what will be required from the successful applicant; this can be effected through a job-description, which can be denoted on a nine-point scale and which includes personal information, education, work experience (essential and preferred), mental ability, physique, social role, emotional stability, initiative and motivation.

Prior to the interview, discussion must take place with the nominated chairman and members of the interviewing panel to enable them to decide the areas which need special emphasis during the interview.

Immediately prior to the interview, it must be ensured that no interruptions are likely to occur during the procedure and so potentially disabling and disadvantaging candidates. A comfortable seat should be available and an advantageous position in the room for the candidate to obviate putting them at a psychological disadvantage.

Conducting the Interview

In the course of the interview one must consider the job, essential and preferred experience, together with entry and statutory qualifications required. Also, if there is an age limit, either minimum or maximum, this must also be considered. Links in the candidate's information should be found to enable the interview to flow by leading into different aspects which require to be discussed. (Long pauses during an interview are disruptive to the candidate and members of the interviewing panel.) Any unexplained gaps in the information need to be explained. The panel should endeavour to avoid asking a question which will produce a negative or positive response, that is 'yes' 'no'. They should endeavour to be objective. Avoid bias. Show interest in what the candidate is saying by following up with further questions. Avoid situations which make the candidate uneasy. On completion of questions by the panel, the candidate should be invited to ask questions or get clarification of points which relate to the job. The panel must inform candidates of the final decision, and offer counselling to unsuccessful candidates if deemed to be appropriate and useful.

Having interviewed and selected the candidate, the next important aspect in their personal development and career direction is to ensure their induction into the organisation. This must be followed by regular monitoring of their progress, in the work situation, ensuring counselling as and when required, and appraising their work performance.

Appraisal

To appraise effectively, one needs to know one's staff individually.

What are the merits on appraisal system? Who should be appraised? By whom? How often? What useful information should the exercise yield? Do managers know sufficient about the staff, their development, expertise, 'pressures', the 'real' self to be able to appraise objectively? Has the average nurse manager (at lower management levels) sufficient time, training expertise and courage to do this job objectively?

What is the purpose, and indeed the value, of a system of appraisal for nurses? What, in fact, are the objectives?

The principal objectives include:

1. To provide, in a systematic way, for performance review and to keep senior officers informed of this, and of nurses' potential for advancement.
2. To provide a specific opportunity for counselling and for the nurse to discuss her progress and to help resolve any difficulties which impede good nursing or management.
3. To identify any need for further training or broadening of experience. To enable more reliable and informative references to be provided.

Merit. What is the merit of a good system of appraisal? Certainly it is important objectively and systematically to review performance, to identify needs and to suggest ways of improving performance. This, clearly, should be done regularly so that mistakes are put right. Also, in this context, counselling is vital if done by the right person at the right time and in the correct setting, otherwise it can be a useless and a time-consuming — even dangerous — exercise.

Performance Appraisal. What, in fact, is performance appraisal? Essentially it is the examination of all facets of the individual, including task performance.

Performance appraisal in nursing raises some important questions: What degree of consultation should there be between those who design the scheme, those who operate it and those who are subject to it, about the type of scheme, design of forms and procedures? If present performance is to be assessed, how can it be measured — against targets set by a manager? A manager and the subordinate? By visible personal qualities, e.g. drive, initiative, etc.,? By critical incidents, or in other ways? If potential is being assessed, can this be done realistically? Are there reliable indicators to future success? Who is the person most likely to be able to assess present and future performance? How, if at all, does it link with the promotion system?

Appraisal Interview

One should make clear the purpose of the interview, which is to help the nurses project themselves.

It is wise to discuss first the job situation, i.e. the nurse's own job and how it fits into the system (and also possible improvements in the job or set-up, if they do not seem satisfactory). This is a better ice-breaking topic than to discuss efficiency. Cover the nurse's normal duties and responsibilities, and special job during the year, what he/she likes most and least about the work, relationships with his colleagues, superior and subordinates.

At this point, if there have been failures in performance, as well as successes, they must be mentioned frankly. This will not necessarily be pleasant, and the interviewer may be tempted to play down these failures. If this were done, however, the interview would fail in its purpose. In addition, the following would need to be discussed: action taken during the year to aid the nurse's development; their interests and motivation, aspirations and plans for the future.

By the end of the interview, the nurse should be quite clear as to how they stand. The interview should be terminated, if possible, with positive suggestions. In any case, ask them if there is anything else *they* wish to mention.

Philosophy and Use of the Interview

The National Staff Committee (N & W), in its concern for ensuring a high standard of nursing appointments, has issued useful guidelines to secure good practice in the course of selecting and appointing candidates to NHS posts.

The guidelines advise; as a prelude to the selection interview, use should be make of the termination interview with the present post occupant to identify reasons for leaving, and to establish, if possible, any underlying organisational problems. The termination interview is seen as being important to assist with the review of key tasks and responsibilities of the post as well as to help the personnel specification for the future post holder. It advises, in the present climate of manpower and economic problems, a conscious decision should be made as to the usefulness and relevance to the organisation of the present post: should it continue? If the post is to continue, then attention should be directed to the potential post occupant: what sort of person is required? The strategies and cost of advertising should be examined, agreed, effected, and most important, monitored.

On receipt of the requisite number of applications, determine a shortlist of candidates, using an appropriate panel (usually two or three persons with a central interest in the post and in personnel), establish the main interviewing panel comprising external assessors as required by procedure, obtain references and notify candidates of date, time, place and nature of the interview (individual or group). On conclusion of the interview the successful candidate should be notified and unsuccessful candidates should be offered, if thought to be relevant, post-interview counselling. To ensure a 'settling-in' period, during which the person is introduced to the organisation, an induction programme should be planned.

Limitations of the Interview as a Means of Selection

In the interview situation there is a tendency to emphasise the job, its nature, requirements and demands rather than to focus on the person, their personality and particularly the abilities needed, together with the potential of the interviewee to do the job efficiently and effectively. Frequently, emphasis on the job, job-analysis or on the task, is done to isolate the skills and knowledge thought to be central to the performance of the job successfully. However, certain commentators (Dinham and Summerhill, 1979) point out the limitations of this approach in so far that it suggests the jobs consist of clearly defined tasks which remain constant; this approach, wrongly, assumes a static view of performance. Also, it is limited to the extent that the effective performance of most jobs requires intellectual, emotional and social abilities in addition to defined tasks. The tendency to place emphasis on formal qualifications rather than on intellectual qualities is basically one of difficulty in identifying and assessing the latter.

Despite the criticisms and the alleged shortcomings of the interview as a device of selection, it is difficult to find a suitable alternative. However, to compensate for the limitations of the interview, and to help establish a fuller profile of the interviewee, additional devices such as aptitude and ability tests may be entertained.

Nurse-Patient/Relative Interview

The nursing interview has important functions which include collecting information and effecting a channel of communication between the patient, the nurse and other health care professionals. Obviously, in this situation, the nurse needs to assess the nature and relevance of the information obtained; but, most important, to note any inflections or emphasis the patient may put on certain statements which denote undue apprehension, fear or anxiety. The channelling of information needs to be a two-way process, i.e. receiving information from the patient to shed light on his physical, social and emotional state, his needs, worries and aspirations, and giving information to the patient on ward procedure, in relation to his care plan, and generally on any related nursing/medical care matters where achieving patients'/clients' co-operation is important.

The interview is an essential instrument in establishing the nurse-patient relationship as it enables the nurse to observe and respond to patients'/clients' verbal and non-verbal responses, to listen and to record data. It enables the nurse to 'draw' out patients'/clients' feelings so that she can become aware of their needs' (Murray, 1980).

Counselling

In addition to their many functions from time-to-time nurse managers may also (most probably will) have to counsel staff and students, either as a preventive measure or when they present with problems. Staff/student problems may have different and many roots and may range from academic, work, social (relationships), emotional (stress-burnout) and domestic. The precipitating causes relating to staff/student problems are many, and include the increasing complexity of medicine and the reduced length of stay of patients in hospital which cause an increase in pressure, of a significant nature, for nurses and midwives.

Anxiety, fear and stress in nursing have also many and varied roots which relate to the nurse's role, its lack of clarity, elements, responsibility, degree of authority and autonomy and its level of accountability. In addition, in relation to the job of the nurse, such things as the status afforded by society, the rewards offered in the way of salary and conditions of employment together with the preparation of nurses, including the nature of their education and training — professional and managerial — career prospects and the level of support afforded can have an effect on the degree and duration of stress produced. Other factors which affect stress include the nature of inter-professional and intra-professional relations, organisational structure and climate — particularly the climate of industrial relations. Clearly, also nurses' activities outside the work situation will have an effect. In this context, the degree of stress encountered in their work may be compounded by problems and conflicts arising from their social-domestic environment.

Nurse managers, at all levels of management, must learn to spot the behaviour clues of their staff, who, very often, may be in a state of frustration, or be showing signs of apprehension, uncertainty and anxiety; and act promptly by giving them support and encouragement — or by taking whatever measures are deemed to be necessary, to obviate or reduce these states. In this respect, managers must acknowledge the sensitivity and needs of their staff and ensure that everything possible is done to promote their personal harmony, satisfaction and fulfilment. The strengths, and the weaknesses, of staff must be identified and acknowledged and any necessary adjustments to workload made as well as affording them support. This support may be usefully initiated through the provision of a formal counselling service to encourage staff to come to terms with their problems and difficulties by getting to know themselves, their make-up, strengths and weaknesses.

Causes for Concern

Rogers (1974) states: 'Below the level of the problem situation about which the individual is complaining, lies a search': a search which has as a central point the desire of the person to know himself. In this respect, Rogers suggests that each person is asking: 'Who am I, really? How can I get in touch with this real self, underlying surface behaviour; How can I become myself?'

The changing nature of medical care as well as repeated changes in the NHS structure has added to the strain imposed on nurses. In addition, the constant tension in ITUs, the ethical problems of abortion, transplantation, resuscitation and euthanasia, uncertainty over rapid decisions to be made in times of crisis, the care of an increasing number of patients with major disorders, anxieties about errors in drug dosage and the constant tension while attempting against heavy odds — particularly financial cutbacks and manpower shortages — to maintain acceptable standards of care, produce stress of an unacceptable level, in nursing. Other aspects of nursing care which make particular demands upon nursing staff include the treatment of drug addiction, care of the elderly, care of the young chronic sick and care of the terminally ill. These facts were highlighted by the Briggs Committee in 1972 (para.581, p.176) as producing added strain on nursing staff.

In addition, nurses like other people may sometimes feel rejected and abandoned — even by their nursing colleagues, and their bosses, (GNC Annual Report, 1979/80). This rejection and apparent abandoment may cause them bewilderment, anger and distress.

In a paper presented to an International Conference (Crawley, 1982, 1983) the situations which give rise to stress, distress, anxiety and depression in nurses were seen to be related to the bereavement of a close relative which, one or two years later, caused the nurse to present with 'difficulties at work, sudden or developing intolerance of certain patients, exhaustion, irritability, anxiety, prolonged distress over the death of patients and threat of disciplinary action because of a drop in standards'.

Mrs Crawley emphasises that the most common causes of concern in nurses include role conflict, removal of traditional defences against anxiety and projection and identification. She puts forward the thesis that, 'nurses develop a system for relating to a colleague who is also a patient.' Nurses evolve systems to provide 'a safety barrier between themselves and their own emotional and physical pain'. This barrier makes it possible for them 'to function without having to confront and resolve much of the conflict which is provoked by their stressful work'.

Clearly, in this situation, there is a need for a service (staff welfare) which would enable nurses to discuss, to externalise their feelings, stress and anxiety in a controlled environment and with confidence.

The Briggs Committee (HMSO, 1972) underlined that counselling is an important function, not just in relation to staff welfare, but in order to achieve an improved standard of care. In saying this the committee has in mind the views expressed by Revans (1959) who found evidence to suggest that 'hospitals able to retain their staff are also able to discharge their patients more rapidly and directly connected recovery rates of patients with nursing staff morale' (para.582, p.176).

However, despite the advice of Briggs, to date only *four* accredited counsellors for nurses exist in the UK (RCN, 1984).

The RCN Counselling Help and Advice Together (CHAT) is a service for nurses which enables them to discuss things that are important to them and which are causing them distress. The service which is based at the RCN in London has *two* counsellors who travel to see clients or to visit nurses in prison or at home. Clearly, despite the excellent work done, this service, with the best intentions, can only deal in a superficial way with the problems — and the results of those problems on nurses.

The demands on trained nurses and nursing students in addition to those already mentioned, include concentrated learning of skills and knowledge frequently in new areas which make additional intellectual demands. Also, the stress associated with having to study and work in an environment which is anxiety-charged as well as the stress which is associated with one's own personal social-emotional development, e.g. students' newly found independence, testing new roles and making new relationships. In addition, issues relating to making personal and career choices as well as the problems produced by constant 'giving' of oneself, intellectually, socially and emotionally to the patient, leads to a drain of one's social and emotional funds, which, at its extreme, produces burnout.

The pressures on trained nurses may be similar but, additionally, are particularly associated with coming to terms with the demands of their profession particularly in the domains of increased responsibility and accountability, frequently in the absence of the necessary authority and autonomy, to enable them make demanding nursing decisions.

Problems also arise because of public demands (patients and relatives), and expectations in relation to their care and the inability, for many reasons, of the health care service to realistically and successfully meet those demands and expectations due to lack of resources. Also there are the increasing problems which confront nurses which are associated with the effects of new technology, often without the necessary education updating, in the management of patients. Most important, there are the virtual unceasing organisational changes for which there is little preparation, although about which volumes of information are made available; but for which little, if any, in the way of educational training, emotional support and understanding is provided.

There are various ways in which nursing in particular and the NHS in general can respond to the many pressures, the great stress and the increasing problems which nurses encounter. These include providing improved training and education, ensuring the necessary resources, monitoring, reducing and/or changing their workload if the situation demands (*Code of Professional Conduct* (UKCC, 1984) paras. 10/11); but, most important, affording them a confidential form or agency where they can externalise their fears and worries and be enabled to come to terms with their problems. In essence, providing a counselling service.

Concept

What is meant by the term counselling? What does counselling staff entail?

Counselling is helping people to make their own decisions — to solve their problems. In effect it is a means of enabling people to help themselves: to know and become themselves.

Couselling is an important function, not just in relation to staff welfare, but in order to achieve an improved standard of patient care. In the latter, Revans (1959) found evidence to suggest that hospitals able to retain their staff are also able to discharge their patients more rapidly, and his research findings directly connected recovery rates of patients with nursing staff morale.

The counselling function has three main elements: an action, a mode of acting; an area, the scope or range of the action; and a clientele, the actual or intended person/group of recipients of the action. In essence counselling is a relationship in which the counsellor empathically understands the client. The scope of counselling action is wide; but central to it is the self-actualisation of the person/group.

In essence, counselling is one of many strategies (others include teaching, giving information and direct action), to help people explore a problem, clarify conflicting issues and discover alternative ways of dealing with it, so that they can decide what to do about it; that is, helping people to help themselves (Hopson, 1981).

Framework: Hallmark

Any person attempting to help another must have a framework, a model, some definite ideas to help themselves first to understand their intentions for wanting to help; and to assist their approach to a clearer understanding of the problem. Brammer (1973) provides the counsellor with a model which embraces an awareness of his own values, needs, communication style, and their effects on others. The model relies widely and is based on the experience of other practitioners who have tried to make sense out of their observations by writing their ideas into a systematic theory. In addition, the work of Loughary and Ripley (1979) provides the following approach to helping.

Essentially, they say where 'helping' is indicated, there first of all exists a problem. Because of this, or arising from it, assistance — help — is signalled. To provide this help various strategies and approaches (plans) are decided. Finally, the strategies are used to transfrom the problem into acceptable, desired outcomes.

Central to the counselling role is negotiation with the person to be counselled together with establishing a relationship in which the counsellor emphatically understands the client. In this respect, the activity of counselling becomes a very personal one, and demands training in special skills of the counsellor which include those of communication, problem solving and interpersonal relationships. The counsellor has to establish a relationship with the person, be sincere, show empathy and, most important, be able to get the person to focus on the central problem. In this way the person is more easily able to establish a strategy to help resolve the problem, move towards a greater and clearer understanding of the problem, and decide, adopt and maintain a course of action.

The essence of counselling is listening to people, and giving them the opportunity to make their own decisions and act upon them. This is needed to help people grow in self-knowledge and come to a realistic understanding of their own powers and limitations.

The scope of counselling action is wide; but central to it is the self-actualisation of the person/group.

Counselling and Nurses

Counselling of nurses was seen as central to student and staff development by the Briggs Committee (1972) which identified a successful counselling scheme as being two-pronged, i.e. academic advice and career guidance, and personal counselling. The committee saw career guidance as 'a function of personnel department and line managers' (para.537). In relation to personal counselling, this, the committee felt 'should be available when needed'. To effect this function satisfactorily, they advised, 'a network of different people and services covering help on a wide range of problems from education and career guidance to health matters, should be established' (para.585).

The Need: Demand

The need for counselling in nursing stems from the necessity to respond to nursing students and trained nurses as complete individuals with actual or potential problems.

Prerequisites to Effective Counselling

If a proper, efficient and usable counselling service is to be adopted, there are certain vital prerequisites to its success. Apart from the provision of trained, experienced and skilled counsellors, it is paramount that the physical conditions for counselling are adequate: a private and comfortable room; the support of colleagues together with a relaxed and secluded waiting area. Essentially what is needed is the provision of adequate staff services and a core of staff with the necessary caring skills with the ability to direct them to themselves and others.

It is most important, where counsellors are an acknowledged part of the organisation, that they be afforded appropriate status and conditions of service. Their interaction with nurse educationists and nurse managers demands equality of status to enable them perform their role and overcome any difficulties.

Role of the Curriculum in the Development of Skills

Finally, the education and training of nurses in inter-personal skills and their integration into the curriculum, at basic and post-basic levels, is essential to enable nurses to provide an acceptable standard of care, to their patients; but also to help in acknowledging the needs of their colleagues.

The nursing curriculum, in reflecting broad categories of skills, should include sound basic preparation which is geared to the needs of patients/clients (WHO, 1966). In this context, the focus should include understanding human behaviour; the development of an alert, questioning, and critical mind of the nurse together with developing the observation, insight, foresight, imagination and creativity abilities and potential of nurses. Also the ability to communicate effectively, to make sound judgements, and sound decisions, in addition to being able to anticipate health needs and institute nursing measures, are all necessary requirements for nurses to grow professionally.

There exists a variety of inter-personal skills whose use, directly or indirectly, underlines the delivery of quality care; these can only be met and developed in a nursing/management curriculum which has an abundance of learning experiences, both theoretical and practical. The value of this form of education lies not only in its effects in developing the individual nurse, but, most important, in helping the nurse to approach patients and their families with greater understanding and sensitivity whilst at the same time enabling them to relate more confidently and effectively with their peers and other health care professionals.

The role of the nurse is both complex in its nature and demanding in its execution in terms of nurse-patient and inter-professional interactions. Therefore, training in the skills and the techniques, which are prerequisites of sound practice, whether this be to patients, clients or colleagues, should form an essential component of all programmes of staff development. But, equally important for interviewees, as most of us find ourselves in this situation sometime, is to inform themselves on the skills needed to 'sell' themselves when being interviewed.

To perform these activities effectively, nurses must, as a prerequisite, acquire relevant knowledge and develop and use appropriate skills. (The knowledge base of nursing will be discussed in the following chapter.) The skills which nurses must acquire, in addition to those already mentioned, include those of:

1. Inter-personal and inter-professional relationships;
2. Decision making — problem solving;
3. Decision taking;
4. Leadership
5. Interviewing, which includes those of appraisal and counselling;
6. Communication; and
7. Study, which includes those of reading — books, articles and reports; writing — reports; and study — the ability to analyse, appraise, assimilate and use information.

Patients, clients, relatives and nurses require information for many reasons but primarily to enable nurses to make realistic and accurate decisions about patient care. Patients and clients require information about their care plan to ensure their interest, understanding and co-operation. In nursing, there continues to be uncertainty about nurses' role and functions. Communication systems in hospital are intended (ought to be used) to provide patients and their relatives with information as well as providing rapid and accurate information about patients, or about services for patients, to staff. In the final analysis, 'the carers' — all nurses — need channels through which they can externalise, in a confidential and/or secure manner, individually or in groups, their fears, anxieties and problems.

References

Argyle, M. (1972) *The Psychology of Interpersonal Behaviour.* Pelican, London
Argyle, M. *et al.* (1958) Supervisory methods related to productivity absenteeism and labour turnovers. *Journal of Human Relations, 28,* 23–45
———— (1972) *The Psychology of International Behaviour.* Pelican, London
Argyris, C. (1967) How tommorow's executives will make decisions. *Think Magazine,* Nov. - Dec., p.18
Blake, R.P. and Mouton, J. (1964) *The Managerial Grid.* Gulf Publishing, Houston
Bowers, D.G. and Seashore, S.E. (1966) Predicting organizational effectiveness with a four-factor theory of leadership. *Administrative Science Quarterly, 11,* 238–63
Brammer, L.M. (1973) *The Helping Relationship.* Prentice-Hall, New Jersey
Cartwright, D. and Zander, A. (eds.) (1960) *Group Dynamics: Research and Theory.* Harper and Row, New York
Cooper, R.C. (1966) Leader's task relevance and subordinate behaviour in industrial work groups. *Human Relations, 19,* 57–84
Crawley, P. (1982) Counselling Migrants and Foreign Workers. (Paper presented at the Tenth International Round Table for the Advancement of Counselling, University of Lausanne, Switzerland). pp.1–9
———— (1983) Counselling and Guidance of Disabled Persons. (Paper presented at the Eleventh International Round Table for the Advancement of Counselling, Vienna). pp.1–7
Davies, I.K. (1967) *The Management of Learning.* McGraw-Hill, New York
DHSS (1972) Management Arrangements of the Reorganised NHS (Grey Book). HMSO, London
———— (1983) NHS Management Inquiry (Griffiths), DHSS
———— (1984) Implementation of the NHS Management Inquiry (HC(84)13). DHSS
Drucker, P.F. (1975) *The Practice of Management.* Heinemann, London
Fielder, F.E. (1967) *The Theory of Leadership Effectiveness.* McGraw-Hill, New York
Fulmer, R.M. (1978) *The New Management,* 3rd edn. Macmillan, New York
Gay, W.A. and Cameron, D. (1967) *A Manager's Casebook.* Heinemann, London
Gibb, C.A. (1954) Leadership. in G.Lindzey (ed.) *Handbook of Social Psychology.* Addison-Wesley, New York
General Nursing Council for England and Wales (1979/80) Annual Report, GNC
Halpin, A.W. (1966) *Theory and Research in Education Administration.* Macmillan, New York
HMSO (1972) Report on the Committee on Nursing (Briggs). Cmnd. no.5115. HMSO, London
Hopson, B. (1981) Counselling and helping. in C.L.Cooper (ed.) *Psychology and Mangement.* Macmillan, New York
Hurley, B.A. (1978) Socialisation for roles. in M.E. Hardy and M.E. Conway (eds.) *Role Theory: Perspectives for Health Professionals.* Appleton-Century-Crofts, New York
Likert, R. (1967) *The Human Organization: Its Management and Value.* McGraw-Hill, New York
Loughary, J.W. and Ripley, T.M. (1979) *Helping Others Help Themselves.* McGraw-Hill, New York
Lyden, F.J., Shipman, G.A. and Kroll, M. (eds.) (1969) *Policies, Decisions and Organisation.* Meredith, Iowa, USA
McGregor, D. (1960) *The Human Side of Enterprise,* McGraw-Hill, New York
Miller, R.G.J. (1960) Information input, overload and psychopathology. *American Journal of Psychiatry, 116,* 695–704
Mintzberg, H. (1973) *The Nature of Managerial Work.* Harper and Row, New York
———— *The Structuring of Organizations.* Prentice-Hall, New Jersey

Mott, P.E. (1972) *The Characteristics of Effective Organisations*. Harper and Row, New York

Murray, M. (1980) *Fundamentals of Nursing*, 2nd edn. Prentice-Hall, Englewood Cliffs, NJ

National Staff Committee (N & W) (1980) *Nursing Appointment Programmes: A Guide to Good Practice*. NSC, London

—— (1980) *Foundation Management Training*. NSC, London

Price, J.L. (1968) *Organizational Effectiveness: An Inventory of Propositions*. Richard D. Irwin, Homewood, Illinois

Revans, R.W. (1959) *The Hospital as an Organism: A Study in Communication and Morale*. Pergamon Press, New York

—— (1964) The morale and effectiveness of general hospitals. in G. McLachan (ed.) *Problems and Progress in Medical Care*. Oxford University Press, Oxford

—— (1964) *Standards for Morale: Cause and Effect in Hospitals*. Oxford Universities Press, Oxford

—— (1972) in Wieland and H. Leigh (eds.) *Changing Hospitals: A Report on the Internal Communication Project*. Tavistock, London

Rezler, A.G. and Stevens, B.J. (1978) The Nurse Evaluation in Education and Service

Rogers, C.R. (1974) *On Becoming a Person*. Constable, London

Royal College of Nursing (1984) A Report on the Effects of the Financial and Manpower Cuts in the NHS. (Nurse Alert). RCN

Secord, P.F.S. and Blackman, C.W.B. (1974) *Social Psychology*, 2nd edn. McGraw-Hill, New York

Sergiovanni, T.J. *et al.* (1969) Towards a particularistic approach to leadership style: Some findings. *American Educational Research Journal, 6*(1), 62–79

Strongman, K.T. (1979) *Psychology for the Paramedical Professions*. Croom Helm, London

Thorndike, R.L. (1967) The prediction of vocational success. *Vocational Guidance Quarterly, 11,* 179–87

Ullrich, R.A. and Wieland, G.F. (1980) *Organization Theory and Design*. Richard D. Irwin, Homewood, Illinois

United Kingdom Central Council for Nursing, Midwifery and Health Visiting (1984) *Code of Professional Conduct*, 2nd edn. UKCC

Weinstein, E.A. (1969) The development of interpersonal competencies. in D.A. Goslin (ed.) *Handbook of Socialization Theory and Research*. Houghton Mifflin, Boston, Massachusetts

WHO (1966) WHO Expert Committee on Nursing (Fifth Report). WHO

Wieland, G.F. (1965) Complexity and Co-ordination in Organizations. Doctoral Dissertation. University of Michigan

—— (1980) Two ways of using behavioural science to improve management. *Health Services Manager,* Feb. pp. 1–4

Advised Further Reading

Adair, J. (1979) *Training for Decisions,* Gower, Aldershot

Argyle, M. (1969) *Social Interaction.* Methuen, London

Ashworth, P. (1979) Sensory deprivation. The acutely ill. *Nursing Times, 75*(7), 290–4

Beveridge, W.E. (1981) Another look at the selection interview. *Nursing Focus, 2*(7), 226–9

Bridge, W. and Macleod Clark, J (1981) *Communication in Nursing Care.* HM+M, Aylesbury

Broadbent, D.E. (1958) *Perception and Communication.* Permagon, Oxford

Cooper, C.L. (1981) *Psychology and Management: A Text for Managers and Trade Unionists.* Macmillan Press, London

Daws, P.P. (1973) Mental health and education: counselling as prophylaxis. *BMT Journal of Guidance and Counselling, 1*(2), 2–10

De Bono, E. (1981) *Management: Problem Solving.* Temple Smith, London
Etzioni, A. (ed.) (1960) *Readings on Modern Organizations.* Prentice-Hall, Englwood Cliffs, N.J.
Faulkner, A. (ed.) (1984) *Communication. Recent Advances in Nursing.* Vol.7. Churchill Livingstone, Edinburgh
French, P. (1983) *Social Skills for Nursing Practice.* Croom Helm, London
Fulmer, R.M. (1971) Crisis management. *Association Management,* Oct., pp.71–4
Further Education Unit (1984) *Common Core Teaching and Learning* Jan., FEU
——— (1984) *Routes to Coping.* April, FEU
Gross, B.M. (1964) *The Managing of Organizations.* Free Press, New York
Hardy, M.E. and Conway, M.E. (1978) *Role Theory: Perspectives for Health Care Professionals.* Appleton-Century-Crofts, New York
Harrison, S. (1982) Consensus decision-making in the National Health Service — a review. *Management Studies (UK), 19*(4), 377–94
Hilgarde, E.R. *et al.* (1981) *Introduction to Psychology,* 8th edn. Harcourt, Brace, Jovanovich, Orlando, Florida
Hollman, T.D. (1972) Employment interviewers' errors in processing positive and negative information. *Journal of Applied Psychology, 56,* 130–34
Kagan, C. (ed.) (1985) *Interpersonal Skills in Nursing: Research and Applications.* Croom Helm, London
Katz, D. and Kahn, R. (1966) *The Social Psychology of Organizations.* Wiley, New York
Kron, T. (1967) *Communication in Nursing.* Saunders, Philadelphia
Lancaster, W. and Lancaster, J. (1969) National decision making: Managing uncertainty. *Journal of Nursing Administration, XII*(9), 23–8
MacLeod Clark, J. (1981) Communication in Nursing. *Nursing Times, 77,* 12
March, J.G. and Simon, H.A. (1958) *Organizations.* Wiley, New York
Rogers, C.R. (1969) *Freedom to Learn.* Merrill, London
Simmons, D.D. (1971) Management Styles. College Management Readings and Cases. Coombe Lodge, vol.1
Stewart. W. (1983) *Counselling in Nursing: A Problem-Solving Approach,* Harper and Row, London
Stoghill, P.M. (1974) *Handbook of Leadership.* Free Press, New York
Strongman, K.T. (1979) *Psychology for the Paramedical Professions,* Croom Helm, London

Audio-visual Aids

Bowman, M.P. (1981) *The Nurse in the 1980s* (A series of programmes which include interviewing, selection, appraisal, counselling, communication, decision making and leadership). Graves Medical Audiovisual Library, Essex

11 CONTINUING EDUCATION: PERSPECTIVES AND OPTIONS

Aims

The aims of this chapter are:

1. To examine the concept of continuing development of nurses generally, and in particular, in management skills and management knowledge.
2. To explore some of the problems which are associated with the provision of continuing education in nursing.
3. To examine different educational options for the development of nurses.

Learning Objectives

The purpose of this chapter is to enable the reader to:

1. Understand the concept of continuing education.
2. Appreciate some of the problems which are associated with the development of post-basic nurse education curricula.
3. Evaluate some options for the professional development of nurses.

Currently, there is much excitement in nursing education. This excitement is precipitated by developments, albeit at present at embryo stage, which have occurred in the wake of the recent nursing legislation. These developments include the recent publications of the RCN on the education of nurses (March 1985), the ENB 'Syllabus and Examinations for Nurses' (April 1985), together with a consultation paper 'Professional Education/Training Courses' (May 1985) and an ongoing UKCC project on education 'Project 2000'.

The literature dealing with the subject of continuing education in nursing is considerable, as indicated by the appended bibliography. However, the fact that much information (advice, suggestions and guidelines) is available is not in any way indicative of it being heeded or used. The use and application of this information will depend on a combination of factors, not least interest, initiative and motivation of nurses, nurse managers and nurse educationists together with the perceived relevance of the literature to nursing practice and the availability of resources.

'The standard of nursing care depends on the commitment, skill and expertise of the individual nurse.' (UKCC, 1982). Therefore, the educational professional and managerial preparation, at all levels, practice, management and education, must ensure that nurses are properly equipped, in their knowledge, skills and sensitivity, to provide a service of quality to which every patient and client is entitled.

Nursing is essentially a practice discipline and, as such, is dependent on society's support; therefore, the nursing goals set and the service offered must be of quality to meet society's needs.

A common problem facing nurses is that of coping with change, which, over recent years has been both frequent and demanding. Change makes many demands on the nurse including that of adjustment, physically, socially and emotionally. These demands require nurses who are intellectually alert, emotionally resilient and socially adept: in essence nurses who have an appropriate knowledge base as well as being accomplished in the necessary coping behaviour (skills). This can only be effected through regular and appropriate development and updating of all nurses in the necessary knowledge and skills. Therefore, it is incumbent on every nurse teacher and nurse manager to identify and develop nursing talent in the interest of identifying, securing and developing the skills and abilities of their staff, at basic and post-basic levels; and, in this way, ensuring nurses' satisfaction and fulfilment; and through this (improved job satisfaction, morale and motivation) enabling improved patient and client care.

Influences: Evidence

Changes to the role of the nurse have either been advised or precipitated through proposals of reports such as Briggs, Merrison and Griffiths; the EEC Nursing Directives and the *Nurses, Midwives and Health Visitors Act* 1979. Also social change and changes in approach to certain categories of patient coupled with variations in morbidity and mortality rates have been instrumental in accelerating nurses to modify and/or change their role, e.g. move towards a specialist/practitioner/consultant role, In addition, the many reports of professional bodies, notably the RCN have advised/triggered change. But have changes in nurses' education and training occurred to match these inevitable new demands? Are nurses confident in facing the reality and practicality of these new demands in specialist care which call for an 'extended' role? Also, do they have the legitimate authority to act as well as the necessary authority and autonomy to make the nursing decisions which form part of this new, anticipated role? New techniques and advances of the twentieth century, which change the treatment and care of patients, together with trends in education and management, necessitate a new approach to staff development.

A report on Continuing Education for Nurses in Scotland (Scottish Home and Health Dept, 1981) states: 'There is limited provision of planned education and training at work', that 'opportunities for qualified staff are haphazard and there is little or no identification of a specific budget or the provision of resources' (para.2.2.1, p.3). That somewhat pessimistic comment also sums up the situation relating to continuing education for nurses in England and Wales. A situation which, despite the publication of a multitude of papers, reports and memoranda, over the past two decades, has remained impotent.

However, nowadays, the question of realistically educating and updating nurses has taken on a new urgency in so far as it is underlined in the *Code of Professional Conduct* (UKCC, 1984) (though from recent evidence this is not legally binding) and will hopefully have considerable impact on the education, training and updating of nurses, midwives and health visitors. (paras, 3, 12). Regrettably, recent research by Brown and Walton (1985) underlines an urgent need for increased in-service education of both qualified and unqualified staff, which the research identifies as 'the main way in which the training of students could be improved'. (*Nursing Standard,* April 1985).

However, the opportunity to increase in-service education is unlikely and cannot be seriously contemplated in the presence of headlines such as: 'ENB to go broke to avoid redundancies'. This headline was precipitated when the ENB chose to go broke rather than make up to 100 nurse teachers redundant (Chudley, 1984). Clearly, any cuts, let alone substantial cuts, to nurse education would further depress already unstable and declining standards of care.

There exists overwhelming evidence which underlines the indispensable place of continuing education and training in the professional development and practice of the nurse. This evidence supports, and strongly advises, the place of continuing, in-service education in maintaining a quality nursing service. This evidence is included in reports of the WHO (1966), Powell (1966), Salmon (1966), Briggs (HMSO, 1972), Merrison (HMSO, 1979), NSC (N&M) (1981), Continuing Education for the Nursing Profession in Scotland (1981) and RCN (1982).

The many useful points made in a WHO report (1966) include a statement on the relationship of in-service education to maintaining a 'high standard of patient care' (para.3.3, p.11). The report also linked the 'developing and grooming of nursing leaders' to a successful programme of post-basic education (para.5.2, p.22).

The Powell report (1966), virtually at the same time, emphasised that 'the training received by student nurses does not of itself prepare them for all the duties a nurse may be called upon to perform throughout a nursing career'. Also, the report made clear that if nurses fail to keep up with new knowledge, the lack of understanding which is sure to follow will lead to 'dissatisfaction, inefficiency and unrest' (paras.8 and 10, p.2).

The Salmon report (1966) recommended that for successful performance of the job, vocational training is necessary; this can be practical — given 'on-the-job' (by precept), or theoretical — through formal instruction (by concept). The formal instruction should be given locally and in immediate preparation for roles about to be undertaken, so as to be economical in time and effort. Practical instruction should also be progressive, nurses being posted to jobs of increasing difficulty within the grade (para.9.11, pp.93–94).

The Briggs report (1972) gave considerable space to in-service education. Among its recommendations were that nurses should be given the opportunity through post-registration courses to 'broaden their education as well as deepen it, thereby enhancing the standard of care given to patients'. And, in this context, the report alluded to the aspect of nurses' preparation which should be acknowledged and developed including 'the cultivation of qualities of personality, i.e. maturity, responsibility, insight, tolerance and the ability to cope with stress in oneself and in others together with employment needs and prospects'. The emphasis should be on comprehensive patient care in so far that nurses need to know and should have discussed, 'the psychological needs of the patient' along with information relating to patients'/clients' 'social aspects including family relationships' (para.253, p.80).

The Merrison report (1979) was emphatic in its recommendation for post-basic education: 'nurses, midwives and health visitors should be adequately prepared for advanced roles in clinical specialties, education, management and research. Health authorities should establish budgets and develop programmes for their nurses' (para.13.52, p.203).

Concept

Continuing education of the nurse spans the period from studentship to retirement. In essence, it is career-long. It has implications for the nurse, nurse colleagues, related health care professionals, the patient/client, the organisation as a whole and the quality of service provided.

Continuing education poses many questions which include: Why?

What? When? How? and Where should education take place?

The central purpose of continuing education is to provide nurses with the necessary equipment, skills, knowledge, competence and security to do their job efficiently and effectively and in so doing to utilise their potential to the full, i.e. enabling their own fulfilment and ensuring improved and enlightened patient/client management.

Continuing education, if it is to be effective, must primarily enable the nurse to acquire, develop and continually update as appropriate, the basic competencies (Nurses, Midwives and Health Visitors Rules Approval Order 1983, paras18, 24, 35 and 39). In addition, continuing education must take account of the special needs of nurses which relate to their career enhancement, special and/or new and more demanding responsibilities and working relationships.

Education and training, to be of value, must be continually developed, appraised, evaluated and updated.

Many modes are available to ensure nurses' updating which include both on and off-the-job development. The spectrum is wide and varied and the ultimate choice will depend on many variables, e.g. availability of resources, suitability of particular mode of development in meeting nurses' and/or organisational needs, age, special requirements in the form of skills and knowledge to be developed, proven effectiveness of mode and the prevailing organisational climate prevailing on staff development, nationally and locally.

Continuing education can be readily depicted by use of a pyramid (Figure 11.1). In the pyramid the base represents the broad-based competencies of the nurse — skills and knowledge which continue to be relevant throughout professional life. These competencies need to be constantly developed and updated, certainly for those nurses who operate at the front-line, at ward and community level. However, they also continue to have relevance and significance for nurses operating at advanced levels, in the clinical environment, in management, in education and research, even though at these levels special competencies need to be acquired, developed and used to ensure the proper fulfilment of one's role. In a staff development programme, scope must be provided within the organisation and with the specialty to ensure manoeuvreability, development and support of staff.

The skills and knowledge involved in personal development are many and varied and broadly include behavioural, social, managerial, interpersonal, inter-professional and legislative competencies.

'Nurse training should enable the nurse to acquire the necessary knowledge and to develop the technical competence and the attitude which

Figure 11.1: Model Depicting an Extension, Development
and Focusing of Competencies for the Nurse, Manager and
Teacher

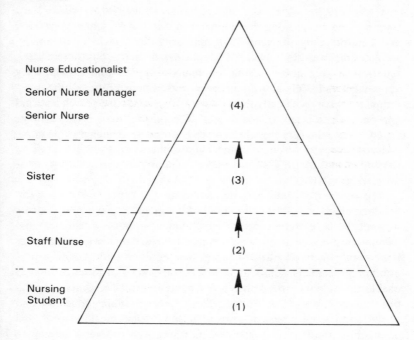

Key:
(1)   Basic competencies.
(2)   Extension and consolidation.
(3)   Updating of basic competencies: development of selective/specific
      competencies.
(4)   Knowledge of nursing competencies relevant, but main focus on
      specific clinical, managerial and educational competencies.
With career progression, education and development continues but in a
narrower, more specialised area.

will make it possible to recognise, understand and respond to the patient's
needs on the basis of an integral human approach' (EEC Advisory Committee on Training in Nursing, 1981). In this context, the committee
underline, the nurse must acquire the ability to identify, formulate and
practice methods satisfying patients'/clients' needs taking cognisance of
and co-ordinating resources. The trained nurse should be adept at planning, organising, implementing and evaluating nursing services. In addition, the trained nurse should have the ability to guide nurses and other

groups; be able to participate in nursing research; and, most important, accept professional responsibility and be willing to pursue further education in nursing.

Continuing in-service education is defined by the NSC (1981) as: 'An aspect of the career-long development of nursing personnel, provided and controlled by the employing authority for which no nationally recognised certificate is awarded.' Fundamental to this philosophy is the requirement that nurses should continually up-date and expand their knowledge and skills as well as accept the responsibility and the commitment to assess critically their own learning needs and search and find appropriate resources to become self-directing for their own learning.

The onus, the report makes clear, is on nurse managers and nurse educationalists to design learning opportunities and to effect teaching methods to ensure the success of adopted approaches in securing continuing education.

The report on Continuing Education for the Nursing Profession in Scotland (1981) has four main aims, which include: 'To prepare nurses to meet the accelerating rate of development in nursing, medical and technological services; to enable nurses to return to work and to function more effectively; to discourage nurses from undertaking a programme in a specialty in which they do not intend to practice; and to enable nurses to meet the demands of a better informed consumer population.' (para.2, p.x). The Working Party view continuing education and professional development in terms of an 'investment for the future', and embracing 'an effective system of staff appraisal', thereby helping to 'reduce the turnover rate significantly' and helping to 'save some expenditure on the administrative work involved in the employment of replacement staff' (para.6.3.1, p.26).

Need and Demand

It is fairly obvious, and indeed educationally undesirable, that all knowledge and skills required by the nurse to do the job effectively, cannot be acquired during the period of basic education. This, in addition to the ever-increasing demands of the job, make it essential that education and training should be on-going, particularly being related to special demands, i.e. skills and knowledge required by the nurse at different stages of development, in different specialties and at different levels of management.

The goals of continuing professional development are basically three, i.e. improving on-going performance through the acquisition and development of skills, knowledge and sensitiveness, the reinforcement of existing already acquired skills and knowledge, and the discovery or uncovering of weaknesses in skills, knowledge, sensitivity — and the mode of instruction or development used (Houle, 1984).

To-day, nurse managers, nurse educationists and nurse clinicians have to work within the framework of complex legislation, including professional (nursing) legislation, industrial relations, health and safety etc. which is having a profound effect on employing authorities, staff, patients and clients. In addition, there is the continuing trend to greater use of nurse specialists which has accelerated as a result of advances in medical technology.

Primarily the aim of staff development, continuing education, is to produce technically and professionally qualified nurses who are capable of interpreting, understanding and adapting to their managerial-professional role and in doing so furthering their own self-actualisation and through this providing a better, more enlightened, service for patients and clients.

Education and training is a dynamic, continuous activity which is carried out against the background of personal and organisational goals and needs of patients and clients and entails primarily identifying these needs; providing relevant training to enable staff to realise those needs and goals; monitoring and evaluating the results of training; and adjusting the training activities to meet the original aims and/or providing further training to meet new or additional goals.

An important aspect of continuing education is to establish links between the learning programme and the work situation through studies derived from 'live' material, job-related project work, or problem-solving exercises based on real situations.

The *Grey Book* (DHSS, 1972) states: 'If the proposed management organisation for the NHS is to be effective in its ultimate aim of securing improvements to health care for patients, highly skilled managers will be needed. The development of managerial skill is a continuous process, involving formal professional management training and experience' (para.3.62, p.64), and 'unless management potential of employees is identified and their development as manager monitored, there is a risk that talent will be wasted' (para.3.64, p.65).

In-service and continuing education for nurses is important for many and varied reasons basic to which is improving/updating their skills and knowledge to enable them to function more effectively in meeting the goals of the NHS and nursing, the needs of patients and clients and to enable their own fulfilment. Imtimately linked to this is that of ensuring their morale, i.e. the degree to which their motives are gratified (Price 1968, 1972), and in this way enhancing their degree of commitment to work, and enabling their own work satisfaction and performance: in essence enhancing the nursing service provided.

A report (NSC, 1981) states that the success of any system of continuing education and staff development relies heavily on the quality of the educational opportunities which are provided at the place of work and upon the effectiveness of the system of staff appraisal and selection for appropriate educational activities (para.3.1.1, p.8). And, that surrounding a formal structure of professional education and development there should be planned identified opportunities at the place of work: the on-the-job elements of continuing education must be closely related to an effective system of staff appraisal and staff development (para.4.1.2, p.16).

Inherent in this philosophy is the principle that nurses must learn and re-learn throughout their professional lives in order to keep pace with modern trends, technology, the changing needs of the service and the new demands of patients, clients and relatives. The nursing competencies which require to be successfully engaged and completed to enable the nursing student to make application for admission to Part 1, 3, 5, or 8 of the Register (RCN, RMN, RNMH and RSCN) only provide, at basic and elementary level, opportunities for nursing students to lay a sound framework for their personal professional development by acquiring basic cognitive, affective, psychomotor and clinical competencies. Also, those competencies which enable application to be made for Part 2, 4, 6, and 7, i.e. EN(G), EN(M), EN(MH) and EN, require the student to undertake nursing care under the direction of a nurse registered in Part 1, 3, 5 or 8, clearly place great demands on a thorough basic and post-basic development of these nurses.

Basic nursing education can only be a foundation. It needs to be followed by systematic updating and more advanced preparation for specialised roles through post-basic educational programmes (Merrison, para.13.51, p.203).

However, the intention of nurse managers and nurse educationists to focus on the most effective and efficient methods of education to enable nurses to acquire the right skills and knowledge, in the most suitable environment and through this to effect the highest standard and quality of patient and client care, has been considerably frustrated and made impotent. In this respect, in a period of rapid change, organisations and managers unable to adapt are soon in trouble; this situation is achieved only by learning, i.e. by being able to do tomorrow that which might have been unnecessary today. 'The organisation that continues to express only the ideas of the past is not learning and training systems intended to develop our young workers may do little more than to make them proficient in yesterday's techniques' (Revans, 1983). Therefore, the preparation of nurses to enable them to function proficiently in meeting their changing role is a major problem that faces nurse managers and nurse educationists.

The education and the up-dating of knowledge and skills, keeping in step with, if not in advance of, new developments, is a prerequisite of any professional, ensuring that they update and develop, and through this understand in a clearer way current needs and demands of their patients/clients, thereby enhancing the quality of their care through improved understanding and practice.

Links between Continuing Education and Quality Care

There is disturbing information in the report of the Royal Commission on the National Health Service (Merrison report), which expresses concern about declining standards of nursing care and which underlines the main areas of risk in hospitals and in the community (para.13.5, p.185). Also, the recent report of the RCN makes uneasy reading in so far as the ability of the NHS to deliver satisfactory care to patients and clients. In this respect, the report states that in 1974 the nursing workforce consisted of 36 per cent trained nurses (registered and enrolled), 33 per cent learners and 31 per cent auxiliaries. Of the trained nurses most were working in the community and some in teaching and administration, so diluting the trained workforce on the wards further. Subsequent to this period (1976) trained nurses increased by 82 per cent; but auxiliaries had increased by 244 per cent. Similarly, consultants had increased by 185 per cent. In the period between 1976 to 1982 a slight change by way of improvement took place (RCN, 1984). However, the compound effect of this was an aggravation of already declining standards of care. In this context, the work of senior nurses at ward and community level in the planning, monitoring and evaluation of care together with enabling the motivation, appraisal, leadership, assessment and counselling of nurses, identifies a situation which is very demanding physically, mentally and emotionally, which warrants a high degree of expertise and which, of necessity, demands close links between professionals in the work situation. To be effective in the management of their patients these links must also be acknowledged, realistically, in the joint preparation of professionals.

The link between education in management skills and management and knowledge with the quality of management practised is made in a report of the NSC (1980) which states: 'unless everyone engaged in, or concerned with training achieve a high standard of managerial ability there can only be a decline in the quality of nurse management' (para.24, p.16).

Why, therefore, in spite of the depth and variety of information, advice and guidelines and the obvious need for both separate and combined development of staff, has the approach to continuing education remained stubbornly blunt? This, in itself, prompts many supplementary questions, in the interest of finding an answer. For example, is there continuing evidence for the place of management skills and knowledge to be more pronounced in the nurse's curriculum — at basic and post-basic levels? Do nurses feel a need for and see the relevance of this type of development? Should more emphasis be placed on 'on-the-job' as opposed to 'off-the-job' training? What should the balance be? In the final analysis is there a tangible link between better education and training and effective patient care? If this is so, what is the evidence? And, most important, why is there only limited activity to help devise suitable curricula?

The hospital, the ward and the community external to the hospital are complex systems of human interaction whose organisation and successful management demand specialist knowledge and skills, in addition to those acquired in basic nursing curricula to enable nurses to lead teams, to solve problems and to make decisions, to manage budgets and to motivate their staff. The need for decision-making to be made close to patients was underlined in *Patients First* which highlighted as a prime objective, that decisions should be taken by those who work directly with patients to enable the meeting of patients' needs (para.3, p.1).

Rationale for Continuing Education

An RCN seminar (March 1982) endorsed the principle that appointment to clinical posts at any level must be in accordance with specified criteria which indicate that the person appointed is suitably qualified in terms of formal qualification, experience and/or other relevant attainments, and advised that opportunities be available, as of right, for regular study leave. It also advised before taking up a post as sister a module on clinical management, based on a training ward, should be undertaken. The seminar participants acknowledged that these proposals, if accepted, would promote and enhance nursing care.

An ongoing project which is being conducted by the King's Fund (1982) and which is associated with two London hospitals, has as its prinicipal aim, 'to prepare registered general nurses to function efficiently as sisters'. The philosophy of the course is, 'that the best and quickest method of preparing the ward sister is in the real life situation'. The intention is that the nurse will encounter problems and challenges and, in doing so, with the support of a tutor, will develop clinical managerial and teaching skills.

There are a variety of management training approaches ranging from individual home study supported by group discussion and teaching and tutorially supported projects or assignments as well as courses of various types and duration run within the NHS either in or away from the place of work to meet the needs, and the convenience, of nurses.

No single learning process for management education seems adequate on its own. In this respect, a number of factors affect the choice of learning methods which include the nature of learning, the learner's learning style, the teacher's learning style, resources available and the environment in which learning takes place. The level of learning e.g. memory, understanding, application and transfer will vary with the learning methods whether these be off-the-job, i.e. lectures, talks, programmed learning, discussion, role play, experimental learning, group exercises and sensitivity training, or on-the-job which include assignments, projects, job rotation, demonstration, supervised practice, counselling and discovery learning.

In addition, people learn in different ways, e.g. individuals have their own favoured learning style which, of necessity, entails the use of a wide ranging of learning methods and teaching strategies to cater for these diverse styles. Regrettably, this philosophy is rarely, if ever, applied to programmes relating to the development of staff.

In order to learn people must want to learn. Essentially, learning is enhanced when people perceive a reason for doing so, therefore, it is of vital importance that nurses are made aware of the significance and of the relevance of continuing education. In everyday life, the chief reason for wanting to learn is the solving of problems either at work or in the home. In this context Professor Revans links learning and management: 'Managers learn as they manage and they manage because they have learned — and go on learning.' (Revans, 1983).

Learning within a large and complex organisation such as the NHS or nursing, if it is to be effective, must include an understanding by nurses of the aims and needs of the organisation, of their own role, and of the roles of other professionals with whom they work.

Clearly, many factors influence training and development and, in this context, are related to the organisation, the job and the nurse (Figure 11.2).
They include:

1. Social climate
2. Economic climate
3. National policies (Government)
4. Policies of Statutory and Professional Bodies
5. New technology demanding new skills and knowledge (learning and unlearning)
6. Staff performance
7. Staff aspirations
8. Staff satisfaction.

In a paper produced by a Working Party on continuing education (1981) several interesting and important issues are raised in relation to managerial development. For example, it emphasises that internal development within the organisation is an important foundation for management development. Also, it advises that the use of courses should represent a conscious and selective building on that foundation. Even though some universities, notably Brunel, Birmingham and Manchester, have engaged in the research of some of the problems which confront nurses, nurse managers and nurse educators in relation to various aspects of post-basic education, enabling them to be used effectively, evaluation of practice to date has been sporadic.

Research carried out by the University of Birmingham Health Services Management Centre (Roberts *et al.*, 1981) supported the fact that management development of staff should be based on a prior analysis of roles involved. In addition, the findings supported the principle that development of staff should be based on a prior analysis of needs carried out in the work situation. Also it recognised that many options are available to in-service training officers to meet training needs, and, most important, that these training needs must embrace problems in both the organisational and the individual aspects of managerial roles.

The authors say that 'to focus on one form of development is both unwise, unrealistic and not wholly rewarding — for the nurse and the organisation, since individual potential may be developed — and

Figure 11.2: External and Internal Factors Which Will Influence Training and Development for Individuals and/or Groups of Staff

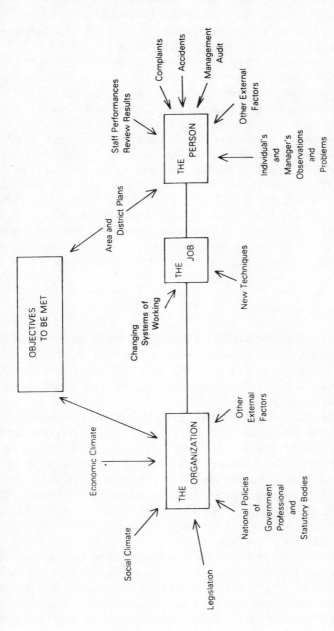

Source: National Staff Committee for Nurses and Midwives (1981) The Organisation and Provision of Continuing In-service Education and Training

demonstrated in different ways'. Therefore, 'particular emphasis should be focused on on-the-job management development which is only possible to effect through an organisational learning climate which seriously entertains the self-development of the nurse'.

The research suggests that internal development of nurses provides an improved and secure base for investment in external courses and, in this respect, non-course methods for developing training and education in management skills and knowledge should be regarded by senior management with interest, enthusiasm and as a priority.

For many years there has been considerable investment (no information on costs and numbers of staff is available) by the DHSS, through the NSC and Health Authorities, on 'courses' essentially as sole agents of staff orientation to new technology and structures. The results of this type of experience found from my own research (Bowman, 1980) for most nurses, is both harassing, unclear and virtually futile. Obviously courses play some part in staff development and must be considered among the general options available to training officers and senior managers; but is enough value placed upon the alternatives to courses?

Non-course Options

On-the-job training which enables staff to come to terms with their own organisation, examine its problems at first hand and develop feasible solutions should be a priority investment for management at any level; the use of courses should represent a conscious but selective building on this foundation.

Non-course options are many and include on-the-job assignments, projects, counselling and supervised practice. The non-course approach underlines the centrality of self-development to enhancing organisational development. In a basic way, this can be effected by using the expertise of specialists within the nurse's own hospital or district and can be pariculary useful in learning the skills and expertise of finance and personnel. However, for results to be effective in terms of useful learning, nurses need to be self-reliant and prepared to believe in the possibility of developing themselves.

The rationale underlying the development of nurses must take account of the aims and needs of the service, the needs of patients and the needs of staff. The effective execution of any programme and/or approach will be governed by such things as the immediate and long-term skills and needs of staff in the efficient performance of their job; the age of the group; their present state of knowledge, together with the availability of an adequate number and suitably qualified and experienced training/supervisory staff.

As a prelude to any staff development programme there needs to be a real commitment and understanding by the NHS, to provide an effective service. Staff must be able to appreciate the relevance of management development, particularly in relation to the productivity and viability of the service offered, to always ensure quality care. Expertise within the profession and the broader NHS organisation should be harnessed, developed and utilised in the development of staff. Apart from the educational value of this approach, it is particularly commendable nowadays in the light of economic stringencies.

The principal steps to be taken when planning a staff development programme include, identifying training needs of different groups and different levels of management, deciding priorities, establishing a plan, and implementing, monitoring and evaluating the plan.

Any successful scheme must take into account such key issues as the nature of the educational experience; the educational preparation must be congruent with the nature of the specialism for which it is attempting to fit the nurse. Also, the facilities (or the lack of them) provided by training institutions will also have an important bearing on the ultimate effects of a particular programme. In this context, the number and the quality of the teachers together with the availability of other relevant resources, e.g. library, educational technology, will affect the learning experience. Also the age, experience and the willingness of nurses to learn will influence the final result.

The position in nursing is additionally complicated by the scale and rapidity of current innovation and change and is aggravated by a critical shortage of nurse teachers. (Present nurse teacher shortage is estimated to be in order of 33 per cent.) This will be further aggravated by the recently announced policy of the ENB to reduce the number of places on future nurse teacher courses by 25 per cent.

What therefore can be done to improve education and training, at post-basic level, to enable nurses to meet their clinical and managerial responsibilities?

Staff development should take place when and where it is most effective and appropriate in relation to the nurse and the organisation, i.e., on-the-job — action-learning, where problems are examined, or off-the-job seminars, discussions and courses. A vital prerequisite in deciding the nature and the time for staff development is that of the level and the extent of nurses' decision-making as well as the urgency for the updating of knowledge and skills.

In addition to the use of formal courses as a means of staff development, non-course options should be given serious consideration by nurse
managers including 'coaching', where managers stretch their subordinates
to higher levels of performance, giving constructive feedback and putting work incidents into a framework from which principles can be drawn
to guide future action. Also in this category are included performance
review, distance learning, study days, additional involvement in organisational management development, tutorial and advisory visits, briefing,
job rotation, and, most important, participation in special projects through
the agency of problem-solving and action learning groups.

Role of Action Learning

At the present time, in the Health Service, there is a growing appeal
for action learning for those involved with the development of staff in
the health care professions, largely one suspects because implicit in action learning is the need to help managers, and all others who engage
in it, by setting them to tackle real problems that have defied solution.

The nurse and the patient are faced with considerable tasks of adjustment, the nurse to a way of life, the patient to a path of recovery. Commenting on this Revans (1976) states that 'patient care is, for nurse and
patient alike, substantially a learning process'. And, 'in this context,
learning processes, at any level, are more than obedience to instructions,
however clear, however appropriate, however authoritative'. Learning
occurs most effectively when the doubts in the mind of the learner can
be spontaneously voiced. Therefore the difference between giving nurses
the opportunity to ask questions and/or of denying this opportunity Revans
equates with, 'the difference between learning and not learning'.

Professor Revans states that action learning enables managers to acquire insight by setting them to tackle real problems that have so far
defied solution.

The action learning approach is problem-centred in so far that a group
of selected managers is set up to work on a range of complex problems.
Forces for personal and corporate development can emerge from the combination of individual effort with group stimulus and support guided by
an outside tutor acting as a 'catalyst' to facilitate the team's potential
and suggest specialist help for participants as required.

Role-based training (already mentioned in Chapter 5) as a contribution to mangement development which focuses on helping nurses to

function more effectively in the role they occupy by providing them with an opportunity to gain greater understanding of that role, particularly in relation to the skills and knowledge needed for its successful occupance, is highlighted by the NSC (1983). This is achieved through linking learning to work-related problems as well as providing a professionally led training by continuous involvement in the planning and implementation of the programme by senior nurse managers who act as professional facilitators with nurses' managers. The NSC advise that role-based training should be adopted throughout England and Wales to meet the training and development needs of nurses, particularly in the grades from ward sister to Director of Nursing Service. However, it also signals the exercise of caution, to avoid following slavishly one form of training and emphasises that multidisciplinary training together with training in special skills, e.g. computer training and industrial relations, should not be neglected.

The Real Issues: Developments

Currently, important developments are taking place in the UK which, hopefully, will enhance the training and development of nurses. These developments include the establishment of the United Kingdom Central Council, the National Boards, the RCN Commission on Nursing Education which has the broad and somewhat demanding terms of reference of examining the whole field of nursing education and of making recommendations. The Commission, which was independent, was chaired by Dr Harvey Judge who hopes the outcome will be to re-shape nursing education on the lines of teacher education. The Commission presented its report in March 1985. In addition, the ENB has recently (May, 1985) published a special paper (Professional Education/Training Courses: A Consultation Paper) which has as its basis a strategy for nursing education. Also, currently the UKCC has an on-going research project (Project 2000). Project 2000 is the name of the review set up by the UKCC to look into the future professional practice for nursing, midwifery and health visiting. It is a 'total and radical review of the professional preparation for nursing, midwifery and health visiting; the purpose is to prepare practitioners for the health care needs of society in the 1990's and beyond'.

The work for Project 2000 has been carried out by sub-groups that have been looking at the organisation of nursing, midwifery, and health visiting in the UK; the recommendations in previous reports on education and training in nursing, midwifery and health visiting; how health care needs are likely to develop over the next 10–20 years and identifying the implications for the development of nursing, midwifery and health visiting; financial and manpower requirements and their implications; the basic principles on which professional education should be founded; and the picture of the ideal practitioner for the 1990s.

Issues that will be addressed in discussion papers will include: student status, levels of practitioner, and generic/specialist preparation. Project 2000 'is not taking the present legislation as a constraint and where necessary will be making proposals for legislative change' (UKCC, 1985). The ENB will subsequently examine the findings of this project and attempt to reform nursing curricula.

Encouraging and developing nursing talent (Code of Professional Nursing Conduct) in nurses' quest for improved quality care can be focused by developing their skills and abilities and improving their knowledge base throught the agency of intentional and continuing education, which as well as focusing on professional knowledge, skills and abilities should encourage what was recommended some quarter of a century (Brotherson, 1960) ago, i.e. the readiness of a profession to 'look analytically at the events or working methods with which it is concerned, a willingness to encourage scientific study and experimentation, and an ability to accept the proven conclusions and act accordingly'. In this context, he emphasises that even though the ability to carry out research as well as the opportunity to undertake research will relate only to the few, 'an urgent and understanding sense of the need for research should be part of the metal equipment of every member of any profession'.

Nursing research is a prerequisite to the viability and integrity of the nursing profession in so far as it is necessary to identify weakness in nursing practice, nursing management and nursing education, to examine problems in these areas and to recommend more suitable approaches and practices. In this respect, nursing research, e.g. research relating to role, communications, inter-professional relationships, nursing manpower, quality care and the curriculum, its findings and recommendations, must be read, discussed, interpreted, examined for validity and, if found reliable and applicable to nursing situations, must be applied. This understanding analysis and application to be effective requires the continuous extension and development in nurses of their intellectual, cognitive, as well as their psychomotor and affective skills and knowledge. This can only be done thoroughly through the proper development and constant updating of the nursing competencies and requires a sound basic and post-basic philosophy and practice of nursing education.

In nursing today there is to be expected much emphasis on information technology, particularly in relation to the increased use of computers in the education of nurses and in assisting nurse managers in streamlining their work. However, nurse education, nurse management and, most important, nursing practice entails much more than the use of mechanical apparatus which at best can save nurses' time on monitoring and carrying out routine tasks and at worst can reduce nurses' contact with patients and clients and as a direct result will limit the ability of nurses to develop and use inter-personal skills. In fact, with nurses carefully monitored and compensated for, the essence of good nursing care may be lost in high technology, and academically orientated approach. In essence, high technology can reduce the caring ability of nurses and as a result directly affect patient/client care and rehabilitation. Therefore, a note of caution must be exercised in the enthusiasm of the caring professions for high technology.

Curriculum Development: Perspectives — Is there a 'Right' Approach?

Hospitals are in reality what Maslow (1972) referred to as 'low synergy institutions' i.e. while the system/s within the hospital are substantially inter-dependent, health care professionals do not act in an inter-dependent way. Health care professionals learn a rigorous scientific discipline as the 'content' of their training. The 'process', not explicit, inculcates a value for autonomous decision-making (marked and allowed in the medical profession, difficult to achieve though in nursing), personal achievement and improving one's own performance (Wiesbord, 1981).

Substantially, to date, the approach to the managerial development of nurses has been 'course' rather than 'job' orientated. Obviously both approaches have merit. But is there an 'ideal' — a 'right' — approach to help staff acquire the requisite knowledge and skills to help them do their job more effectively? What, in fact, are the criteria of sound, realistic and appropriate continuing education and training development of nurses?

Essentially and substantially, the development of nurses should be planned in relation to the needs, goals and demands of their patients/clients, i.e. the service to be performed, nurses' special responsibilities and their particular need to acquire specialist skills and knowledge at any given time, e.g. in relation to the budget, decision making, etc., and their career aspirations. The approach, in the main, should relate closely to the special problems and responsibilities which are encountered by staff in their work situation: in essence nurses' role expectations and the related training/education needs.

To attempt to suggest a proposed curriculum for front-line nurses, and indeed nurses at any level of the NHS, and to do so with an element of accuracy, in the prevailing situation of organisational change and uncertainty, is difficult. The present demanding professional and organisational climate with its roots in technology and legislation necessitates a more decisive, realistic and relevant approach to the development of nurses to ensure the viability and enhancement of nursing practice.

In-service training and education for nurses should be planned in relation to the goals of the NHS in general and nursing in particular and, in this respect must meet the ever-changing and more demanding needs of patients and clients, as well as reflecting the needs of staff by using their potential, abilities, aptitudes, aspirations, skills, knowledge and creativity optimally. Training and education, in meeting these needs, must ensure nurses' knowledge and skills are kept at peak performance and up-to-date and, in this way, their training education and development needs to be continuous.

When designing and planning the curriculum, the objectives, content, teaching methods and methods of evaluation must be clear, specific, positive and relevant and attainable to the organisation, the patient/client and the staff. In addition to the structure and approach to the teaching of the curriculum, i.e. whether training is to be done on-the-job or off-the-job; whether the agencies of teaching are to be seminars, discussions, conferences, tutorials, workshops or lectures, whether action-learning or distance learning approaches are to be used, additional though central factors such as the age, ability, special needs and experience of the proposed target group, must be considered.

Curriculum Integration

Arguments for an integrated curriculum include the following.

1. Integration counteracts the compartmentalisation of knowledge which is the result of a 'subject-centred' view of knowledge held by 'experts'.
2. Integration, especially of the inter-disciplinary type, allows a more comprehensive view to be developed of a broad study area than is usually possible through the pursuit of individual subjects.
3. Integration, especially of the inter-disciplinary type, allows problems

and issues to be explored in a holistic way, through bringing to bear upon them the perspectives of different subjects.

4. The explosion of knowledge and rapid social change have been reflected in increasing emphasis, in both general and vocational education, on a more active preparation of the learner for the modern world. The development of personal, social and 'coping' skills is seen as being of particular importance in this context. It has been argued that such skills are best arrived at through an inter-disciplinary scheme of themes and problems which relate 'real life' or vocational issues. And

5. From a pragmatic point of view, curriculum packages based on integrated knowledge can (a) facilitate a higher degree of 'balance' in the curriculum and (b) lead to a saving in teaching time.

Arguments against integration include the following.

1. In moving away from the division of knowledge in terms of the established subjects, one moves towards fields of studies which lack established enquiry modes and academic standards. And,

2. Integrated courses ignore the conventional divisions and distinctions between such areas.

To enhance staff development, the expertise which is available within the profession, should be harnessed, developed and utilised optimally in the supervision, support and training of staff to achieve stated objectives.

Clearly, if nursing is to meet its primary objective of ensuring effective patient care nurses will require to be made aware of the existence, and use, of new and related technology and practices.

In-service training and education should take place when and where it is most appropriate and effective in meeting organisational and individual needs. In this respect, decisions must be made by nurse managers on whether the apporach being considered should be based on broad principles and/or on specific skills and education. Most important, the approach which is adopted must align with the nature and extent of decision-making by the nurse at the appropriate managerial level, which, in turn should mould the course/approach, i.e. whether uni-disciplinary, uni-professionally and/or multi-disciplinary, multi-professionally.

Wherever in-service development is engaged, vital prerequisites to success include, pre-course/activity briefing and explanation to reduce unnecessary fear and anxiety as well as to make clear the purpose of the development; ensuring a flexible approach to enable participants to examine and discuss issues of interest and importance to them as well as to the organisers; use of the more participative methods of teaching to allow optimum engagement of the group; and to ensure post-course discussion to facilitate comment, evaluation and feedback.

To enable nurses to learn on-the-job as well as off-the-job, a variety of educational opportunities must be made available. To ensure a balance of the educational experience, tuition at the place of work could be provided in the form of workshops, seminars, study days, meetings and peer group discussions. In addition the provision of useful educational activities outside of the work place might include attendance at conferences, refresher courses, specialist short courses, study tours and sabbatical leave.

Where formal courses are entertained a 'modular' approach could be usefully considered to enable the regular updating of information as well as taking cognisance of the learning problems of individuals which may be associated with such things as age and level of experience.

Staff development, whether job-linked or course-aligned, should be seen as a stimulating and rewarding experience for nurses; but, most important, it must be accepted as an inevitable and vital agency/resource ensuring the integrity and viability of nursing while simultaneously securing the status and role of the nurse: in essence securing the professionalisation of nurses which is long overdue.

In caring, helping others (patients, clients and colleagues), to grow nurses must learn both specific and general knowledge, to the degree that they are able, 'Caring includes both explicit and implicit knowledge i.e. knowing that something is so and knowing how to do something.' (Mayeroff, 1971).

The philosophy of a recent report (RCN, 1985) on nursing education, if accepted and implemented, shall, in conjunction with vigorous activity of the statutory bodies for nursing, without a doubt progress nursing practice and nursing education into the year 2000.

The report is clear as well as being evolutionary and revolutionary, and, if accepted by the nursing profession, shall substantially change nursing education.

In this respect, the report makes many important points and says that the problems of nursing education, though not new have progressively become more urgent; the report proposes, that 'nothing less than fundamental reform can now be effective' (para.1.1, p.7). To effect this reforming and re-shaping, nursing education must be disentangled from the 'organisation of the services which nurses deliver' (para.1.4, p.8).

The report underlines the 'uneasy relationship' that exists between nurse educators, nurse managers and ward staff. In essence, the correct situation — a correction long overdue — is for nurse education to be shifted outside the NHS (para.2.7, p.17).

How can this radical change, the separation of nursing education from nursing practice, be achieved?

The approach to the future education and training of nurses, to be effective, should include changes which embrace giving trainee nurses student status; integrating nursing education with further and higher education; ensuring a single basic nursing qualification; and reducing the number of care assistants. In addition, the report advises the creation of a new independent body to advise the Secretaries of State on the supply and education of nurses. Also, the report states that all nurse teachers should be graduates and, most important, carry clinical responsibility (something long overdue).

If the recommendations can be successfully implemented, the presumption of the Commission is 'the nation will enjoy a system of nurse education' which is 'effective in generating quality and less wasteful in consuming resources' (para.5.13, p.50).

It is sincerely hoped that the government of the day, the nursing statutory bodies and, most important, the profession as a whole will ensure that these long-awaited reforms will unhesitatingly and unstintedly be implemented.

Finally, in Drucker's (1974) view 'Only if targets are defined can resources be allocated to their attainment, priorities and deadlines set, and somebody held accountable for results.' In this respect, unless clear goals are set, and made known to staff, subsequent and appropriate training and education of staff is reduced in value, if it is not entirely impossible.

References

Bowman, M.P. (1980) The Management Education and Training Needs of First-line Nursing Officers in the Gateshead Area Health Authority. Unpublished MEd. Thesis. University of Newcastle upon Tyne.

Brown, J. and Walton, I. (1985) *How Nurses Learn: A National Study of the Training of Nurses in Mental Handicap.* DHSS

Brotherson, J.H.F. (1960) Research-mindedness and the health professions. in *International Council of Nurses. Learning to Investigate Nursing Problems.* (Report of an International Seminar on Research in Nursing). London

Chudley, P. (1984) ENB to go broke to avoid redundancies. *Nursing Standard, 356,* 1

DHSS (1972) Management Arrangements for the Reorganised National Health Service

(Grey Book). DHSS, London

———— (1979) Patients First (Consultative Paper on the Structure and Management of the NHS in England and Wales). HMSO, London

Drucker, P.F. (1974) *Why Service Institutions do not Perform — Management Tasks, Responsibilities and Practices,* Harper and Row, New York

EEC Commission of the European Communities (1981) Advisory Committee on Training in Nursing. Report of the Training of Nurses Responsible for General Care (R82/5/A). EEC

English National Board for Nursing, Midwifery and Health Visiting (1985) The Syllabus and Examinations for Courses in General Nursing Leading to Registration in Part I of the Register (1985(19)ERDB, April). ENB

HMSO (1972) Report of the Committee on Nursing (Briggs). Cmd. no. 5115. HMSO, London

———— (1979) Royal Commission on the National Health Service (Merrison). Cmnd. no. 7615. HMSO, London

Houle, C. (1984) Overview of continuing professional education. in S. Goodlad (ed.) *Education for the Professions.* SRHE & NFER-Nelson, Windsor

Kings' Fund Centre (1982) Ward Sister Preparation: A Contribution to Curriculum Building. (Project Paper no. 36). King' Fund Centre

Maslow, A.H. (1972) *Synergy in the Society and in the Individual. The Further Reaches of Human Nature.* Chapter 14. Viking Press New York

Mayeroff, M. (1971) *On Caring.* Harper and Row, New York

Ministry of Health Central Council (1966) The Post-certificate Training and Education of Nurses (Powell). HMSO, London

Ministry of Health Scottish Home and Health Dept (1966) Report of the Committee on Senior Nursing Staff Structure (Salmon). HMSO, London

National Staff Committee for Nurses and Midwives (1980) Foundation Management Training. NSC

———— (1981) Recommendations on the Organisation and Provision of Continuing In-service Education and Training. NSC

———— (1983) Role Based Training as a Means of Developing Nurse Managers. NSC

Nurses, Midwives and Health Visitors Rules Approval Order 1983, HMSO, London

Price, J.L. (1968) *Organizational Effectiveness: An Inventory of Propositions.* Richard D. Irwin, Homewood, Illinois

———— (1972) *Handbook of Organizational Measurement.* D.C. Heath, Lexington, Massachusetts

Revans, R.W. (1976) *Action Learning in Hospitals: Diagnosis and Therapy.* McGraw-Hill, New York

———— (1983) *The ABC of Action Learning.* Chartwell-Bratt, Bromley

Roberts, J.N., White, D.K. and Thompson, D.J.C. (1981) Change Strategies for Health Authorities: The Contribution of Organisational Development. (Special Paper: Workshop for Senior NHS Managers). Health Services Management Centre, University of Birmingham

Royal College of Nursing (1982) Seminar: Advanced Clinical Roles. RCN

———— (1983) Towards a New Professional Structure for Nursing (Report of the Working Group on a Professional Nursing Structure for the NHS). RCN

———— (1984) A Report on the Financial and Manpower Cuts in the NHS. (Nurse Alert) RCN

———— (1985) The Education of Nurses: A New Dispensation. (Commission on Nursing Education). RCN

Scottish Home and Health Dept (1981) Continuing Education for the Nursing Profession in Scotland. (Report of a Working Party on Continuing Education and Professional Development for Nurses, Midwives and Health Visitors). Scottish Home and Health Dept

United Kingdom Central Council for Nursing, Midwifery and Health Visiting (1982)

Education and Training (Working Group 3). UKCC
—— (1984) Code of Professional Conduct, 2nd edn. UKCC
—— (1984) Teachers of Nursing, Midwifery and Health Visiting: A Consultation Paper. UKCC
—— (1985) Project 2000. A Review set up by the UKCC to Look into the Future Professional Practice of Nursing, Midwifery and Health Visiting. UKCC
Weiland, G.F. (ed.) (1981) *Improving Health Care Mangement.* Health Administration Press. Ann Arbor, MI
Weisbord, M.R. (1981) Why organization development hasn't worked (so far) in medical centres. in: G. F. Weiland (ed.) *Improving Health Care Management.* Health Administration Press. Ann Arbor, MI
World Health Organisation (1966) WHO Expert Committee on Nursing (Fifth Report). WHO
—— (1977) The Nursing Process. (Report on the First Meeting of the Technical Advisory Group). WHO

Advised Further Reading

Alkin, M.C. and Fitz-Gibbon, C.T. (1975) Methods and Theories for evaluating programs. *Journal of Research and Development in Education, 8*(3), 2–14
Ashton, D. (1974) The trainer's role in project-based management development. *Journal of European Training, 3*(4), 206–13
Baquer, A. and Revans, R.W. (1973) 'But surely, that is their job? A Study in Practical Co-operation through Action Learning. International Publications, London
Bowman, M.P. (1979) Why this dilemma; *Nursing Mirror, 155*(13), 32–3
—— (1982) Forward thinking. *Nursing Mirror, 154*(5), x-xxi
Burgoyne, J.G. and Stuart, R. (1978) *Management Development: Context and Strategies.* Gower, Aldershot
Cang, S., MacDonald, I., Melia, A. and Ovretveit, J. (1981) *An Emerging Model for Sister Roles in General Hospitals.* Health Services Organisation Research Unit, Brunel University
Cropley, A.J. and Dave, R.H. (1978) *Lifelong Education and the Training of Teachers.* Pergamon, Oxford
DHSS (1973) Personnel Management in the National Health Service No. 1. Management Education and Training. DHSS, London
—— (1975) Management Education and Training in the NHS: Review of Guidelines (RSC/IS/189). DHSS, London
—— (1981) Seminar: Professional Development in Clinical Nursing — The 1980s. DHSS, London
—— (1983) NHS Management Inquiry, DHSS, London
Dimarcol, N. (1976) Predictors of management: training effectiveness for nursing supervisors, *Journal of Continental Education Nursing, 7*(4), 38–46
Edwards, M. (Chairman) (1976) Front-line Management. (Report of BIM Working Party). BIM, London
Elgood, C. (1981) *Handbook of Management Games,* 2nd end. Gower, Aldershot
Farnish, S. (1983) Ward Sister Preparation: A Survey in Three Districts (NERU Report no.2). Nursing Education Research Unit, Dept of Nursing Studies, Chelsea College, University of London
French, P. (1983) *Social Skills for Nursing Practice.* Croom Helm, London
Gane, R.M. and Briggs, L.J. (1979) *Principles of Instructional Design.* Holt, Rinehart and Winston, New York
Hamblin, A.C. (1974) *Evaluation and Control of Training.* McGraw-Hill, New York

McClusky, H.Y. (1974) The coming of age of life-long learning. *Journal of Development in Education, 7*, 97–106

Myers, M.T. and Myers, M.G.T. (1982) *Managing by Communication: An Organizational Approach.* McGraw-Hill, New York

National Training Council for the National Health Service (1974) Preparation and Follow-up for Management Training Courses. NTC

———— (1980) Making Use of the Further Education System: A guide for NHS Managers. NTC

Nelson, D.F. (Project Leader) (1970) *Enquiry into Management Technician Roles in the Construction Industry.* Construction Industry Training Board

Pedlar, M. (1974) Learning in management education. *Journal of European Training, 3*(4), 182–95

———— et al. (1978) *A Manager's Guide to Self-development.* McGraw-Hill, New York

Revans, R.W. (1964) *Action Learning in Hospitals: Diagnosis and Therapy.* McGraw-Hill, New York

———— (1982) *The Origins and Growth of Action Learning.* Chartwell Bratt, Bromley

Royal College of Nursing (1981) A Structure for Nursing (Report of the RCN Group on a Professional Nursing Structure for the NHS). RCN

Steed Henderson, M. (ed.) (1982) *Nursing Education.* Churchill Livingstone, Edinburgh

Tanner, D. and Tanner, L. (1975) *Curriculum Development: Theory and Practice.* Collier Macmillan, London

Thompson, D. (1983) Perception, power and responsibility in management development: A study of the implications for change in the National Health Service. *Management Education and Development, 14*(3), 212–32

Ullrich, R.A. and Weiland, G.F. (1981) *Organization Theory and Design.* Richard D. Irwin, Homewood, Illinois

Weiland, G.F. (ed.) (1981) *Improving Health Care Management.* Health Administration Press, Ann Arbor, MI

12 LEGISLATION AND KEY REPORTS: A FRAMEWORK FOR CHANGING NURSING EDUCATION AND NURSING MANAGEMENT

Aims

The aims of this chapter are:

1. To examine the structure and consequences of the *Nurses, Midwives and Health Visitors Act* 1979, on nursing education.
2. To examine the effects of the EEC Nursing Directives on the nursing profession.
3. To assess the impact of recent reports and legislation on the care of patients and clients.

Learning Objectives

The purpose of this chapter is to enable the reader to:

1. Establish the relevance of current nursing legislation to:
   a. The preparation of the nurse and
   b. The care of patients and clients.
2. Appraise the effects of current nursing legislation on changing nursing.
3. Assess the impact of nursing legislation on the quality of patient/client care.

The main legislation and reports which substantially form the framework for the future development of nursing, nursing education and nursing management in the United Kingdom, include:

1. The EEC Nursing Directives.
2. The Briggs report (HMSO, 1972).
3. *Nurses, Midwives and Health Visitors Act* 1979.
4. The Merrison report (HMSO, 1979) and the Consultative Paper, *Patients First* (DHSS, 1979).

Many other equally important reports which will shape the future of nursing, including Griffiths (DHSS, 1983), Körner (NHS/DHSS, 1984), have already been discussed.

251

The Treaty of Rome

The Treaty of Rome (1957) enabled the setting up of the European Economic Community (1958). Even though the original membership was six states, i.e. Belgium, Luxembourg, Netherlands, France, Germany and Holland, the Community has since expanded to include additionally Denmark, Ireland, the United Kingdom, Greece, Spain and Portugal.

The central intention underlying an integrated community was primarily to ensure economic viability and integrity of member states. Essentially (in theory if not in practice) an important objective is that of ensuring closer working bonds and relationships between the peoples of the member states.

The basic organisational structure and functions of the Community consists of the Council of Ministers which is the principal, if not the only, decision-making body together with the Commission whose function is virtually exclusively related to policy making. The European Parliament consists of elected representatives of member states. The decisions (some) of the Council are conveyed in the form of Directives which are legally binding in the context of their intentions — aims. However, member states do have flexibility as to the achievement of these aims.

The primary objectives of the EEC are:

1. The harmonious development of economic activities;
2. Continuous and balanced expansion; and
3. Closer relations between member states.

To achieve these objectives several obstacles had to be overcome — several conditions had to be achieved. The principal obstacle which concerns nursing education relates to 'Abolition of obstacles to freedom of movement for persons, services and capital'. In this context, the situation as it affects the nursing profession relates to:

The abolition of restrictions, e.g. work permits, the mutual recognition of certificates, diplomas and degrees; the co-ordination and the standardization of nursing education, particularly in relation to the common minimum programme which is intended to include requirements for entry to training, the subject matter of training together with specialist forms of training.

EEC Law and Professional Freedom of Movement

By the Treaty of Rome, accepted by the United Kingdom by the Treaty of Accession in January 1972, Regulations of the EEC have the force of law in member countries while Directives override national governments as far as policy aims are concerned, though the choice of the exact method of implementation is left to the individual government. EEC Regulation 1912/68 is, therefore the law in Britain and provides that all EEC nationals in all matters concerned with employment have exactly the same rights as British people in Britain and elsewhere in the Community nationals of the UK must receive equal treatment to that accorded to the nationals of other EEC countries. Thus, work permits are not required and where residence permits are applicable these are automatically granted once a job is obtained. Any trade union agreement, administrative ruling of a government department or other authority which discriminates against EEC nationals is illegal but the EEC regulations do permit exclusion on the grounds of health, public security or public policy or lack of a professional qualification recognisable by the particular nation. Therefore, the establishment of common standards for reciprocal recognition of qualifications is necessary and regulations and directives to that end were actually being drafted at the time of the accession of the UK but difficulty is still being experienced in reaching agreement. One problem is the question of the balance to be struck between practical work and experience on the one hand and academic achievement on the other and another difficulty being the question of the status of various examining bodies. In addition, exemption from the free movement of labour provisions is permitted as regards 'state employees', who are differently defined and include different categories in some of the member nations (for instance teachers are within the category in France, but not in England) and the position is further complicated by 'self employed' being defined so as to include persons here regarded as 'employees'. Other bars to full mobility are differences in social security systems within the member states (though community nationals must be afforded the same benefits as are available in a member state to its own nationals) and in administrative structures.

The EEC Nursing Directives were signed in June 1977. Some major effects arising from the signing relate to the mutual recognition of diplomas, certificates and other evidence of final qualifications, including measures to facilitate the effective exercise of the right of establishment and freedom to provide services; the co-ordination of provisions laid down by law, regulation or administrative action in respect of activities of nurses responsible for general care, including training requirements;

and the setting up of an Advisory Committee on Training. (The Nursing Directives affect only the 'nurse responsible for general care'.)

The aspects of the legislation which directly or indirectly affect nursing education relate to the rationalisation of nursing educaion at basic level; the mutual recognition of certificates, diplomas and degrees; and the abolition of work permits. These changes are embodied in the EEC Nursing Directive and are legally binding on all member states of the European Community. The principal Directives relating to nursing include:

1. Directive 77/452/EEC.
2. Directive 77/453/EEC.
3. Directive 77/454/EEC.

Directive 77/452/EEC. This concerns the mutual recognition of diplomas, certificates and other evidence of the formal qualifications, together with measures to facilitate the effective exercise of this right of establishment and freedom to provide services. Under this directive, nurses of member states have 'acquired rights', i.e. nurses whose qualifications do not satisfy all the minimum training required by Article 1, Directive 77/453/EEC and wish to have their qualifications accepted must supply to the appropriate member state the nurse's qualifications accompanied by a certificate (by the competent authority, i.e. authorities awarding diplomas/certificates of competence to practise) stating that the nurse has been engaged as a nurse responsible for general care for at least 3 years during the 5 years prior to the date of issue of the certificate. Most important, these activities must have included 'taking full responsibility for the planning, organisation and carrying out of the nursing care of the patient' (Article 4).

Directive 77/453/EEC. This concerns the co-ordination of provisions laid down by law, regulation or administrative action in respect of the activities of nurses responsible for general care. In essence, this directive specifies that the final award is subject to 'passing an examination which guarantees that during training the nurse acquired knowledge of the sciences on which general nursing is based', i.e. anatomy, physiology, psychology, sociology, ethics, principles of health and nursing, clinical experience (gained under the supervisor of qualified nursing staff) and where the number of qualified staff and equipment are appropriate for the nursing care of patients together with an acknowledgement of the ability of the nurse to participate in the practical training of health

personnel as well as to experience working with other health care pro-
fessionsal.

On entry to a school of nursing candidates must provide evidence of
a general school education of 10 years' duration attested by a diploma,
certificate or other formal qualification awarded by the competent
authorities or bodies in a member state, or a certificate resulting from
a qualifying examination of an equivalent standard for entrance to a
nurses' training school. Also, full-time training must cover the subjects
of the training programme and comprise a 3-year course or 4600 hours
of theoretical and clincal instruction (Article 1, paras. 2(b) to 4).

Directive 77/454/EEC. This directive is concerned with the setting up
of an Advisory Committee on Training in Nursing.

In June, 1974, Council passed a resolution in 'favour of the establishment of Advisory Committees'. The Advisory Committee on Nursing
was set up in 1978.

The task of the Committee is to help to ensure 'a comparably high
standard of training of the various categories of nursing personnel
throughout the Community', by the exchange of comprehensive information on the training methods and the content, level and structure of
theoretical and practical instruction provided in the Member States
together with developing common approaches to the standard to be attained in the training of nursing personnel, and, as appropriate, to the
structure and content of such training.

The Committee has an 'advisory function' to the Commission in con-
nection with the training of nurses.

Midwifery Directive 80/155/EEC. This concerns the co-ordination of provisions laid down by law, regulation or administrative action relating
to the taking up and pursuit of the activities of midwives. The kind and
standard of training for admission to Part 10 of the Register must meet
the requirements of the Midwives Directive and, in addition, consist of
theoretical, clinical and practical instruction together with practical experience in the nursing and care of the mother and baby.

Two important Committees relating to nurses in the community include, 'The Standing Committee of Nurses of the European Community' (1971) whose terms of reference include those of education, nursing
service working conditions and a monitoring role. The 'Advisory Committee on Training in Nursing' (1977) has the principal role to help to
ensure a high standard of training of nurses in the community.

The Treaty of Rome enables the free movement of workers (EEC,

No.1612/68). This total freedom for professionals to practise in Member States and the potential effects on patients and clients arising from the inadequate command of language of practitioners, the lack of proper understanding of specific legal requirements of member states together with variations in the standards of education, training and subsequent qualifications awarded, could bring many problems in its wake. To obviate and/or limit these effects, the EEC Council (which has major responsibility for policy and decision making) issue appropriate Nursing Directives with the intention of regulating factors such as standards of entry, programme of training (Article 3, Directive 77/452/EEC); linguistic knowledge (Article 15, Directive 77/452/EEC); the mutual recognition of the final award, certificate, diploma or degree (Article 57, Directive 77/452/EEC) and co-ordinating the conditions governing training (Directive 77/453/EEC).

Nurses wishing to work in another member state must have a certificate issued by 'a competent authority' in their own country attesting to their character (Article 6, Directive 77/452/EEC).

In the case of nurses who through no fault of theirs are unable to meet the requirements of Nursing Directive 77/453/EEC, i.e. their training was completed prior to the implementation of the directives, a certificate, from the competent authority, must be submitted stating that these nurses have 'been responsible for general care for at least three years during the five years prior to the issue of the certificate' and that these activities have included, 'taking full responsiblity for the planning, organisation and carrying out the nursing care of the patient' (Directive 77/452/EEC, Article 4).

For midwives to practise in member states, different approaches to training are entertained, e.g. those who are general nurses, to comply with the nursing directives, must have undertaken full time training of either 2 years or 3600 hours; or 18 months training or 3000 hours, in addition to one year's practice post-qualification. Direct entrants to midwifery require the minimum of a 3 year training.

The General Trained Nurse (Nurse Responsible for General Care): Education and Training

The EEC legislation states that the general trained nurse exercises in conformity with the national legislation the following essential functions:

1. Giving skilled nursing care to persons as required in accordance with the physical, emotional and spiritual needs of the patient, whether

that care is given in Health Institutions, homes, schools, places of work.

2. Observing physical and emotional situations and conditions which have significant bearing on health and communicating those observations to other members of the health team; and

3. training and giving guidance to auxiliary personnel who are required to fulfil the nursing service needs of all health agencies.

This involves an evaluation of the nursing needs of a particular patient and assigning personnel in accordance with the needs of the patient at a particular time.

The task of ensuring the uniform education and training of nurses, in all member states, is difficult to achieve. The problem is compounded by differing approaches to training in different states. This situation poses a major problem to effecting and maintaining the standard and quality of education and training.

The rationalisation of nursing education, despite the industry of professional and statutory bodies, at national and international level is difficult. The attempt at rationalising nursing education in the UK has its roots in the Briggs report.

The Briggs Report: Preamble to Rationalising Nursing Education

To effect the rationalisation of nursing education in the UK a committee, under the chairmanship of Professor Asa Briggs, was established in 1970 with the intention of bringing nursing 'into line' with and to speak with 'one voice' in Europe (paras.294, 305, 307, 619).

The terms of reference of the Committee were:

To review the role of the nurse and the midwife in the hospital and in the community and the education and training required for that role, so that the best use is made available manpower to meet present needs and the needs of an integrated Health Service.

The report underlined the need to rationalise nursing in so far as the existence of 'a single organisation would guarantee that an authoritative voice for British nursing and midwifery would be heard outside the profession within this country, and in the long term, of equal importance, within the EEC' (para.619, pp.185–186). The Committee recommended changes to the statutory framework in which nursing is practised together with examination and modification of the prevailing nurse education system and an examination of nursing manpower.

Changes in the statutory framework advised by the Briggs Committee included setting up a single central body (now known as the United Kingdom Central Council for Nursing, Midwifery and Health Visiting) with the responsibility for professional standards, education and discipline in nursing and midwifery in Great Britain, The Central Nursing and Midwifery Council together with three distinct Nursing and Midwifery Education Boards (now known as National Boards) for England, Scotland and Wales, responsible to the Council and three Area Committees for Nursing and Midwifery Education. The report advised that education should be regarded as a continuing process under unified control and, in this respect, the setting up of a number of Colleges of Health Studies should be explored. Also, there should be close liason for recruitment purposes between the Colleges and Schools and the Youth Employment Service.

The Committee advised that there should be one basic course of 18 months for all entrants to nursing which would lead to the award of a statutory qualification, the Certificate in Nursing Practice, and a further 18 months training would lead to a second statutory qualification, Registration. In addition, Registration would include or be followed by courses leading to the award of a Higher Certificate (non-statutory) in a particular branch of nursing or midwifery.

On manpower issues, the Committee underlined the importance of 'special attention' to increasing male recruitment, and the recruitment of more A-level undergraduate students and graduate entrants. Also, they advised the setting up of manpower and personnel departments at regional and central levels. Most important, they advised identifying long-term and short-term objectives in order that the quality of patient/client care could be improved and that resources could be used to good effect.

The Problems

Having spent several years 'gathering dust' many senior nurses felt a number of the detailed recommendations made in the Briggs report were overtaken by events — in short they were outdated by the time the Briggs Bill became law in 1979. Clearly, there is considerable truth in this as borne out by the retrospective legislation and framework for education. In addition, the proposed structure caused concern among professionals.

Sadly, from the date of publication of the report to effecting the appropriate legislation (1979) 7 years elapsed. Despite this shortcoming the report marked a turning point in the history of nursing education in that it recommended a broad-based nursing profession which would include a commmon core of training for all types of qualification together with a common portal of entry for enrolled and registered nurses. Most important, the Committee emphasised the importance of continuing education throughout the nurse's career.

Even though the proposals were warmly received by the profession, when it came to reality, i.e. to implementing the recommendations, the Briggs Bill ran into trouble; the trouble in part was due to the potential/inevitable unification of existing statutory bodies which would have meant a loss of authority, influence and power for the principal independent controlling groups in nursing, midwifery and health visiting. The midwives underlined their unease about their potential lack of influence; subsequently the provision of a Standing Committee on Midwifery was established.

The health visitors who were not recognised in the original Bill as a separate profession, demanded equality. This recognition was achieved through the inclusion of Health Visitors in the subsequent legislation, i.e. the Nurses and Midwives Bill became the Nurses, Midwives and Health Visitors Bill, subsequently becoming the *Nurses, Midwives and Health Visitors Act*. The continuing influence of health visitors continued throught the establishment of a Joint Health Visiting Committee of the National Boards and Central Council.

The district nurses protested that no special provision was made in the Bill for them. However, an attempt was made to allay their fears by the assurance that the Secretary of State would be empowered to establish a Committee for District Nursing — albeit by subsidiary legislation. Ultimately district nursing was given a voice through the establishment of a Joint Committee on District Nursing.

The Way Forward

The Briggs report apart from indicating the future framework for nursing, also gave important guidelines on education and nursing manpower. For example, the report stated that education should be regarded as a continuing process under unified controls. It also advised close liason for recruitment purposes between colleges, schools and the Youth Employment Service. (Advice, that after 13 years, now seems to have become alive through the initiative of the ENB to establish links with polytechnics through the use of nurse education 'pilot' studies). The framework proposed included a basic course of training of 18 months duration for all entrants which would lead to the award of a statutory qualification, the Certificate in Nursing. It also proposed a further 18 months which would lead to a second statutory qualification and registration. Following registration the report advised that the nurse could undertake courses leading to the award of a Higher Certificate (non-statutory), in a particular branch of nursing or midwifery.

Basically, the Briggs philosophy, together with its proposed framework for nursing education attempted to move nurses out of the closet of tradition to face the reality of the twentieth century and in doing so to come to terms with national and international influences relating to change. And so, following a prolonged period of gestation, new nursing legislation was born in the form of the *Nurses, Midwives and Health Visitors Act* 1979.

Nurses, Midwives and Health Visitors Act 1979

It has been stated that nurses' knowledge base, largely because of the increased sophistication in medical science and technology, is inadequate, thereby reducing or obviating nurses' ability and competence 'to prescribe nursing care or complement doctors' (Professor Baroness McFarlane, 1983). To-day, the opportunities, and the challenges, presented to nurses are many, great and demanding; but does education theory and practice, nursing research and the environment in which nursing is practised optimise these opportunities, meet these challenges? Is the training and education of nurses adequate to meet nurses' needs in caring satisfactorily for their patients and clients while meeting their own developmental needs? These are questions — dilemmas — which face nurse educationists, nurse managers and nursing statutory bodies in the 1980s. But, of course they are not unique, presenting problems and dilemmas previously unrecorded. In fact, as far back as four decades ago an RCN Committee (1943) was set up with the terms of reference: 'to consider how best to model nursing education so as to ensure the preservation of the highest professional standards'.

At the end of June 1983 the statutory bodies responsible for the education and training of nurses, midwives, health visitors, district nurses and clinical nursing studies, were dissolved. The functions previously undertaken by these statutory bodies now became the responsibility of the United Kingdom Central Council for Nursing, Midwifery and Health Visiting together with the National Boards for Nursing, Midwifery and Health Visiting for England, Scotland, Wales and Northern Ireland.

The Act of Parliament which enabled this change is the *Nurses, Midwives and Health Visitors Act* 1979. The Act, in addition to enabling the establishment of these bodies also makes new provision with respect to 'the education, training, regulation and discipline of nurses, midwives and health visitors and the maintenance of a single professional register'. In essence, the 1979 Act sets up a new structure.

The 1979 Act is intended to enable the nursing profession to control its own standards and practice to a much greater extent than did (for many reasons) the divided former statutory bodies.

Through the agency of the Nurses Act three main branches of the nursing profession and four countries are brought together under one umbrella.

The Act is a direct result of the Briggs report (1972) which was developed in concert with the report on the National Health Service (*Grey Book*, 1972) as well as having close links and alignment with the nursing policy of the European Community.

The broad concerted goals of EEC nursing policy in conjunction with the UK new nursing structure includes: a correction of nursing 'apprenticeship', promotion, development and improvement of nursing education at basic and post-basic levels together with enabling nurses' competence and confidence, through improved preparation to provide a quality nursing service. In this way, the UKCC and the National Boards co-ordinate the education, training and regulation of nurses, midwives and health visitors.

On July 1st 1983, new statutory rules concerned with the education and training of nurses, midwives and health visitors replaced the old statutory rules. In the words of the UKCC, 'Far from "new" meaning "different", the 1983 rules closely resemble the old ones.' However, three aspects of the nurses' rules are different from the previous ones:

1. The age on entry: the minimum age is now 17½ years of age, except in Scotland where 17 years is acceptable.
2. Terminology: the profession has agreed to use the terms First Level and Second Level Nurse, and
3. Academic requirements: the new rules allow whatever practices currently exist in each country to continue — until January 1986, when the requirement of all first level entrants will be 5 O-level GCE passes, alternative qualifications, or success in Council's Test.

Council is responsible for the formulation of rules on training which the National Boards must follow, but the Boards are 'allowed to add their own education flavour by producing their own guidelines'.

Statutory Bodies

United Kingdom Central Council for Nursing, Midwifery and Health Visiting

The UKCC, even though formally established in November 1980, together with the four National Boards, assumed their full functions and responsibilities on 1 July 1983. (Figure 12.1). The UKCC replaced nine statutory and training bodies for nursing.

The UKCC and the four National Boards are five independent bodies but they work closely together. Central Council is responsible for the policy and the drafting of the rules to govern training and education, registration and professional conduct and, in this way, its work can be summarised as maintaining the professional register of all nurses; developing standards of education and training and establishing and improving standards of professional conduct, and protecting the public from unsafe practitioners.

The UKCC has a membership of 45 which comprise 7 members nominated by each National Board and 17 members appointed by the Secretary of State. The Council has a chairman appointed (initially) by the Secretary of State and a deputy chairman appointed by the Council.

The principal function of the Council is to establish and improve standards of training and professional conduct for nurses, midwives and health visitors, and in this context, by means of rules, determine conditions of entry to training and the standard of training with a view to registration. Also, the Council has power to provide advice for nurses, midwives and health visitors on standards of professional conduct. (This is exemplified in the Code of Conduct for Nurses, Midwives and Health Visitors.) In addition, Council is empowered to make provision in relation to the type and standard of training for nurses already registered. More generally, Council must have regard for the interests of all groups within the professions.

In practice, these objectives are realised in different ways and by many means. For example through improved education and training, and by carefully monitoring the professional conduct of nurses. In addition the Council must ensure that standards of training meet EEC regulations.

Committees. The Standing Committees of the UKCC include those of Midwifery and Finance, Education Policy Advisory Committee,

Figure 12.1: The National Boards and the UKCC

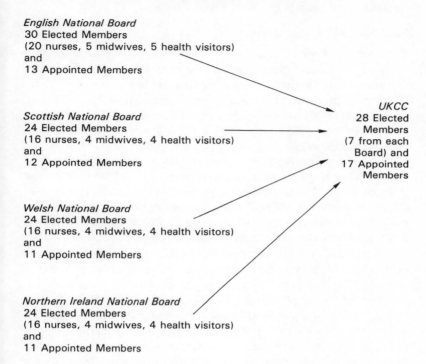

English National Board
30 Elected Members
(20 nurses, 5 midwives, 5 health visitors)
and
13 Appointed Members

Scottish National Board
24 Elected Members
(16 nurses, 4 midwives, 4 health visitors)
and
12 Appointed Members

Welsh National Board
24 Elected Members
(16 nurses, 4 midwives, 4 health visitors)
and
11 Appointed Members

Northern Ireland National Board
24 Elected Members
(16 nurses, 4 midwives, 4 health visitors)
and
11 Appointed Members

UKCC
28 Elected
Members
(7 from each
Board) and
17 Appointed
Members

Source: Reproduced by Permission of the United Kingdom Central Council for Nursing, Midwifery and Health Visiting.

Research, Registration, Professional Conduct, and Health. As well there are the District Nursing Joint Committeee and the Health Visiting Joint Committee.

The overall functions of the committees are embraced under the broad headings of advice, guidance, initiation and enquiry, and, in this way the UKCC is helped in carrying out its principal functions in a thorough and effective way by getting advice on financial matters, personnel, accommodation and equipment; taking guidance on matters relating to the education and training of nurses and the initiation and facilitation of research in and for the profession; and enquiry is conducted on matters as professional conduct and health as a possible cause of the 'unfitness' of nurses to practice. Most important, the Council consults the Midwifery committee together with the District Nursing and Health Visiting Joint committees on matters relating to their functions.

Functions and Responsibilities

Registration (Single Professional Register). The UKCC under Section 10 of the 1979 Act is obliged to draw up rules determining the criteria that are to be met to prove a nurse's entitlement to practice. In essence, the Council must maintain a register of nurses, midwives and health visitors and, in this context, make provision for the evidence to be produced, fees to be paid together with criteria for registration to remain effective for those applying for registration as well as for those whose names are on the register. The rules applying to nurses, midwives and health visitors to gain registration to different parts of the register, are included in the Nurses, Midwives and Health Visitors Rule Approval Order 1983 (HMSO, 1983). The present register has 11 parts which embrace the qualifications of RCN, EN(G), RMN, EN(M), RNMH, EN(MH), EN(Scotland/Northern Ireland), RSCN, RFN, RM, and RHV.

Every nurse has one entry on the SPR which will include every qualification of that nurse. All records are brought together to form the SPR.

The important implications for nurses, midwives and health visitors relating to organisation under the new legislation include: registration and practice are separate, i.e. registration does not necessarily mean entitlement to practise. Entitlement to practise is dependent upon factors such as age, licensing, which is linked to the payment of a fee, evidence of professional enhancement, and, where required, reorientation training.

The *Nurses, Midwives and Health Visitors Act* 1979 permits one register only (Section 10). The new single professional register was formed by the merger of the registers, rolls and records created and maintained by the former statutory and training bodies. The register includes the names of all nurses, midwives and health visitors who are entitled to practice in the UK.

Entitlement to Practise. The UKCC maintains a single professional register and, in this respect, prerequisites to maintaining the right to practise by nurses include the central issues of periodic relicensing, an upper age limit, payment of a periodic registration fee and, most important, mandatory re-training, to ensure a continuing competence of nurses in the skills and knowledge of nursing as well as change and innovation in technology in general and their effects on the practice of nursing.

Entitlement to practise under the Act is based upon:

1. *Age*. The present upper age limit is 70 years. Exceptionally beyond that age nurses might be allowed to practise, but only with the approval of the UKCC.
2. *Reorientation*. From January, 1985, nurses will lose their entitlement to practise if they have been absent from the profession for five years or more, unless they undergo a period of reorientation by undertaking a refresher course in the form of in-service training courses, full or part-time courses, study days or involvement in some other forms of education and training. Other forms of education and training remain unspecified but in reality are wide and varied (see Chapter 11).
3. *Updating*. From January, 1990, entitlement to practise will depend on whether nurses can satisfy the Council that they have kept up with developments in nursing. Despite the fact that the onus for updating is on individual nurses (Code of Professional Conduct, para.3), in practice this may prove difficult in view of the scarcity of resources both within and external to hospitals. In practice, one suspects the major responsibility for ensuring the education and training of staff will remain with senior nurse managers in general and nurse teachers in particular; the latter whose numbers are much depreciated and already fully committed.
4. *Relicensing*. The 1979 Act gives the UKCC power to institute a periodic relicensing fee for all nurses, midwives, and health visitors in order that they remain entitled to practise. Relicensing will also have other important off-shoots, e.g. the introduction of a periodic fee would, in itself, enable an effective register to be maintained, reviewed and updated as well as ensuring regular contact with the members of the professions and would facilitate the ready revision of the register which, if required, could become the basis for a future nurses' electoral role.

The conduct of nurses in relation to the patient and to themselves and to their colleagues, is a vital one. It is at the root of providing a satisfactory service for the patient. The first edition of the Code was published in July 1983: a second edition was published in November 1984.

Each of the National Boards have their own Investigating Committee to consider cases of alleged misconduct by nurses, midwives and health visitors. These Committees may then refer cases to the Professional Conduct Committee or Health Committee of the UKCC. Both Committees hear cases to determine whether or not a nurse, midwife or health visitor should be removed from the register or part of it. The Health Committee particularly enquires into cases of alleged unfitness of nurses due to ill-health which may interfere with their ability to practise.

Are the underlying demands of the Code realistic? Feasible? Can the inevitable demands placed upon nurses through it (and if they deviate from which, may incur disciplinary action) be taken seriously, particularly in the vagueness of such vital prerequisites as the authority, responsibility, accountability, and autonomy for nursing decision making by nurses?

The National Boards

In essence, there is a basic legislative structure for all National Boards with some differences in practice. Each National Board has Midwifery and Finance Standing Committees which they must consult on matters relating to midwifery and finance. Also, the Secretary of State, 'May, by order, constitute other Standing Committees', 'Joint Committees of the Central Council and the National Boards' and 'Local Training Committees' (Schedule 2, Section 6, paras 4, 7 (2) (5), 8 (1) and 9 (1) *Nurses, Midwives and Health Visitors Act* 1979.) In addition, some committees are also governed by additional legislation in the form of statutory instruments, eg. S1 1983 No 1219, S1 1982 No 1568 and S1 1983 No 1219.

The functions of the National Boards generally are many, and include responsibility for providing courses leading to registration, providing courses for those already on the Register, and ensuring that all courses are of a satisfactory standard. The Boards also arrange for examinations in nursing and midwifery in appropriate institiutions where such training is undertaken and must monitor standards both in hospitals and in Institutes of Higher Education conducting courses in nursing, midwifery, health visiting and district nursing. They must also record additional qualifications on the Professional Register maintained by the UKCC. They are responsible for the investigation of alleged professional misconduct ('conduct unworthy of a nurse, midwife or health visitor, and includes obtaining registration by fraud') of qualified staff.

To assist the work of the National Boards there may be a range of specialist panels, liaison committees and working groups. In addition, in Scotland, local training committees have also been established in each mainland Health Board area to assist the National Board in the exercise of its training functions.

Through this network of committees, and in conjunction with the UKCC, the Boards discharge their functions by preparation and control of nurses and, in this way, improve standards of patient/client care.

England, Wales, Scotland and Northern Ireland each has a National Board. The National Boards have a numerically differing membership, e.g. the maximum being for Northern Ireland 35, and for the other National Boards 45. In fact the ENB has 30 elected members (20 nurses, 5 midwives and 5 health visitors) and 15 appointed members. The SNB has 24 elected members (16 nurses, 4 midwives and 4 health visitors) and 12 appointed members. The WNB and the NINB each have 24 elected members (16 nurses, 4 midwives and 4 health visitors) and 11 appointed members.

The National Boards are responsible for ensuring that the policies of the Council in respect of education and training are carried out and in this way provide or arrange for others to provide at institutions approved by the Board courses/training for qualification as a nurse, midwife or health visitor. The Boards must ensure courses meet the requirements of the Central Council, and must hold examinations for the Register, and additional qualifications. In practice this means providing courses of training with a view to enabling persons to qualify for registration as nurses, midwives and health visitors as well as to provide courses of further training at post-basic level. In this context, the Boards must ensure that courses are satisfactory in their content and standard. In addition to arranging training, Boards must ensure that examinations are arranged to enable nurses to satisfy requirements for registration and/or to obtain additional qualifications. They must also collaborate with the UKCC to promote improved training methods and, most important, investigate cases of alleged misconduct, and, if the case is sufficiently serious to refer it to the UKCC Professional Conduct Committee.

Committees. The Standing Committees of the Boards include those of midwifery and finance. The Joint Committees of the ENB include those on midwifery, health visiting and district nursing which, in addition to having an advisory function, also have some executive functions. In addition to these Committees there is a Committee on education policy, investigating and approvals/applications: the last two in addition to the finance committee have executive functions. Most important, the Board has advisory committees on mental illness, mental handicap, general/paediatric and occupational health.

The important implication for nurses of the composition, i.e. the balance in the membership, of the UKCC and the National Boards arises from the fact that approximately one-third of their membership are appointed. In effect, the profession has no control over a substantial proportion of the membership of statutory bodies which are ostensibly provided to represent the views of nurses.

The EEC Directives and the 1979 Nurses Act: Curriculum Implications

The general curriculum objectives made known by the UKCC are: to equip the nurses to work in a team with social, medical and paramedical staff; to prepare them for a professional qualification; to develop students' awareness of their own needs and the needs of others; to develop an ability to be self-critical and analytical and to equip nurses to provide the highest possible standard of care.

In the context of the EEC Nursing Directives, Directive 77/453/EEC concerns the 'co-ordination of the provisions laid down by law, regulation or administrative action in respect of activities of nurses responsible for general care'.

Developing Standards of Education and Training (See also Chapter 11).

The training leading to the award of a formal qualification must include a section on nursing comprising the nature and ethics of the profession; general principles of health and nursing and nursing principles which relate to general and specialist medicine; general and specialist surgery; child care and paediatrics; maternity care; mental health and psychiatry, and the care of the old and geriatrics. The section on the Basic Sciences must embrace anatomy and physiology; pathology; bacteriology; virology and parasitology; biophysics, biochemistry and radiology; dietetics; hygiene; preventive medicine; health education; and pharmacology. The Social Sciences curriculum must include sociology; psychology; principles of adminstration; principles of teaching; social and health legislation; and legal aspects of nursing.

Clinical instruction must reflect general and specialist medicine; general and specialist surgery; child care and paediatrics; maternity care; mental health and psychiatry; care of the old and geriatrics; and home nursing.

Award of Certificates/Diplomas for General Care

The final award, certificate or diploma is based on criteria to be met by the student and obligations to be met by the training institution. These obligations are specified in Article 3 of Directive 77/452/EEC and are subject to nurses passing an examination which guarantees that during their training they have acquired:

1. Adequate knowledge of the sciences on which general nursing is based, including sufficient understanding of the structure, physiological functions and behaviour of healthy and sick persons, and of the relationship between the state of health and the physical and social environment of the human being.
2. Sufficient knowledge of the nature and ethics of the profession and of the general principles of health and nursing.
3. Adequate clinical experience; such experience, which should be selected for its training value, should be gained under the supervision of qualified nursing staff and in places where the number of qualified staff and equipment are appropriate for the nursing care of the patients.
4. The ability to participate in the practical training of health personnel and experience of working with such personnel. And
5. Experience of working with members of other professions in the health sector.

Member states must also ensure that the institution training nurses co-ordinates theory and practice throughout the programme. In this respect, the theoretical and technical training must be balanced and co-ordinated with the clinical training of nurses in such a way that the knowledge and experience may be acquired in an adequate manner. Clinical instruction in nursing must take the form of supervised in-service training in hospital departments or other health services, including home nursing services, approved by the competent authoritites or bodies. During training student nurses must participate in the activities of the departments concerned in so far as those activities contribute to their training. They must be informed of the responsibilities of nursing care.

Variations on Minimum Training Requirements

Member states whose diplomas, certificates and other evidence of formal qualifications do not satisfy all the minimum training requirements (Article 1 of Directive 77/453/EEC), must recognise, as being sufficient proof, evidence of the formal qualifications of nurses awarded by those member states before the implementation of Directive 77/453/EEC. This evidence must be accompanied by a certificate stating that those nationals have effectively and lawfully been engaged in the activities of nurses responsible for general care for at least 3 years during the 5 years prior to the date of issue of the certificate. These activities must have included taking full responsiblity for the planning, organisation and carrying out of the nursing care of the patient.

Change: Implications of New Legislation for Practitioners, Managers and Educationists

It is hoped that the changes which are being effected will, without doubt, provide a better educated and more intellectually, socially and attitudinally improved nurse, with a corresponding improvement in the care and management of patients and clients.

However, as in all forms of change, irrespective of their magnitude, certain requirements have to be met if the change is to be effective. The general implications of the new legisalation are far-reaching, if implemented, in improving the education of nurses at basic and post-basic levels as well as having a positive effect on patient care. The implications concern such central issues as:

1. The nursing student.
2. The single professional register.
3. The grade of nurse.
4. The development of Colleges of Nursing and Midwifery.
5. Nursing curricula.
6. The nursing budget, and
7. The nursing service.

The Nursing Student

The term 'nursing student' refers to a nurse who, in preparation for a statutory qualification is in a controlled learning situation and who, while never being in a position of professional accountability, nevertheless is required to assume increasing responsibility for the care of his/her patient/client. Is it feasible, given the present situation in nursing, where so-called senior nursing students may be given responsibility for a ward on night duty (albeit with trained nursing cover — somewhere) to focus purely on the responsibility element rather than on both? Clearly it is incumbent on nurse managers to ensure wards are properly and adequately 'covered'; but, in my view it is extremely doubtful if this can be realistically effected in the present situation. Perhaps more important, is it right and proper that any member of the health care team let alone a nurse professional should be deemed to be wholly devoid of accountability while operating at this level of practice? These are issues that have been raised by the profession, but, as yet, no answers have been found. In addition, the student has 'protected employee' status which, hopefully, will ensure fewer hours committed to the work in the clinical setting during the first year, but with increasing hours of work and increased responsibility during later years of training. This concept was challenged by the Royal College of Nursing which saw it as, 'weakening the position of the nurse, and the nurse educationist by emphasising the dominance of nurse management in relation to the nursing student' (Ellis, 1982; Editorial, 1982).

Grade of Nurse: Status of Enrolled Nurse

The grade of nurse, first level and second level nurse, has produced some consternation in the profession. The views expressed by many nurses indicate that the new terminology (even though the profession agreed to the use of these terms (UKCC Review, Handover Special No.6, 1983), will cause an extension of the gulf already in existence, between the student and pupil nurse and the registered and enrolled nurse, particularly in their status and worth to the profession. Nobody doubts the real worth of enrolled nurses, although clearly their future is unclear. The evidence is inconsistent, despite many reassurances by the UKCC to its commitment to maintaining the enrolled nurse.

In January 1982, UKCC Working Group 3, following discussion and debate with the National Boards, released a consultation paper, 'The Development of Nurse Education' for discussion and comment by the profession. This paper recommended 'that there should be one basic level of qualification as a nurse'. And, 'the position of existing enrolled nurses should be protected'. More recently (1983) the unclear policy of the UKCC on the issue of the enrolled nurse has heightened enrolled nurses' doubts, following the publication of a UKCC circular (Admin/84/03), the purpose of which was to summarise its policy about enrolled nurses. The paper provoked intense discussion and considerable confusion within the profession. However, in view of the complexities of the issues involved (one such issue being that of a decision on one or two levels of nurse), and the absence of a clear, mandate, it was decided, 'that Council should not immediately proceed on any of the matters raised'. And, in this respect, the circular (Admin/84/03) concludes: 'No further study on one or two grades of nurse has been possible and the matter stands referred for Council consideration at some future date.'

Regrettably, such indecision caused considerable consternation in the profession as exemplified by the RCN Council: 'the statement was unhelpful and did nothing at all to reassure enrolled nurses about their future' (*Nursing Standard*, 15 Mar, 1984). The Chairman of the RCN's Committee on Labour Relations, reporting to the RCN Council, expressed the views of its members thus: 'Members of the CLR said it was morally wrong to continue to train SENs if there was no role for them in the future.'

'The greater flexibility and interchangeability in having one grade of nurse, and the provision of updating and refreshment courses should help to offset the effect on the nursing service.' (Working Group 3).

The reality and validity of this statement is difficult to appreciate in view of the mammoth task of reorganisation and re-education of nurses facing nurse managers and nurse educationists. However, at this critical time, when nursing education is at the crossroads, it is vital that the profession as a whole is optimistic and constructive about the present exciting developments and their potential reforming effects on nursing education and nursing practice; though retaining a realism about the practicalities of such redirection and reform.

Establishing and Improving Standards of Professional Conduct: Protecting the Public

The chief implications of the new legislation relate to the regulation and rationalisation of nursing education, primarily enabling nurses to speak with one voice in Europe; to improve the education of nurses; and, most important, through improved education and enlightenment, to ensure a high standard of nursing care for patients.

There is separation between the award of a qualification (the responsibility of the National Boards) and registration (the responsibility of the Central Council). The UKCC and the National Boards are required by the 1979 Act to establish and improve standards of training for nurses, midwives and health visitors and, in this respect, all nurses, midwives and health visitors are required to maintain their professional competence to enable them to continue to practise. This is both laudable and necessary; but also has inherent weaknesses which are related to the number of nurses to be educated and updated, and, very often most probably the sheer practical problems of coping with so sizeable a group without the necessary resources, particularly nurse teachers and, because of these the UKCC which is responsible for establishing and improving standards of professional conduct, no doubt will encounter many problems.

The Professional Code of Conduct underlines clearly that the protection and safeguarding of the patients/clients through the promotion of high standards of professional conduct and practice together with the support and development of colleagues rests not only with the appropriate nursing statutory bodies; but, most important, with nurses themselves.

The nature and quality of nurse education are vital elements and determinants of enabling a high standard of practice, and, in this context, the UKCC: 'is committed to work to improve standards of professional conduct as one of its major objectives' (Dame Catherine Hall, 1985).

In practice, any person could allege that an action and/or omission by a registered nurse, midwife or health visitor is misconduct in a professional sense. As a result, the appropriate statutory bodies must consider such allegations. In this situation it is a requirement of law (Rule 4 (1) Statutory Instrument 1983, number 887) that the National Boards 'investigate such cases with a view to proceedings before the Council or a Committee of the Council for the practitioner to be removed from the Register or part/s of it'.

The UKCC and the National Boards are required by law to establish and improve standards of training for nurses, midwives and health visitors. Because of this legal requirement the UKCC is responsible for establishing and improving standards of professional conduct and formulating the rules to determine the circumstances under which a person's name may be removed from or restored to the register.

The Code of Professional Conduct was first published in July 1983 (1st edn. UKCC, 1983). a revised Code was issued in July 1984.

The areas of practice which are defined in the Code are deemed to be central to the 'proper fulfilment of professional responsibility and professional accountability of the nurse, midwife and health visitor'. The Code gives 'guidance and advice' to practising nurses on areas such as complying with the country/state, province/territory in which the nurse works, having due regard to their custom and practice (Code of Conduct 1983/EEC Nursing Directives).

In respect of nurses' accountability and responsibility for practice, they must 'sustain and improve their knowledge and competence' (para.3). Also, they must have regard to the values and beliefs of patients/clients and avoid abuse of their special nurse-patient-client relationship in relation to confidentiality together with access to patients'/clients' 'property, residence or workplace' (paras.3, 11). Also, nurses, midwives and health visitors must safeguard the interests, ensure the well-being and have regard for the customs of their patients/clients and ensure the environment in which they are nursed enables safe practice (paras. 2, 6, 8 and 10).

To ensure protection of the patient/client nurses must ensure their own updating while simultaneously having due regard for their colleagues and subordinates in terms of helping them to develop (become professionally competent) and by ensuring their 'workload and pressures' are not excessive and intolerable (paras. 3, 4, 7, 11 and 12).

The Code of Professional Conduct is intended to help nurses to 'perform their professional duties in accordance with nationally improved guidelines or codes of practice' and if such practices, codes or law are found to conflict with safe practice, appropriate change should be initiated 'throught the appropriate channels'.

The onus is on nurses (as well as the UKCC) to 're-appraise continuously the relevance of the ˙Code to the social and professional context in which nurses, midwives and health visitors must practice' (p.4.) The philosophy of the Code of Professional Conduct is 'to promote high standards of professional practice and conduct on the part of nurses, midwives and health visitors, to ensure that justice is done, in respect of those who are brought within this function and that every encouragement is given to the individual practitioner to re-establish himself or herself, if it can be demonstrated that this is not contrary to the public interest'. Obviously, a code of conduct is central to any profession; but many questions have been raised by professional bodies and nurses in relation to the reality and the validity of certain aspects of the code (Pyne, 1983, Howard, 1983, Storey, 1985). More recently, in a case of law, the judge rejected any legal significance of the code.

Issues

Some issues that have been raised as to the applicability of the code relate to paragraphs 1, 2, 10 and 11. For example, if it becomes impossible to promote and safeguard (as a professional would like) the well-being and interests of patients/clients (paras.1, 2 and 10) because of the lack of resources (much discussed), what can really be done to remedy the situation, particularly at a time when resources are just not available? Likewise, even though clearly important to the physical, social and emotional sustenance of one's colleagues, what can really be done throughout the profession, to obviate or reduce an inappropriately high workload and/or undue pressures on colleagues, knowing the reality of the impoverishment of staff numbers, lack of a counselling service and an increasing lack of real recognition by Government and the public at large of the real issues facing nursing? Does the Code exclusively focus on safety but not on the now vital issues of human rights, the promotion of personal well-being together with inter-professional relationships?

Colleges of Nursing and Midwifery

The official policy (Working Group 3) underlined the need for Colleges of Nursing and Midwifery: 'There is a virtue in the nursing students being able to see and inhabit an institution dedicated to their learning and where registered nurses pursue further studies.' Each College was seen as having a separate identity, guided and regulated by an independent governing body, responsible to a National Board. The concept of College is seen as, 'central to an educational structure'.

Initially, a view expressed was that Colleges would be based on Health Districts and would replace existing nursing and midwifery schools. However, the proposal was not exactly clear, central to which was that there are 186 Health Districts: the anticipated number of colleges was 100 to 120. If this situation were to prevail it is clear that some district schools of nursing would have to amalgamate in an effort to meet the educational needs of their nursing students. In theory, this provision might help to economise on tutorial staff, but clearly many additional problems could emerge in relation to such things as logistics and the accountability of students.

In management terms the College would have a governing body accountable to the National Board: the Chairman of the governing body would be appointed by the National Board. National Boards would have the responsibility of ensuring that the preparation of students was of a standard necessary to comply with the requirements of professional qualification in accordance with the rules of the UKCC.

The ENB's plan relating to the number of colleges of nursing and midwifery was criticised by the RCN in that the proposal would reduce the number of nursing and midwifery schools by almost one-third. Current information states that the development of colleges of nursing is in abeyance; but district schools of nursing are being encouraged to develop educational initiatives with Institutes of Education. In fact, these initiatives have already taken root and recently (March 1985) the ENB approved six pilot schemes on basic general nurse education.

The Curriculum

In relation to curricula initiatives and requirements, the demands on nurse educationists (because of lack of numbers) and nurse managers (because of the numbers of staff involved) are many. In the context of curriculum development and implementation, the education and development of staff, even though a priority, will encounter many impediments and give rise to numerous problems, not least of which is the magnitude of the requirement of providing a satisfactory programme of basic education together with ensuring the updating of staff at post-basic level through the provision of reorientation courses, conversion courses, courses for care assistants and ensuring a programme of continuing education. This, in the view of many educationists and managers, in view of the magnitude of the task, will produce intolerable pressures for them, many of whom are already disadvantaged through impoverished resources.

Manpower

A prerequisite to the successful education of nurses is the correction of the long-standing shortage of nurse teachers.

Working Group 3 was particularly hazy on the manpower implications of the proposed educational system, particularly in relation to the extra provision of trained nurses and nurse supervisors with appropriate supervisory and teaching skills, to ensure its success and, in this respect stated: 'It is impossible to quantify precisely the staffing levels that will enable nursing students to contribute to the work of the ward in a manner which would maximise the learning nature of the experience.' However, it also stated, 'there will be a need for nurse teachers to plan and provide the educational element'.

The present obvious dissatisfaction of nurse teachers with their status, authority, working conditions and great responsibility together with the reduction of teacher courses by 25 per cent (*Nursing Standard*, April 1984) on preparatory courses and the long-standing imbalance in the ratio of teachers to students, must inevitably (despite the enthusiasm of some teachers) have at least a limiting effect and, at the most, a crippling effect on the educational initiatives being considered and ultimately further aggravate declining standards of care. The regrettable fact relating to nursing manpower is that present 'care' is provided largely by a workforce who are in the main either untrained or unqualified. If enrolled nurse training is discontinued it is estimated that eventually such a shortfall in qualified nurses, by 1994, would force the profession to resort to untrained manpower by as much as 50 per cent to cope with service demands (Chudley, 1984).

In the opening chapter of this book I discussed innovation and change together with the many and varied precipitating factors of change. The real issue is: are nursing and nurses capable of real change? Will the enabling legislation in the form of *Nurses, Midwives and Health Visitors Act* 1979 together with the EEC Nursing Directives propel the profession successfully into the next century, safeguarding as it does nursing's treasured traditions, standards and ethics? Clearly, the exciting occurrences that are currently taking place in nursing practice and nursing education must be matured, exploited and used optimally, wisely and creatively. Nursing is a great profession of which all nurses must be proud. To enable this they must become emancipated through education, training and the acquisition of the authority and autonomy which will enable them to plot their future wisely and usefully and utilise change positively when the profession not only becomes aware of its problems, but, most important, critically and objectively examines the real issues — the demands made upon it by society, technology, education and in doing so reorganises and re-establishes its priorities, identifying its strengths and weaknesses and moves smoothly and effectively into the next century.

The broad approaches to the education and training of the nurse responsible for general practice are sound and clear. Attempts are being made to change nurses in a thinking as well as a caring profession. The roots of these approaches are dated; but wisely recently revived in EEC documents (April 1981), the publication of the ENB (1985) and in the acceptance by the RCN of the report by the Commission on Nursing Education (1985) which recommends making schools of nursing part of the higher education system. Even though moving nurse education out of the domain of nursing and into the domain of higher education will not in itself solve all the problems facing the nursing profession, it will go some way towards resolving such long-standing traditional issues in nursing as the education versus service debate which, over the years, has been a source of smouldering conflict between nurse educationists and nurse managers. However, it may accentuate other equally important issues as providing the necessary workforce of trained and qualified nurses to fill the vacuum thus created, and ensure the care of patients and clients.

The ENB (1985) publication (Guidelines for Courses leading to Part 1 of the Register) even though novel in its layout and concept, emphasises patient-centred care and encompasses the nursing competencies for the theoretical foundation for nursing practice, expects nurse educationists (probably rightly) 'to translate the existing syllabus into a very broad-based curriculum' i.e. fulfilling the needs of nursing students and the respective institutions within a varied social and economic structure. This, in my view, presents a major task for nurse educationists and nurse managers: one which demands closer understanding and co-operation than at present on matters of the education and training of nurses as well as establishing close links and activity with institutes of higher education. Links and activity which, as yet, in the majority of situations remain unestablished. Philosophies of education and training which remain purely theoretical.

If the new legislation coupled with recent initiatives are to be successful in providing nurses who are equipped to take their rightful place and to work effectively in a multi-professional team, to improve their critical faculties and conceptualisation thus enabling them to be more analytical in their viewing of situations, then a concerted agreement must be reached, acknowledged as being relevant and implemented in relation to the improved education and training of nurses.

Clearly, there are many variables related to the development and the provision of a quality service; the key variables being the nurse, nurse teachers, nursing curricula, the extent of the nursing budget, the nature of nursing manpower, the attitudes and values of staff together with their status, rewards, motivation and leadership.

The central objective of any legislation and/or reports on the health care professions, of which nursing is predominant because of its size, special closeness and relationship with the patient, must be focused on raising the standard and quality of care. Therefore, the events discussed, to have value, must be seen within the context of the National Health Service and in the context of the complexities of delivering care in a multi-professional context with its many inherent problems of differing priorities, values, attitudes, goals, training and development; as well as the anomalies of status, authority, responsibility, power and influence within the various professional groups.

The question that arises in my mind is this: will the nursing legislation create a straitjacket for nurses, in essence fixing their working parameters which, if they breach them, will subject the nurses to punitive measures, instead of first of all resolving the key problems that bedevil the proper working and self-actualisation of nurses and which relate to status, salary and working conditions, inter-professional working relationships, education and training, retraining and updating and, most important, the ever-present problem of their unclear and ambiguous role.

Legislation must not be regarded as an end in itself but a means to an end, that of ensuring the development and working of efficient and safe professional practitioners thus securing and enabling a quality service to the patient.

Finally, it is difficult to prophesy, with even a degree of accuracy, the ultimate effects of the legislation on the re-shaping, the changing, of nursing management and nursing education, not because of the weaknesses or the inappropriateness of the guidelines and framework provided; but because of the lengthy catalogue of potential historic and traditional impediments.

References

Chudley, P. (1984) Grim protection at ANB conference. *Nursing Standard, 335,* 1
—— (1984) *Nursing Standard, 344,* 1
DHSS (1972) Management Arrangements for the Reorganised National Health Service (Grey Book). HMSO, London
—— (1979) Patients First (Consultative Paper on the Structure and Management of the NHS in England and Wales). HMSO, London
—— (1980) Summary of Comments Received on the Consultative Paper. DHSS, London
—— (1983) NHS Management Inquiry (Griffiths) DHSS, London
Editorial (1982) *Nursing Standard, 246,* 2
Ellis, S. (1982) Mixed feelings on education paper. *Nursing Standard, 246,* 1
EEC (Commission of the European Communities) (1977) Legislation. *Official Journal of the European Communities, 20* (L176), 1–11
—— (1981) Advisory Committee on Training in Nursing (Report on the Training of Nurses Responsible for General Care, in Particular on the Balance to be found Between Theoretical and Clinical Instruction for this Category of Nurse). (EEC 111/D/76/6/80-EN). EEC
—— (1984) Advisory Committee on Training in Nursing (Report on Psychiatric Nursing in the European Community) (111/D/700/7/82-EN). EEC
English National Board (1983) The End of the Beginning. Sept. 1980–Sept. 1983. ENB
—— (1983) The English National Board and Change in Statutory Bodies. ENB
—— (1985) The Syllabus and Examinations for Courses in General Nursing Leading to Registration in Part I of the Register. ENB
General Nursing Council for England and Walesp (1977/78) Annual Report. GNC
Hall, Dame C. (1985) The way forward. *Senior Nurse, 2*(1), 16–18
HMSO (1972) Report of the Committee on Nursing (Briggs). Cmnd. no. 5115. HMSO, London
—— (1979) Royal Commission on the National Health Service (Merrison). Cmnd. 7615. HMSO, London
Howard, G. (1983) Nurses who refuse to work may not be on strike. *Nursing Mirror, 157*(16), 9
McFarlane, Baroness (1983) Nursing Mirror Lecture 1983. *Nursing Mirror, 156*(23), 17–20
National Board for Scotland (1985) How We Work. NBS
NHS/DHSS (1982/1984) Steering Group on Health Services Information (Five reports) (Körner). HMSO, London
Nurses, Midwives and Health Visitors Act 1979 (Chapter 36). HMSO, London
Nurses, Midwives and Health Visitors Rules Approval Order (1983) No. 873, HMSO, London
Pyne, R. (1983) Misconduct risk. *Nursing Mirror, 157*(16), 9
Royal College of Nursing (1943) Nursing Reconstruction Committee (Horder). RCN
Storey, M. (1985) Managers are ignoring the Code. *Nursing Standard, 383,* Feb. p.1
United Kingdom Central Council for Nursing, Midwifery and Health Visiting (1981) The Single Professional Register. (Consultation Paper, Working Group 2). Nov. UKCC
—— (1982) Education and Training (Consultation Paper 1, Working Group 3), Jan. UKCC
—— (1982) Professional Conduct (Consultation Paper, Working Group 4), April. UKCC
—— (1982) UKCC Review, UKCC
—— (1983) Code of Professional Conduct for Nurses, Midwives and Health Visitors. UKCC
—— (1983) How the UKCC Works for You. July. UKCC
—— (1983) Notices, Concerning a Midwives Code of Practice for Practising Midwives in England and Wales. UKCC

────── (1984) Code of Professional Conduct for Nurses, MIdwives and Health Visitors (Revised). UKCC

────── (1984) The Central Council and the Future (Circular: Admin/84/03). UKCC

────── (1984) Teachers of Nursing, Midwifery and Health Visiting. (Consultation Paper). UKCC

Welsh National Board (1985) Committee Structure. WNB

Advised Further Reading

Henderson, M.S. (ed.) (1982) *Nursing Education.* Churchill Livingstone Edinburgh

HMSO (1970)European Agreement on the Instruction and Education of Nurses (Treaty Series no.92, 1970), Cmnd. no. 4495. HMSO, London

────── (1972) Report on the Committee on Nursing (Briggs). Cmnd. no. 5115. HMSO, London

Lyman, K. (1961) Basic nursing education programmes: A guide to their planning. WHO Publication. Health Paper, no.7, pp.10–24

Maynard, A. (1975) *Health Care in European Community.* Croom Helm, London

Quinn, S. (ed.) (1980) Nursing in the European Community. Croom Helm, London

Ross, T. (1982) UKCC Special. *Nursing Mirror, 155*(15), iii-viii

Steed Henderson, M. (ed.) (1982) *Nursing Education,* Chapter 7, Churchill Livingstone, Edinburgh

United Kingdom Central Council for Nursing, Midwifery and Health Visiting (1983) Handover Special (no.6), July, UKCC

────── (1983) Code of Professional Conduct for Nurses, Midwives and Health Visitors, July, UKCC

INDEX

Abel, P.M. 177
Aberdeen Formula 165, 174
   see also information, manpower
    and productivity
accountability 11, 39, 44, 52, 58, 59,
   113, 114, 115, 116, 120, 142, 154
action learning 240
aim of nursing 86
aims of staff development 231
   see also education
Alkin, M.C. 149, 248
Alonso, R.C. 125
alternating rhythms 54, 123
Althaus, J.N. 177
Altman, J. 88
anxiety 30, 190, 202
Argyle, M. 192, 220
   see also interpersonal skills
Argyris, C. 201, 220
Ashton, D. 249
Ashworth, P. 222
Athlone report 153, 175
Atkinson, R.C. 222
Atkinson, R.L. 222
authority 11, 16, 31, 52, 58, 59, 114,
   116, 120
autonomy 11, 16, 31, 52, 58, 59, 113,
   114, 116, 117, 120, 142
   see also professionalism; Code of
    Professional Conduct

Backman, C.W.B. 203, 220
Bacquer, A. 249
Ball, J.A. 147, 148, 149, 177
   see also Criteria for Care
Barnard, K. 62, 79
Barr, A. 163, 166, 174
   see also manpower
Batey, M.V. 115, 116, 117, 124
Batten, J. 177, 186
Bennett, M. 50, 54, 79, 104, 149
   see also nursing structure and
    functions
Bennis, W. 15, 21, 23, 25
Beveridge, C. 158, 174
Binsted, D. 22, 25

   see also innovation and change
Blanchard, K.H. 88, 177
Blake, P.R. 201, 202, 220
   see also leadership, productivity
Block, D. 104, 118, 124, 135, 147
Bosanquet, N. 56, 125
'Bottom-up Approach' 163
   see also manpower
Bowers, D.G. 203, 220
Bowman, M.P. 57, 58, 75, 104, 125,
   222, 238, 247, 249
Bramham, J. 177
Brammer, L.M. 214, 217, 220
Briggs, L.J. 249
Briggs report 6, 7, 8, 56, 57, 60, 71,
   75, 76, 78, 83, 87, 92, 94, 96, 97,
   111, 115, 117, 122, 124, 127,
   148, 151, 179, 185, 214, 215,
   217, 220, 225, 226, 227, 251,
   261, 279
   see also reports-key
Brown, N. 46
Brown, R.G.S. 46
Brunel University 58, 59,
   see also nurses' role
Burgoyne, J.G. 97, 103, 249
burnout 178, 180
burnout defined 178–86
   see also stress
burnout, signs of 182
   see also stress
Burns, T. 153, 174
Bussey, A.L. 158, 174
Butcher, R. 107, 124

Cang, S. 58, 61, 62, 79, 125, 249
Cameron, D. 197, 220
   see also problems — concept
Campbell, D.T. 147
care
   declining standards 77, 127
   delivery 48
   evaluation 86, 143–5
   impediments; *see also* Merrison
    report; Nurse Alert
   management 89–125

nursing philosophy 54
standards 18, 118, 126–49, 147–8;
    see also quality of care;
    references
systematic approach 134
caring and care 110, 134, 142
    see also Standards of Care
caring and professionalism 111
caring role 109
    see also Mayeroff, M.
Carlson, D. 104
Cartwright, D. 201
causes of declining standards 127
    see also references 46, 79, 80
challenges to the NHS 29
change 5–27
    approaches 15, 16
    assumptions 12
    effects 24
    motivation for 20
    multiple factors 132–3
    research findings 22
    resistance and restraints 21
    role models 12
    technological 130
    themes 16–17
    see also references 25–7;
        innovation
change agents 13, 14, 20, 21
change in clinical practice
    effecting change 20, 22, 23, 24
change in nursing 17
Chapman, C. 55, 125
Christman, L. 177
Chudley, P. 226, 247, 276, 279
Clare, C.C. 80
Clark, C.C. 104
client system 21
Code of Professional Conduct 55, 99,
    114, 116, 119, 135, 136, 138,
    148, 185, 186, 207, 242, 272,
    273, 274, 279
    see also professionalism, standard
        of care, UKCC
cognitive redefinition 17
Cogwheel reports 9, 25, 26, 31, 46,
    79, 177, 185, 186
Cohen, M.A. 108, 124, 125
Colavecchio, R. 104, 142, 148
Cole, G.A. 88
Colleges of Nursing and Midwifery
    275
Collier, M.M. 147

Commission on Nursing Education 6,
    26
    see also education and training
Committees of UKCC 262–4
    see also legislation
communication 13, 20, 189, 192
    concept of 190–3
    impediments to 193
    and morale 190
    in nursing 191
    process 192
    see also interpersonal skills,
        references 220–1
Community Health Councils (CHCs)
    39
components of caring 122, 123
    see also Mayeroff, M.
concerns of the manager 92
conflict 16
consensus management 41, 77, 195
Consultative Paper on the Structure
    and Management Arrangements
    of the NHS (Patients First) 31,
    33, 35, 36, 77, 79, 95, 103,
    251
continuing education 223–50
Continuing Education for the Nursing
    Profession in Scotland (report)
    6, 9, 226, 230, 248
controlling practice 108, 117–22
Cooper, C.L. 13, 25, 186, 222
Cooper, R.C. 201, 220
counselling 213, 218
counselling concept 216–18
    see also references 220–1,
        Crawley, P.
    causes for concern 214
Counselling, Help and Advice
    Together (CHAT) 215
courage 55, 123
    see also Mayeroff, M.
Craska, N.L. 125
Crawley, P. 214, 220
Criteria for Care 145
critique of NHS management 40
    see also Griffiths, Merrison and
        Taylor reports
Cropley, A.J. 249
Crosby, P.B. 104
curriculum implications of EEC
    nursing directives and Nurses Act
    1979 268–72; *see also references*
    279–80

role in the development of skills
218-20, 220-1, 247-8; *see
also references*
developments, perspectives 243-6,
275, 276, 223-50
see also education

Daily Telegraph 43, 74
Dave, R.M. 249
Davidmann, D. 46
Davies, I.K. 207, 210
Davis, C.K. 105
Daws, P.P. 222
De Bono, E. 222
decisions
concept 194
strategies for decision-making 200
see also references 220-1
De Geyndt, D.W. 149
De Greene, K.B. 105
De Young, L. 125
delegation of tasks 61
demands on nurse
trained and students 215
Democracy in the National Health
Service (consultative paper) 36
Dennis, L.C. 141, 148, 170, 171
see also standards, quality of care
Dent, H.E. 125
Department of Health and Social
Security (DHSS) 13, 44, 76, 85
seminar 64, 95, 120, 121, 138,
142
see also nursing structure and
functions
Diekelman, N. 88
Dimarcol, N. 249
Draper, P. 46, 47, 76, 79
Drucker, P. 23, 25, 47, 88, 92, 104,
194, 196, 220, 247
Duffy, E. 186

education
rationalising nursing education
257-74
links with quality of care 233-4
see also references 279-80
education and training 63, 64, 94,
96-124, 223-50
see also the National Health
Service and Care Management;
references 247-8
education, continuing

concept 227-30
rationale 234
Edwards, M. 249
effects of burnout 182
effects of NHS Act 1980 37
Elgood, C. 249
Ellis, S. 279
Employment Protection Act 6, 164
Engel, G.V. 107, 117, 124
English National Board (ENB) 134,
223, 226, 239, 247, 253, 260,
263, 264, 267, 279
entitlement to practise 263
see also education
ethical dilemmas of nursing 51
Etzioni, A. 222
European Economic Community (EEC)
Nursing Directives 8, 10, 13, 15,
18, 20, 25, 52, 54, 79, 87, 95,
104, 149, 185, 225, 229, 251,
252, 254-6, 279
law 253
see also legislation 251-80;
references 279-80
euthanasia 18
evaluation 115, 135, 143
Evans, T. 46, 47

factors that influence training and
development 236, 238
factors which affect the provision of
care 132
factors which affect the supply of
nurses 152
Farnish, S. 249
Faulkner, A. 222
Fayol, H. 89, 99, 104, 105
Fiedler, F.E. 201, 202, 220
see also leadership
financial cutbacks in the NHS 19
see also Merrison report, Taylor,
D., Nurse Alert
Finch, J. 19, 25
Fink, S. 21, 24, 25
see also innovation; change
Fitz-Gibbon, C.T. 149
framework for helping 217
see also Mayeroff, M.
framework for nurse manpower 162
see also references 174-5
Franken, R.E. 88
French, P. 222, 249
Fulmer, R.M. 20, 25, 88, 105, 177,

194, 220
function of nursing management 86
functions and responsibilities of the
    UKCC 264–7
functions of Personnel Director 171
    see also Griffiths report

Gane, R.M. 249
Gay, W.A. 197, 220
General Manager 171
general management defined 40
    see also Fayol, H., Griffiths report
General Nursing Council for England
    and Wales 105, 125, 131, 148,
    185, 215, 220, 279
General Trained Nurse — education
    and training 256–62
    see also education, ENB, UKCC
Gibb, C.A. 202, 220
    see also leadership
goals of continuing education 229–30
    see also education and training
Godber report 102, 103
Godfrey, M. 183, 185
Goldstone, L.A. 147, 148, 149, 177
    see also 'Monitor', criteria for care
Goode, E. 113, 124
Goodland, S. 106, 124, 149
good management 75
Gordon, G.K. 105
Grace Reynold's Application and Study
    of Peto (GRASP) 166, 167, 175
Gregory, J. 88
Greiner, L. 22
Griffiths, R. interview 43, 48, 78
Griffiths Inquiry 40–5
Griffiths Report 6, 8, 11, 16, 18, 25,
    28, 30, 31, 40, 42, 43, 44, 45, 50,
    64, 76, 77, 79, 80, 87, 95, 103,
    151, 168, 171, 179, 191, 195,
    210, 206, 207, 208, 224, 251
Gross, B.M. 222
Grusky, O. 80
guidelines for better management 76

Hafer, J.C. 177
Hall, Dame Catherine 119, 124, 131,
    148, 279
    see also Code of Professional
        Conduct
Hall, R.A. 117, 124
Halpin, A.W. 201, 220
Hamblin, A.C. 249

Hancock, C. 125
Handy, C. 47
Harries, C. 158, 175
Harrison, S. 222
Harrison, W.D. 180, 185
Haussman, R.K.D. 177
Health and Safety at Work Act 164
health care system 49
Hegvary, S.T. 134, 148, 177
Heirs, B. 47
helping relationship 112
    see also Rogers, C.R.
Henderson, M.S. 280
Henderson, V. 50, 79, 105
Hersey, P. 88, 177
Herzberg, F. 88, 90, 91, 104, 172,
    175
Hilgarde, E.R. 222
Hingley, P. 61, 79, 119, 124, 148,
    185
    see also stress
holistic approach to care 134
Hollander, E. 17
Hollman, T.D. 222
Homans, G. 16
honesty 55, 123
    see also Mayeroff, M.
hope 55, 123
    see also Mayeroff, M.
Hopping, R. 125
Hopson, B. 217, 221
Horder report 126, 148, 153, 175,
    260, 279
Houle, C. 248
Howard report 102, 104, 274, 279
human purpose 50
human system 49
    see also Revans, R.
humanising care 134
humility 55, 123
    see also Mayeroff, M.
Hunt, J.W. 177
Hurley, B.A. 188, 221
Hurka, S.J. 169, 175

implications of new legislation for
    nurse practitioners, managers and
    educationists 270–4
incentives 78, 172
influencing the organisation of health
    care 170
information 150–77
    as a preparation to manpower

planning 150–77
see also manpower, productivity;
   references 174–5
innovation 5–27
see also change; *references* 25–7
International Council of Nurses (ICN)
   54, 79, 105
interpersonal skills 187–222
   importance 188–9
   see also references 220–1
interview
   appraisal 209–10
   counselling 218
   philosophy and use 211
   selection 208
interviewing
   concept of 207–8
introducing innovation into clinical
   practice 23
issues relating to nursing legislation
   273–8
   nurse/patient/related 211–12
   nurse practitioners, managers and
      educationists 270–4

Jelinek, R.C. 141, 148, 170, 171,
   175, 177
   see also standards; quality of care
job complexity 190
job of managers 98
job-satisfaction 107
Johnson, M. 177, 180, 186
Joiner, C. 177, 186
Joint Committee on District Nursing
   259
Joint Health Visiting Committee 259
Jones, E. 125

Kagan, C. 222
Kahn, R. 12, 14, 26, 222
Kalish, R. 83
Katz, D. 12, 14, 26, 222
Keighley, T. 175
Kenny, J. 153, 175
Kilbrick, A. 23
King's Fund Centre 248
Klein, R. 46, 47
knowledge 54, 56
   see also Mayeroff, M.
Körner reports 6, 15, 26, 31, 154,
   156–62, 175, 251, 279
   see also information, manpower,
      productivity; *references* 175–6

Körner Working Groups 9
Kramer, M. 14, 20, 26, 105, 107,
   121, 124
   see also professionalism
Kroll, M. 221
Kron, T. 222

Lader, M. 186
Lancaster, J. 23, 24, 26
   see also innovation; change
Lancaster, W. 23, 24, 26
   see also innovation; change;
      references 220–1
Larsley, I. 149
Latham, G.P. 177, 186
Leader Behavioural Description
   Questionnaire 204
   see also Halpin, A.W.
leadership 41, 201–7
   concept 201–2
   continency theory 204
   implications for nurses 206
   role 205
   styles 203
   see also interpersonal skills
learning
   action 239–40
legal constraints 19
legislation 251–80
   see also references 124, 279–80
Levitt, R. 47
Lewis, F.M. 115, 116, 117, 124
Lewin, K. 17, 26
   see also innovation; change
Likert, R. 201, 221
links between continuing education and
   quality of care 232, 233
   see also standards; quality of care
links between management and care 74
Linkwood, M.E. 148, 149
Linwood, M.E. 149
Lyden, F.J. 194, 221
Lyman, K. 280
Lyons, T.F. 169, 175

McCarthy, M. 105
   see also Whitley Council
McCloskey, J.C. 125
McClusky, H.Y. 249
MacDonald, I. 249
McFarlane, Professor Baroness 10, 26,
   51, 55, 79, 102, 104, 106, 120,
   122, 124, 279

McGregor, D. 90, 104, 200, 221
    see also motivation, patients' needs
MacGuire, J.M. 105
McLachlan, G. 47, 80, 136, 148, 149
MacLeod Clark, J. 222
Maanem, Th. van 135, 148
Maillart, V. 122, 124, 148
Management Arrangements for the
    Reorganised NHS (Grey Book) 46,
    76, 78, 79, 94, 95, 103, 129, 148,
    155, 174, 185, 195, 220, 290, 291
management education 71–5, 78,
    235–8
    see also education
management structure 66
managing the clinical environment 28,
    92
    see also care
Managerial Grid 202
    see also Blake, R.R.; Mouton, J.
Manpower 129, 142, 150–77, 275
    budgets 154
    estimation 164
    see also information; productivity;
        references 175–6
March, J.G. 46, 222
Marshall, J. 186
Martin, A. 19, 26, 60, 79, 125
Maslow, A.H. 84, 87, 243, 248
    see also patient's needs
Mauksch, I. 11, 15, 26
Mayeroff, M. 54, 80, 83, 87, 105,
    111, 112, 122, 123, 124, 246,
    248
    see also caring role
Maynard, A. 280
Mayston report 6, 7, 18, 25, 31, 57,
    63, 77, 79, 94, 103, 127, 148,
    179, 185
Meadows, A. 106, 124
'measuring' care 133, 139
medical power 78
Melia, A. 249
Meltzer, H. 177, 186
Merrison report 6, 18, 25, 33, 36, 46,
    60, 72, 73, 77, 81, 87, 101,
    104, 115, 117, 127, 129, 136,
    139, 140, 141, 148, 168, 179,
    225, 226, 227, 233, 247, 251,
    279
Meyer, D. 166, 175
    see also GRASP
Miller, M. 11, 15, 26

Miller, R.G.J. 190, 221
Milligan, B. 177
minimum data sets 156
Mintzberg, H. 201, 202, 221
    see also leadership
Mitchell, J. 19, 26, 62, 81
    see also nursing process
Moloney, M.M. 80
'Monitor' a tool for managers 147
    see also Goldstone, L.A.
motivation 41, 83, 172
    see also McGregor, D., Herzberg,
        F., Maslow, A.H.
Mott, P.E. 188, 221
Mouton, J. 201, 202, 220
    see also leadership, productivity
Murray, M. 212, 221
Myers, M.G.T. 249
Myers, M.T. 248

National Boards 260, 266
    specialist panels 266
    Standing Committees 267
National Board for Scotland 279
National Health Service Management
    Board 171
    restructuring 32
    restructuring (1974) 33–6
    restructuring (1982) 36–9
National Health Service 8, 28–47
National Health Service Act
    (1946) 32
    (1972) 1, 33
    (1980) 1, 36
    see also references 46
National Staff Committee (NSC) 95,
    97, 100, 104, 187, 226, 230,
    232, 238
National Training Council for the
    National Health Service (NTC)
    249
needs concept 82
    see also reference 87
needs' fulfilment theory 84
needs of patients 35, 76, 81–8
needs' satisfaction 83
    see also Mayeroff, M.; Maslow,
        A.H., McGregor, D. and
        Herzberg, F.
negative images of the nurse 50
Nelson, D.F. 249
Newman, J.F. 177
Nightingale, F. 71, 80, 105

Nite, G. 50, 105
non-course training options 238–40
Nord, W.R. 177
Northern Ireland National Board 260, 263, 264, 267, 279
Nurse Alert 7, 26, 31, 46, 77, 79, 105, 129, 148
nurse/patient/relative interview 211–12
nurse-patient relationship 89, 137, 188, 189, 191, 207, 212, 219
nurses'
  dissatisfaction 94
  problems 73, 131
  role 19, 31, 52, 56–62, 66, 85–7, 91, 97
  status 142
  see also references 87
Nurses, Midwives and Health Visitors Act 1979 8, 10, 13, 15, 20, 26, 95, 104, 110, 124, 186, 248, 259, 260, 261
Nurses, Midwives and Health Visitors Rules Approval Order 1983 99, 124, 148, 225, 228, 248, 251, 279
nursing competencies 109
  objectives 131
  a philosophy 54–5
  process 52–3, 86–7
  productivity, concept of 167; *see also* Griffiths, R., Merrison and Weiland, G.
  structure and functions 48–80
  see also education; *references* 79–80

Oates, J. 177
objectives of staff appraisal 209–10
observations on the Griffiths Inquiry 42
O'Connor, J.G. 106, 124
Office of Health Economics (OHE) 26, 33, 46
O'Hanlon, J.F. 186
Olsen, M. 16
Operational Research Service (ORS) 164
organisation — gap 14
Oskins, S.L. 183, 186
Ovretveit, J. 249
Ozimek, D. 177, 186

Paine, W.S. 180, 186
patience 54

  see also Mayeroff, M.
patient dependency 163
Patients First: Summary of Comments received on the Consultative Paper 46, 76
Peplau, H. 125
planning process 89
Platt report 5, 6, 26, 94, 127, 148
practice
  controlling 108, 117–22
  safe 61
problems, concept of 194–200
problems that confront health care professionals 29
problem-solving 14
  see also interpersonal skills
problem-solving framework 196–9
  see also references 220–1
productivity 16, 49, 91, 150–77
  see also information, manpower, Griffiths, R; Merrison and Körner reports; *references* 174–5
professional audit 140
professional development 64, 107, 109, 122
professionalism 11, 106–25
  see also Code of Professional Conduct, Kramer, M., Mayeroff, M., UKCC
professionalism
  paradoxes 122
  index 121
  see also references 124
professionals and power 93
protecting the public 272–4
  see also Code of Professional Conduct
Powell, M. 75, 80, 226, 227, 248
Price, J.L. 221, 232, 248
Pyne, R. 125

Quinn, S. 43
quality of care 82, 118, 126, 133, 137
  research 144
  see also standards of care; *references* 147–9
quality service
  impediments 72, 126–47, 137–8
  see also references 147–9

randomised controlled trial (RCT) 139, 140

Rayner Scrutinies 31
  see also Taylor, D.
Reconstruction Committee 5, 124
'refreezing' 17
  see also change
registration 264
Regan, D.E. 28, 46
reinforcement 17
reorganisation of NHS
  (1974) 32–6
  (1982) 36–9
reports — key 251–80
  see also references 26, 46, 79, 124
Resource Allocation Working Party
  (RAWP) 144, 174
resources 19, 56, 81
  see also Griffiths, R., Merrison,
    Nurse Alert and Taylor, D.
responsibility 11, 31, 51, 52, 58, 59,
  93, 112, 113, 114, 120, 142
Revans, R. 6, 25, 26, 30, 46, 49, 50,
  74, 76, 77, 80, 83, 87, 92, 94, 99,
  104, 107, 149, 180, 186, 188,
  194, 221, 248, 249
Rezler, A.G. 148, 188, 221
Rhys-Hearn, C. 163, 165, 175
  see also manpower
Roberts, J.N. 236, 248
Robinson, J. 125
Rogers, C.R. 112, 124, 214, 221, 222
Rogers, E.M. 15, 23, 26
role-based training 101, 241
  see also education 223–50
role-expanded 19, 59
  see also nurses' role
Rose, M.A. 177, 186
Rosenbaum, B.L. 177, 186
Ross, T. 280
Rowbottom, R. 105, 107, 113, 114,
  115, 116, 117, 124, 125
Royal College of Nurses (RCN) 15,
  20, 29, 31, 46, 56, 58, 65, 69, 73,
  77, 80, 86, 87, 95, 104, 105, 107,
  111, 113, 114, 116, 117, 118,
  119, 120, 124, 129, 131, 136,
  137, 141, 149, 153, 221, 223,
  226, 233, 234, 238, 246, 248, 249
Rush Medicus Methodology 146
  see also Goldstone, L.A.

Salmon report 6, 7, 16, 25, 52, 56,
  60, 63, 75, 94, 98, 102, 104, 126,
  148, 179, 186, 226, 227, 248

Sanders, A.F. 186
Schweiger, J.L. 105
Scottish National Board 260, 263, 266,
  267
Seashore, S.E. 203, 221
Secord, P.F.S. 203, 221
self-actualisation 14
  see also Mayeroff, M.
Selye, H. 178, 186
  see also stress
Seminar (DHSS) 64, 103
Sergiovanni, T.J. 201, 203, 221
Service at a professional level 121
  see also Code of Professional
    Conduct
Shipman, G.A. 221
Shoemaker, E.F. 23
Shubin, S. 180, 186
Simmons, D.D. 222
Simon, H.A. 222
Smart, T. 76, 81
Smith, J. 83, 87
Smith, R. 32, 46
social-professional norms 17
Standards for Morale: Cause and
  Effects in Hospitals 6
standards 136–9
Stalker, G.N. 153, 174
Stanley, I. 125
statutory bodies 262
  see also UKCC, National Boards
Steed Henderson, M. 249, 280
Stevens, B.J. 149, 188, 221
Stewart, J. 28, 46
Stewart, W. 222
stress 19, 82, 178–85
  concept 178
  management 183
  see also references 185–6
Stoghill, P.M. 222
Storey, M. 274, 279
Strongman, K. 83, 87, 88, 203, 221,
  222
Stuart, R. 97, 103, 249
systematic approach to care 134

Tanner, D. 249
Tanner, L. 249
Taylor, D. 29, 36, 39, 40, 44, 46, 76,
  80, 88, 149, 153
theory 'X' 90, 200
  see also motivation
theory 'Y' 90, 200

see also motivation
Thompson, D.J.C. 236, 248, 249
Thorndike, R.L. 188, 221
'Top-Down' approach 163
Towards a New Professional Structure
9
   see also nurses' role; *references*
   79–80
Towards Standards 6, 9, 26
   see also standards of care;
   references 147–9
Trade Union and Labour Relations Act
1974/76 129, 148, 164
training requirements, innovations 269
   see also education
Treaty of Rome 252
trust 55, 123
   see also Mayeroff, M.

Ullrich, R. 12, 14, 24, 27, 201, 221,
250
'unfreezing' 17
   see also change
United Kingdom Central Council for
Nursing, Midwifery and Health
Visiting (UKCC) 106, 114, 115,
120, 122, 124, 186, 223, 225,
248, 260, 261, 279, 280
   see also legislation; reports;
   references 279–80
unlearning 23
updating 93
   see also education

Vernon, M.D. 84, 87, 88

Walsh, M.B. 149, 177, 186
Walton, I. 226, 247
Webster, X. 158, 175
Weisbord, M.R. 243, 248
Welsh National Board 260, 263, 266,
267, 280
White, D.K. 236, 248
   see also education, training
Whitley Council 78, 79, 80
   see also McCarthy, M.
Wieland, G. 12, 14, 24, 27, 41, 105,
124, 175, 177, 190, 195, 201,
221, 250
Williams, D. 59, 75, 80, 102, 104,
106
   see also nurses' role
Williams, J. 159, 175
Willis, L.D. 148, 149
Wilson-Barnett, J. 163, 175, 177
Wimbush, F.B. 180, 182, 186
Wolfe, L. 84, 87, 105
Wong, R. 88
World Health Organisation (WHO) 51,
80, 86, 87, 107, 108, 118, 122,
124, 131, 135, 137, 144, 189,
218, 221, 226, 248

Yates, J. 155, 175
Youth Employment Service 259
Yura, H. 149, 177, 186

Zander, A. 201